Praise for *THINK Like a Nurse*

From Nurse Educators:

"This book would really be helpful to newly graduated nurses as well as senior nursing students. Keith gives a great example of situated coaching on electrolytes, cardiac preload, and afterload. I commend Keith on his scholarship and heart in this work."

–Patricia Benner, RN, PhD, FAAN, FRCN
Professor Emerita, University of California, San Francisco
Author of *From Novice to Expert* and co-author of *Educating Nurses: A Call for Radical Transformation*
Living Legend of the American Academy of Nursing

"'THINK Like a Nurse' provides relevant information in an easy-to-read, clear, and focused manner along with helpful advice from an expert nurse and teacher. This book is a powerful resource for nursing students. They can read/review this book each semester and subsequently improve their ability to 'think like a nurse' with each clinical experience as they progress through their nursing program and even their first year of nursing practice."

–Shirlee J. Snyder, EdD, RN
Co-author of Kozier & Erb's Fundamentals of Nursing

"Our clinical faculty appreciate 'Think Like a Nurse' and use it in the first semester clinical week one! The medication and lab references are very helpful in narrowing the amount of information students need to digest. The 'Clinical Reasoning Questions to Develop Nurse Thinking' is an excellent tool for the clinical instructor as they guide their students to begin to think like a nurse."

–Janet Wessels, MSN, RN, PHN
Director, Entry Level Masters Program, School of Nursing
Azusa Pacific University
San Diego, California

"As an experienced bedside nurse and educator, I have always tried to help the brand-new nurse understand how to prioritize what actions are most critical. 'THINK Like a Nurse' puts all of those concepts into clear, logical, and usable steps. My students really appreciate the clinical 'pearls,' the lab overviews, and the cardiac medication reviews. I will be using this book for all my new grads transitioning into practice."

–Willi Ellison, MSN, RN, CEN, CCRN
Residency Coordinator
Dignity Health/St. Rose Hospitals, Las Vegas, Nevada

"In nursing education there is the ideal we strive for and the real world of current clinical realities. There rarely exists a resource that bridges the two so honestly and powerfully as 'Think Like a Nurse.' In nursing education we strive to impart knowledge, but knowledge without wisdom and insight will leave the student nurse struggling to integrate the art of nursing into practice. I recommend this book to

nurse educators, nursing students, and anyone who wants to deeply understand the profession of nursing."

"I highly recommend 'THINK Like a Nurse.' This book is perfect for student nurses in the last semester of their nursing program and for new graduate nurses. Keith takes the common core knowledge and skills that the new nurse needs and drills them down to the nuggets of wisdom needed to be successful in practice. His thoughts and experiences in practice are insightful and easy to apply. A great resource for nurse educators too!"

"Keith has masterfully presented the true essence of nursing including the 'art' with relevant historical perspective. Students will discover what is needed to become an excellent nurse. The strength of this book is the emphasis on how to practically transition successfully to real world practice."

"This book offers the novice nurse guidance and wisdom in a unique resource that is unlike any other student textbook. The author pours his heart and soul into making nursing education logical and fun. This resource should be utilized with students during their final year in nursing education."

From New Nurses:

"'Think like a Nurse' will help students realize their calling and presents a clear path to practically live out the vocation of caring and to do it with joy. Keith's book is like a map in the desert of nursing school by providing needed direction. Those who read it will not be same and as a result will make a difference in all they do as a nurse."

"After reading this book, I am more confident to go into my nursing practice. The wealth of practical information in this short read is like having a year's worth of nursing experience under my belt. I highly recommend this valuable book for new grads!"

"Nursing school has limitations to what can be taught before you graduate and enter the profession. 'THINK Like a Nurse' addresses this and provides the new nurse with need-to-know content, along with Keith's clinical pearls, to help you see the 'big picture' of patient care. I strongly recommend this invaluable book for all nursing students and/or new graduates."

–Andrea Baland, RN

"This is a must-read for all nursing students and new graduates. The content is invaluable and will encourage you to live up to your full potential as a new nurse!"

–Desiree Rohling, RN

"I found 'THINK Like a Nurse' very helpful in getting me to think MORE like a nurse, and LESS like a nursing student...think- less deer-in-the-headlights!"

–Claire Schuchard, RN

"'THINK Like a Nurse' helped me with my job as a newly graduated RN. I truly enjoyed reading and reflecting upon your nursing experiences. I found it particularly helpful that you considered holistic nursing in chapter 1. I also liked how you organized your book starting from the foundation then building up to the applied sciences and critical thinking."

–Renate Jeddahlyn P. Depuno, RN

"When I read 'THINK Like a Nurse,' my first thought was, 'Wow! Where was this book when I was in nursing school?' I enjoyed how much of a condensed version of nursing school this book was. I would definitely recommend this book to my friends who are still in nursing school because I feel it would help benefit them a lot and better prepare them for the 'real' nursing world."

–Samantha Fernando, RN

"As a new grad on the floor, I've come to realize that because I am so focused on doing all the tasks, I sometimes forget to stop and take my time to think about why I am doing what I'm doing. Reading this book made me aware of this and aware of the fact that I can change. I am happy to say that I feel that I've improved my abilities to think like a nurse with the help of this informative book."

–Marian Maniago, RN

"Overall, 'THINK Like a Nurse' definitely prepares new grads for their role as an RN. I benefited most from the content on lab values. This content opened my investigative approach to nursing as well as helping me to become more aware of my patient's situation."

–Jean-Claude Perrenoud, RN

"I liked that the book was very personal, as if Keith was speaking directly to you. This book condensed and summed up a lot of important information used in nursing that allowed me to easily recall and apply to practice such as lab values, common disease processes and what to expect. I feel 'THINK Like a Nurse' should be utilized not only by new grads, but also nursing students."

–Jerisha San Sebastian, RN

THINK

Like a Nurse

Practical Preparation
for Professional Practice
SECOND EDITION

Keith Rischer, RN, MA, CEN, CCRN

KeithRN
Clinical Reasoning Resources

Though there is an almost limitless number of topics that could be covered in nursing education, there are fewer concepts that must be mastered to prepare students for professional practice. I have created a workbook with twelve case studies that cover the most important concepts to practice. If your program uses a concept-based curriculum, these 12 case studies serve as examples that will provide the hook of contextualization that students require to acquire deep learning of what is most important. My store has additional clinical reasoning resources to strengthen student learning.

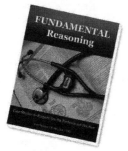

FUNDAMENTAL Reasoning (263 p.)

FUNDAMENTAL Reasoning is a basic introduction to clinical reasoning that is best suited for the fundamental level in registered nurse programs or practical nursing programs. It emphasizes application of the applied sciences of pharmacology, dosage calculation, and F&E. Recognizing clinical relationships and identifying the nursing priority to establish a plan of care are situated with a salient clinical scenario.

RAPID Reasoning (281 p.)

RAPID Reasoning is a "just right" length for most students and educators, best suited for basic med/surg content. Each RAPID Reasoning case study situates essential content to the bedside, and incorporates my step-by-step template of clinical reasoning questions that allows thinking to be practiced in the safety of the classroom.

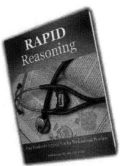

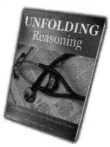

UNFOLDING Reasoning (377 p.)

UNFOLDING Reasoning is an advanced/synthesis level of case studies that contextualizes essential content to the bedside, and incorporates my step-by-step template of clinical reasoning questions. In addition, evaluation is integrated into the scenario with a clinical change of status that must be recognized as the scenario unfolds over time.

Clinical Dilemmas: Case Studies that Cultivate Caring, Civility & Clinical Reasoning (182 p.)

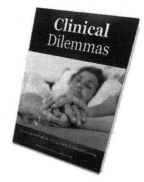

Clinical dilemmas are a series of 15 clinical reasoning case studies that emphasize the "art" of nursing. Each study has an emphasis that integrates aspects of caring, spiritual care, nurse engagement/presence, and ethical decision making and its relevance to nursing practice. Categories include patient, treatment, ethical, and nurse dilemmas that address incivility.

Think Like a Nurse
Practical Preparation for Professional Practice
Second Edition

Author: Keith Rischer, RN, MA, CEN, CCRN

To request a review copy for course adoption, or to inquire regarding speaker availability, email Keith:
Keith@KeithRN.com

Dedication

This book is warmly dedicated to Patricia Benner, RN, PhD, FAAN, FRCN and her ongoing influence to leave the profession of nursing better than when she entered it. Her work as an educator, author, researcher, and scholar has impacted the nursing profession in this generation as well as my own practice as a clinician and educator. It is my desire to honor and practically situate her work that spans over 30 years for the next generation of caregivers in this book. Her emphasis on the importance of caring as well as clinical reasoning and thinking like a nurse in practice makes her work timeless and relevant to all participants in the nursing profession today.

Reviewers

Dean Arnott, RN, BSN, MA, LICSW has 38 years of experience as a hospital nurse, educator, and as an outpatient mental health counselor. Dean works as a staff nurse in the critical care float pool nurse, which involves working in critical care, cardiac telemetry, and circulating/rapid response teams as well as a clinical adjunct.

Georgia Dinndorf-Hogenson, PhD, RN, CNOR is a nurse with 30 years of clinical experience in obstetrics, labor and delivery, nursery, post anesthesia care unit (PACU), trauma, and operating room where she is certified. She has taught as a nurse educator the past 10 years and is currently an assistant professor in the department of Nursing at the College of St. Benedict/ St. Johns University in Collegeville, Minnesota, where she teaches advanced medical/surgical nursing, trauma, and ethics.

Catherine Griswold, EdD, MSN, RN, CLNC, CNE has 20 years of nursing experience as a clinician, administrator, educator and legal nurse consultant. Her background includes psychiatric mental health nursing (children and adults), school health, older adult health working with clients with Alzheimer's disease, and consulting on legal cases involving nurses. As the president of her company, Health Care Educators and Legal Nurse Consultants, Inc., she authored the book *I'm Not Just A Patient...I'm A Health Care Consumer* and has written over a dozen articles related to legal issues in nursing practice.

Barbara Hill, RN, MSN, CNE, CMSRN has 35 years of clinical experience as a nurse practitioner in acute care in med/surg, emergency department, critical care, and home care. Barb has been teaching med/surg and community nursing the past 20 years as both a clinical adjunct and full-time professor at the Community College of Baltimore County in Maryland. For the past 10 summers, Barb has been a camp nurse and has published several articles as well as a regular column for the Association of Camp Nurses (ACN).

Carol Huston, MSN, MPA, DPA, FAAN has been a professor of nursing at California State University, Chico the past 33 years. She is the co-author of five textbooks on leadership, management, and professional issues in nursing (a combined 16 editions) and has published more than 100 articles in leading professional journals. Her co-authored book, *Leadership Roles and Management Functions in Nursing* has been translated into six languages and *Management Decision Making for Nurses* was an AJN book of the year. Dr. Huston served as the 2007–2009 President of the Honor Society of Nursing, Sigma Theta Tau International.

Karla Larson, PhD, MSN, RN has practiced as a geriatric nurse practitioner, parish nurse, and served in medical missions at a remote jungle hospital in Honduras. She has served as a director of nursing, associate dean of faculty at the national corporate level, and faculty development coordinator. She has also helped write nursing curricula at both the program and national level. She has 15 years of experience as a nurse educator in a wide variety of levels including community college, baccalaureate, RN to BSN, masters and DNP.

About the Author

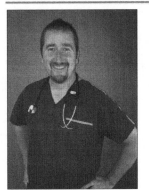

Caring in crisis attracted me to nursing over 30 years ago. I wanted to be a flight nurse/paramedic and chose to get my nursing degree right out of high school. I completed my EMT after my first year of nursing school and began to volunteer as an EMT in our community. I was so traumatized by getting lost on the back country roads with a critical patient in the ambulance, that I re-routed my career path and completed my two-year nursing degree in 1983 at a local community college and entered a very tight job market as a registered nurse.

I started my nursing career as a psychiatric nurse at the local state hospital and went on to pursue my passion for emergency nursing. I then went into long-term care, pediatric home care, step-down NICU, cardiac telemetry, cardiac ICU, and finally, after 16 years, the emergency department (ED). I currently work in the critical care float pool of a large metro hospital and float between the ED, med/surg neuro ICU, cardiac medical ICU, cardiac surgical ICU, cardiac telemetry and circulating/rapid response team. I am currently certified in my practice specialties of critical care and emergency department.

Ten years ago, I realized I enjoyed mentoring new nurses and guiding them in their professional development. I completed my BSN and went straight into a masters in nursing education program so I could pursue teaching at the collegiate level. I have been able to keep current in both clinical practice and nursing education the past several years. This bi-focal lens as a nurse educator and clinical expert nurse has allowed me to remain current in practice and draw from my experience to create salient resources, including this book, that reflect current best practice and the inherent challenges of clinical practice. I have created numerous tools and innovative strategies to strengthen student learning through an emphasis on clinical reasoning that will develop students' ability to think like a nurse.

I have had the opportunity to present my strategies to integrate clinical reasoning in the classroom and clinical settings at national and regional nurse educator conferences across the United States and Canada. I have created a unique template that breaks down the theoretical construct of clinical reasoning into 12 sequential questions that nurses can use in any patient care setting to identify relevant information and establish care priorities. I have created numerous case studies that are derived from themes I have seen in clinical practice. These case studies integrate my template of clinical reasoning questions so students are able to practice the thinking that is required for safe nursing practice. Some of these case studies are also included in this book.

My applied strategies to teach clinical reasoning to nursing students have been recently published in the nursing literature. They are featured in the current 10th edition of *Kozier & Erb's Fundamentals of Nursing,* the upcoming 4th edition of *Professional Issues in Nursing* edited by Carol Huston with a chapter titled "Can Clinical Reasoning Be Taught?" and an article on clinical reasoning for *Innovations in Nursing Education, Volume III* published by the National League for Nursing.

I am passionate about transforming nursing education by integrating clinical reasoning throughout the curriculum. I have created practical tools to help realize this transformation. My website, clinical reasoning resources, and blog are committed to be a part of the solution and to strengthen and support this needed change. I also have a passion to serve the poor through medical missions by using nursing and nursing education to share God's love and improve the quality of health care in the developing world.

Contents

Appendices

Foreword

I have known Keith from my first year of nursing school; he was one of my fundamental nursing instructors and is now a nursing colleague in the float pool at the hospital we both work at. Keith's passion for nursing is evident not only in his practice at the bedside but also through his teaching. The clinical reasoning case studies that he created and presented to our class challenged us to think in a way that we had not experienced to this point in nursing school. His objective was to get us to "think" like a nurse. As his students in lecture, we had to take a step back and look at the bigger picture of what was truly going on with the patient in the clinical scenario. As a class, we had to identify what the clinical data represented and as nurses, the interventions we should implement to intervene and prevent a worst possible scenario from happening. Keith constantly challenged and encouraged us.

Keith had faith in us, and laid a foundation of knowledge that was applied at the bedside. Keith pushed us to start utilizing the same clinical reasoning questions during clinical. Not only did this prepare us before caring for our patients, but it also helped us to be more proficient and consistent with our skills. On a personal level, Keith cares. He was present during a crisis in my life during nursing school. He not only showed compassion for my situation and care as a friend, but his knowledge and grasp of nursing was evident.

This book has been extremely helpful to me in many ways. Not only did it remind me of all the clinical handouts Keith created that I relied on during clinical (i.e., most commonly used medication, clinical reasoning questions, etc.), but also reminded me of the living "house" nursing represents…the foundation, walls, and roof. Keith also reminded us of the centrality of caring to nursing. The content in chapter 3 on the foundation of nursing must be carefully read and not overlooked or missed by the reader. Keith goes into further detail on how to pull what we have learned from the classroom and apply it to the bedside, and how trending data is essential in practice. Keith uncovers the clinical pearls that are relevant to practice. This is something every new graduate entering the workforce should review and apply. The content on bullying is a must-read as well. I highly recommend this book to be read by new graduate nurses and applied at the bedside to help prepare you for practice.

–Heather Squillacioti, RN
Normandale Community College graduate
Minneapolis, Minnesota

Introduction

Why This Book Was Written

Are You Afraid to Be a Nurse?

Though the title of my book is "Think Like a Nurse," would you be surprised to discover that fear is one of the most prevalent emotions that most nursing students experience when they contemplate the reality of being an autonomous professional nurse in practice? Fear that they don't have what it takes. Fear that they may hurt their patients. Fear that they might miss something. In addition to fear, new nurses admit to being unsure of themselves, uncomfortable, and nervous once they are off orientation and are now on their own for the first time. My goal in creating this resource is to empower any student or new nurse to face and conquer their fears. It comes to you from a nurse educator who remains current in clinical practice.

These emotions are not unusual but are normal. But like any emotion, fear, anxiety, and lack of self-confidence can also be debilitating if not faced head-on. In addition to this cauldron of emotions, depending on the shift you work and the clinical setting, you may be responsible for four to eight patients in an acute care setting (double this in transitional or skilled care setting). In nursing school, you were typically responsible for one to two patients in the clinical setting. How will you set priorities and manage your time to accomplish patient care needs with this new reality?

As a result of feeling unprepared for real-world practice, new nurses encounter high levels of stress, anxiety, burnout, and turnover in the first year of practice (Cho, Laschinger, & Wong, 2006). Many new graduate nurses leave the profession in the first year because of job stress, lack of organizational support, poor nurse-physician relations, unreasonable workloads, uncivil work environments, and difficulty transitioning to practice (Clark & Springer, 2012).

A Practical Guide and Mentor

Every new nurse needs a mentor to guide and smooth the often bumpy transition from nursing school to clinical practice. I have written *THINK Like a Nurse* to be this mentor and help students or new nurses transition successfully from academia to clinical practice and not only survive but THRIVE in the process! Knowing that too much information (TMI) is an ongoing concern in nursing education, the last thing nursing students need is another book! But the essence of *THINK Like a Nurse: Practical Preparation for Professional Practice* is very different from any other textbook you may have already purchased. It is not written as a textbook, but in an easy-to-read first-person narrative that will provide practical strategies and approaches to prepare and help you transition successfully to autonomous professional practice.

To prevent you from being a workplace casualty and prepare you for real-world practice, I have written *THINK Like a Nurse* to highlight clinical reasoning and the most important content relevant to the bedside and why this information must be mastered and understood. Clinical reasoning is the nurse's ability to think in action and reason as a situation changes (Benner, Sutphen, Leonard, & Day, 2010). It is the essence of how a nurse thinks in practice, but it is not currently and consistently taught in nursing education. To develop this skill in your practice, I break down the complexity of clinical reasoning so you can understand this nurse thinking skill and incorporate it into your practice.

Building the "Living House"

To help you visualize the professional development you need as you transition to the responsibilities of the professional nurse, I will use the metaphor that student development while in nursing education mirrors the building of a house. This house is not a static structure, but a unique, vibrant "living" house that is a reflection of how you choose to build and add to it over time.

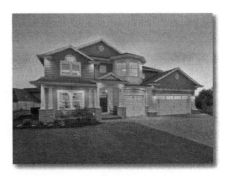

Nursing is a living and vibrant practice that requires your personal involvement and engagement to promote the well-being of those you care for. Just as a home often undergoes remodeling as a family grows over time, the same is true for the professional nurse. You may change practice settings or advance your education to "remodel" your practice setting to management, education, or nurse anesthesia. The "living" house of professional practice will be developed in the following chapters of this book.

A house must have a firm and stable foundation. The ethical comportment or the art of nursing is this foundation. Caring behaviors, nurse engagement, and professionalism in practice must be present or your nursing practice could be on shaky ground before it even begins. Once the foundation is laid it is time to build. The walls of professional practice are the applied sciences of nursing: pharmacology, fluid and electrolytes, and anatomy and physiology.

I will contextualize these essential sciences to the bedside so you can see the relevance of mastering this content and enhance your ability to recognize potentially dangerous clinical trends and provide the best possible care for your patients. Finally, the roof of professional practice consists of how a nurse thinks which includes critical thinking and clinical reasoning, which complete the house and tie everything together.

Though most students can write a three-part nursing diagnostic statement and use this as a priority for a written care plan, this emphasis will not always prepare you to transition to thinking like a nurse in practice. As a nurse in practice, you must be able to THINK IN ACTION, especially when the status of your patient changes. This is the essence of clinical reasoning and is an essential thinking skill that must be understood, incorporated, and practiced. The more you practice these activities you develop muscle memory and are able to react consistently and appropriately in the clinical setting.

The house of professional practice is in need of supporting structures that include safety, education, and expert practice. Safety is practically situated in all that a nurse does at the bedside. The nurse must also embrace the role of educator and realize how patient education can positively affect patient outcomes and even prevent readmissions. Though it takes time to progress to expert practice, I will identify what it takes to get there so that you can be the best that you were trained and created to be!

Finally, I will tie the house together with real-world clinical scenarios to apply all that you have learned in your nursing education. You will be able to practice clinical reasoning by using the unfolding clinical reasoning case studies on COPD/pneumonia, heart failure, and sepsis, which place basic concepts and content in context for practice. Each case study has a fully developed answer key that thoroughly explains the rationale to promote your learning. This allows you to PRACTICE nurse thinking before you enter into practice.

Unique Content

Other books that I have read by clinical nurses to help prepare students for clinical practice emphasize their personal approach to nursing and what they have learned with almost no references from the nursing literature to support their perspective. *THINK Like a Nurse* is grounded in the literature of what is best practice with over 200 citations. I incorporate the theory and best practice recommendations from the literature and through my lens and filter as an expert nurse, as well as a nurse educator, make it practical and easy to apply and integrate into your practice.

The highlights of this unique resource include:

- Practical application exercises that will help make needed connections to strengthen understanding of essential content.
- Emphasis on the most important content and information. Reflection questions at the end of each chapter to facilitate professional growth.
- Additional resources at the end of each chapter that will encourage professional development.
- Clinical reasoning case studies that will strengthen your knowledge and help you practice nurse thinking on the topics of COPD/pneumonia, heart failure, and sepsis.
- Emphasis on real-world clinical practice derived from my more than 30 years of experience in the clinical setting.
- Clinical tools and handouts that will strengthen your knowledge of pharmacology, labs, and clinical reasoning that include:
  - ✓ Worksheet: Medications That Must Be Mastered
  - ✓ Handout: Most Commonly Used Categories of Medications
  - ✓ Worksheet: Lab Planning
  - ✓ Handout: Clinical Lab Values and Nursing Responsibilities
  - ✓ Handout: Clinical Reasoning Questions to Develop Nurse Thinking
  - ✓ Worksheet: Patient Preparation

Students who are ill prepared to think like a nurse will likely struggle once in clinical practice. This struggle can impact patient outcomes. If a new nurse is unable to think in action and clinically reason by recognizing a change in status, what will be the ultimate consequence if, for example, sepsis progresses to septic shock before it is recognized? A patient could die as a result.

I See Dead Patients

"I see dead people" was a famous quote by Cole Sears from the hit horror movie *The Sixth Sense* in 1999. Fortunately, it was only a movie. Unfortunately, I have seen clinical situations as a rapid response nurse that foreshadowed a patient's death as a result of the primary nurse's "failure to rescue" because they did not recognize a change of status until it was too late. This is one scenario I will never forget.

Jenny was a newer nurse who graduated a year ago (some details changed to protect patient confidentiality). She had an elderly male patient named Ken. He had a perforated appendix, but it had been removed successfully two days prior and he was clinically stable. Around midnight, he became restless. His BP was slightly elevated at 158/90 and his HR was in the 100s. He had a history of mild dementia and was not able to readily communicate his needs, so Jenny gave him 1 tablet of Percocet, assuming he was in pain. Two hours later, he continued to be restless and Jenny thought that she heard some faint wheezing. She noted that he was now more tachypneic with a respiratory rate of 28/minute. He had a history of COPD and had an albuterol nebulizer prn ordered, so that was given.

Two hours later, Jenny called me as the rapid response nurse to come and take a look at her patient. She was concerned, but was unable to recognize the problem and wanted a second opinion. After Jenny explained the course of events that transpired to this point, I took one look at Ken and realized that he was in trouble. He was pale, diaphoretic, and his respirations had increased to 40/minute despite the nebulizer two hours ago. He was not responsive to loud verbal commands. The last BP was still on the screen and read 158/90. I asked, "When was the last BP checked?" Jenny stated it was four hours prior. While obtaining another BP, I touched Ken's forehead. It was notably cold, as were his hands. The BP now read 68/30.

Recognizing that Ken was in septic shock, and that IV fluids and vasopressors would be needed emergently, I looked for an IV and found only one, a 24 gauge catheter in the left hand. This is the smallest size IV catheter and is typically used with infants and small children. Realizing that Ken needed a central line and that there was little that could be done to initiate even the most basic life-saving treatments to rescue Ken on the floor, he was emergently transferred to ICU. Within thirty minutes Ken was intubated, a central line was placed, and three vasopressors; norepinephrine [Levophed], phenylephrine [Neosynephrine] and Vasopressin were required to get his systolic blood pressure greater than 90 mmHg.

After this transfer was completed, I asked Jenny a simple clinical reasoning question: "What was the most likely complication that Ken could experience based on his reason for being hospitalized?" Jenny admitted that she hadn't thought about it because she was so focused on getting all of the tasks done with her four other patients.

Had Jenny asked herself this question while caring for Ken – and more importantly – answered it, she would have been thinking like a nurse. She would have vigilantly looked and assessed for EARLY signs of the most likely complication Ken could experience because of his perforated appendix…SEPSIS. Although early signs of sepsis were present at midnight, it was not recognized until it was too late for Ken. He died the next day.

I share this illustration not to frighten you or cause you to reconsider your choice to become a nurse, but to sober you with the incredible responsibility that is inherent in working as a nurse. Though I am in the twilight years of clinical practice, I remain passionate and highly engaged in caring for others because I continue to see the difference that excellent nursing care makes. This book is a labor of love to communicate to the next generation what is absolutely foundational and nonnegotiable to nursing care and practice.

It is only recently that I pursued my passion to teach and became a nurse educator. I care deeply about your professional success and want to do what I can to establish you on a rock-solid foundation as you transition to professional practice. One of my greatest frustrations as a nurse educator has been the inherent difficulty of sharing the depth of my clinical experience with my students because I have been spread so thin as a clinical educator. Though I enjoy the dynamics of clinical education, I felt like a ping-pong ball bouncing from one "crisis" to the next. Now that I have put my thoughts in writing, I invite you to pull up a chair and let me share information that will help you to be practically prepared for professional practice.

Whether you are considering the nursing profession or are a student who has fulfilled all required prerequisites and have been admitted to the nursing program of your choice, in the next chapter, I want you to carefully reflect and take a simple quiz to help determine if you have what it takes to be a nurse.

Part I

Is Nursing for You?

If you are considering entering the nursing profession or have already started nursing school, it is imperative to reflect and determine if nursing is a good fit for your personality and temperament. Chapter 1 contains a 25-question quiz that highlights the essence of the values and traits essential to nursing and enjoying what you do as you serve and care for others. This quiz will serve two purposes: determine your general aptitude as a nurse, and identify your strengths and weaknesses. Your objective is to make any areas identified as a weakness into a strength by the time you graduate from your nursing program.

Chapter 2 addresses some key attitudes and practical strategies to help you be successful as a nursing student. Though nursing education is inherently stressful, by following these simple strategies, you do not have to merely survive your time in nursing school, but you can thrive and maximize your learning in the process!

Chapter 1

Do You Have What It Takes to Be a Nurse?

According to the Bureau of Labor Statistics' employment projections, nursing is listed among the top occupations in terms of job growth through 2022. The nursing workforce will need to increase 19 percent over the next eight years (526,800 additional nurses needed). Because of retirement and transitions in the profession, an additional 525,000 replacement nurses will be need to be added to the workforce, bringing the total number of new nurses needed to 1.05 million by 2022 ("Nursing Shortage," 2014)!

This is an opportunity for many to enter this honorable and highly respected profession and make a difference in the lives of patients and their families as well as increase the gender and ethnic diversity in the nursing profession. Just as the Marines are famously known as looking "for a few good men," nursing is also looking for a "few good men and women," NOT just warm bodies to fill a vacant position. The nursing profession is in need of highly motivated, engaged nurses who are passionately committed to serve others.

Take the Quiz!

Complete this quiz to reflect and discover the aptitudes and traits essential to nursing and see if you have what it takes to be a nurse. There are certain characteristics foundational to nursing that you need to embody by the time you graduate (remember the old Gatorade commercials: "Is it in you?"). Once you determine that nursing is a good "fit" for you, you will be much more likely to persevere and successfully complete nursing education. If, on the other hand, most of these reflections do not resonate with you or are a current weakness, then consider this a red flag, and carefully consider your motivation to become a professional nurse. If you know that you want to be a nurse, use any areas that are identified as a weakness and work hard to make them your strength by the time you graduate from your program!

Take just a moment to write down your answers before proceeding any further. Only one thing is required…be completely honest in your response! Then write down an example that illustrates the response you chose. Compare your answers with my reflections at the end of this chapter and see for yourself if you have what it takes to be a nurse!

Quiz: Do You Have What It Takes to Be a Nurse?

1. What is your passion in life?

2. Why do you want to be a nurse?

3. How do perceive nursing? Is it a job or a profession?

4. What kind of character do you possess?

5. Do you easily identify with the feelings of others?

6. Do you enjoy and find fulfillment in serving others?

7. Is spirituality important to you and how comfortable are you discussing this with others?

8. What biases and attitudes may you have toward those of other cultures?

9. Do you possess a strong work ethic?

10. Are you inwardly motivated to take responsibility for your own learning?

11. Do you feel that your college owes you a degree because you paid for it?

12. Do you consider yourself a lifelong learner?

13. Are you naturally inquisitive about how things work?

14. Do you have a natural aptitude for science?

15. What are you willing to give up to make school a priority?

16. Do you have strong attention to detail?

17. When you make a mistake, do you learn from it or do you try to cover it up?

18. How well do you perform under stress?

19. How well are you able to multitask?

20. Do you readily recognize your limitations and what you do/don't know?

21. Are you comfortable asking questions about anything that is unfamiliar to you?

22. Are you comfortable doing intimate cares and handling body fluids while maintaining privacy and dignity for the patient?

23. How well do you handle responsibility?

24. How well do you communicate with others?

25. How well do you handle conflict with others?

Reflections

Were you surprised and wondered what some of these questions had to do with nursing? This book will go into additional detail to identify the relevance and significance of each of these questions to nursing. To see how your answers compared to my reflections, each question in the quiz, with my responses, is provided below.

1. What is your passion in life?

Because of the sacrifice of time, energy, and money required to become a nurse, most nursing students are motivated and willing to do whatever is needed because they have a personal passion to see it realized. One practical way to determine your personal passions in life is to ask yourself, "What would I be willing to do for free because I enjoy doing it?"

For example, many nurses choose to become a nurse educator because of their passion for teaching and developing others, even though it pays substantially less than clinical practice. As I look back on my journey in nursing, this is what led me to become a nurse educator. I had applied for a local nurse anesthetist program 10 years ago because I felt it was the next logical step after 20 years of clinical practice and I could earn an annual salary of more than $150, 000. I shadowed a nurse anesthetist for a day to see what this scope of practice would involve and at the end of the day it left me relatively uninterested. Though nurse anesthetists are a valued and needed member of the health care team, it was not a good fit for me.

At this same time, I was reading *Wild at Heart* by John Eldredge when this quote literally jumped off the page:

> *"Don't ask yourself what the world needs. Ask yourself what makes you come alive, and do that. Because what the world needs are people who have come fully alive."*
>
> (Eldredge, 2001, p. 200*).*

I realized how much I enjoyed mentoring new nurses in the emergency department and watching the "lightbulb" turn on when what I shared was understood and incorporated into practice by other nurses. This quote gave me permission to pursue what I believe is my God-given passion and talent in nursing, the ability to teach. So after completing my BSN, instead of pursuing the path of what I thought was

NEEDED as a nurse anesthetist, I pursued my PASSION and entered a master's in nursing education program. I have since been blessed to make many contributions to not only my students' learning, but through my writings and website have made a difference with students and educators across America. When you, too, pursue your passion, there is no limit to what you can achieve and do!

What about you? What makes you come alive as you consider becoming a nurse? Is it the opportunity to care for others, or having a good job with benefits? If serving and caring for others is an internal passion of yours, this is an indicator that you are clearly on the right path in your decision to become a nurse.

2. Why do you want to be a nurse?

If you know anything about therapeutic communication, you know that this question is NOT therapeutic, because it starts with a "why." But in the context of your decision to consider or enter nursing, it must be asked because it addresses your primary motivation to become a nurse. Dig deep and look within. You know what the expected and "right" answer is: "Because I want to care for others." But is this really true for you? What really gets you excited about nursing? The ability to care for others, or making good money in a job that is recession-proof, portable, and has numerous opportunities for overtime?

Thirty years ago, beginning nurses made less than $10 an hour. Because the pay was not exceptional, the majority of those who entered the profession were primarily attracted to nursing because they were motivated to care for others. Times have changed. According to the Bureau of Labor Statistics, registered nurses average $31.48 per hour and have an average annual salary of $65,470 ("Registered Nurses," 2014). In addition, there will be ongoing opportunities to work additional overtime, double time and bonuses for extra shifts.

Once in practice, some new nurses become focused on the numerous financial and other benefits. A slow fade can take place that can impact any new nurse regardless of their motivation. The nurse can drift from being patient-centered to self-centered by focusing on what they can get from being a participant in the profession rather than serving others and improving patient outcomes by providing excellent care. This is another reason why motivation matters.

Thankfully, there is an increase in compensation that reflects the worth of the professional nurse. Observant nurse educators have noticed that the altruistic motivation to care for others has been replaced in some by a stronger appeal of how much money they will make as a nurse. Because of instability and resultant layoffs during economic decline in other industries, the realization that nursing pays well, is stable and recession-proof has been the deciding factor for some students to enter nursing.

If the amount of your salary is your primary motivation to consider nursing, please carefully examine your choice to become a nurse. Studies have shown that the caring, patient-centered engagement of the nurse has a direct correlation to patient safety and better patient outcomes. In other words, when the nurse is focused on what he or she gets out of nursing (salary, benefits, etc.) and the patient is secondary, patient safety is affected and adverse outcomes, including death, are more likely to occur.

3. How do you perceive nursing? Is it a job or a profession?

Have you had firsthand experience with nurses who made a difference caring for you or others close to you, or family members who role-modeled what it means to be a nurse? These experiences will likely influence your perception of nursing as a job or a profession. There is a significant difference between the two.

We all know what a job is. In exchange for time worked, one receives a paycheck. It is something that you do and is something that typically is endured, not enjoyed. Think back to your first job in high school. In contrast, to be a nurse is something that you *are*. It is not just something that you do. That is why your personal character is relevant regarding your choice to enter the nursing profession. It is who you are and present with you whether at work or home.

Members of a profession such as nurses, physicians, and lawyers are also defined by the following unique characteristics that are not found in a typical job or occupation:

- They have a specialized body of knowledge
- They must pass a licensing or credentialing examination to participate
- They follow a code of ethics that guides behavior of the profession's members

The ethical standards that guide the nursing profession are found in the American Nurses Association (ANA) Code of Ethics. Specific professional behaviors include relationships with colleagues and others:
"The principle of respect for persons extends to all individuals with whom the nurse interacts. The nurse maintains compassionate and caring relationships with colleagues and others with a commitment to the fair treatment of individuals, to integrity-preserving compromise, and to resolving conflict" ("American Nurses Association," 2015).

The foundational professional behaviors that nursing students must be able to consistently demonstrate can be boiled down to CARING, COMPASSION, and RESPECT toward other students, faculty, and their patients. Read the ANA code of ethics and the values it calls each nurse to embody, and see if you can align yourself with these timeless values and live out what it takes to be and act like a nurse!

4. What kind of character do you possess?

Character matters. Florence Nightingale, the founder of the modern era of the nursing profession, recognized the importance of personal character and virtue to those who would aspire to become a nurse. Nurses at the time of Nightingale had little to no training. Women who were caregivers included alcoholics and prostitutes who routinely came to work drunk, and immoral conduct was not uncommon on the wards where patients received care.

Nightingale identified truthfulness and sympathy as central to nursing (Woodham-Smith, 1951). Though written more than 150 years ago, these values remain relevant today. Honestly reflect on the questions with each essential character trait below and see if these values are established and part of who you are:

- **Truthfulness/honesty.** Academic dishonesty is an ongoing concern in nursing education as students resort to doing whatever is necessary including cheating to pass a class. This places students in a position of moral distress that will follow them into practice ("Moral Distress in Academia," 2015).
  The greater concern that this represents to the nursing profession is that a nursing student who is willing to cut corners in academia will likely do the same in clinical practice. The difference is that in nursing school, the student who cheats is only hurting themselves. In clinical practice cutting corners will adversely impact another human being.

✓ Do you consistently tell the truth regardless of the consequences or only when it's convenient?

✓ Are you willing to cheat on an exam to get a passing grade?

- **Sympathy.** Are you able to identify easily with the pain and suffering of others, or are you distant and aloof?

Building on Nightingale's legacy, the American Nurses Association has identified the following values and character traits as essential to the professional nurse ("Code of Ethics for Nurses," 2015):

- **Integrity.** What are you like when nobody is watching? Are you the same or different?
- **Compassion.** Do you identify with the sufferings of others in such a way that you "suffer together" with them? This is the essence of what it means to be compassionate.

According to the current Gallup poll (2015), nurses continue to have the highest level of honesty and public trust (80%) of all professions the past 13 years, outdistancing physicians (65%) and pharmacists (65%) ("Honesty/Ethics in Professions," 2015). We must guard and value this public trust. Nursing is largely done behind closed doors or a curtain. We need to have nurses who are motivated to uphold the public trust confidence by living out the values that the nursing profession embodies.

5. Do you easily identify with the feelings of others?

How you honestly answer this question is one of the strongest predictors if nursing is truly a good "fit" for you. Remember the old Gatorade commercials with Michael Jordan? Images of athletes sweating Gatorade correlated with the commercial message, "Is it in you?" Do you easily identify and feel the pain and difficulties of others? Or are you aloof and indifferent? This is the essence of empathetic caring.

Caring has traditionally been viewed as the essence of nursing practice and the most important characteristic of a nurse (Leininger, 1988). The essence of caring is that you recognize the value and worth of those you care for and that the patient and his or her experience MATTERS to you (Benner & Wrubel, 1989). In one study, students who scored higher on affective empathy reported being more satisfied in their work (Baldacchino & Galea, 2012).

The centrality of caring to nursing is not new. It was emphasized at the beginning of the modern era by influential nurse educator Isabel Hampton Robb, who later went on to found the American Nurses Association in 1897. In 1900, she wrote in her textbook, *Nursing Ethics*:

> *The spirit in which she does her work makes all the difference. Invested as she should with the dignity of her profession and the cloak of love for suffering humanity, she can ennoble anything her hand may be called upon to do, and for work done in this spirit there will ever come to her a recompense far outweighing that of silver and gold* (Hampton Robb, 1900).

Leading nurse educator and scholar Patricia Benner also affirms that caring remains central to nursing practice. "Nursing can never be reduced to mere technique…the nature of the caring relationship is central to most nursing interventions" (Benner & Wrubel, 1989, p.4). "The nurse is both a knowledge worker and one who cares…knowledge is dangerous if it is divorced from caring" (Benner & Wrubel, 1989, p. 400).

6. Do you enjoy and find fulfillment in serving others?

Nursing is serving others in a time of need. It involves doing whatever is needed to ensure that patient needs are fully met. Serving others is not highly valued in our culture yet it is the essence of the mindset of the professional nurse. Serving is not about a position or what you do. It is an attitude. The best nurses have a strong desire to serve their patients, not themselves. Do you have the heart of a servant? A nurse who is motivated to serve demonstrates the following characteristics (Maxwell, 1999):

1. **Puts the patient first.** This means that the nurse remains aware of the patient's needs, is available to help them, and recognizes that their needs must always come first.
2. **Possesses the confidence to serve.** A true servant is secure and does not feel that it is beneath them as a person to serve others, but embraces and enjoys meeting the needs of the patient and their family. The value you give to others is a reflection of the value you ascribe to yourself.
3. **Is not position-conscious.** Though you are or will soon become a nurse, this title does not encourage you to see serving as beneath you, but you possess a greater sense or obligation to serve.
4. **Serves out of love.** A true servant leader is not motivated by what they can get from their work but is fueled by a love and empathy for others. The nurse that will make a difference will have the highest level of concern for others. It is true that those who would be great must be like the least and the servant of all.

The ability to serve must also be present regardless of how the patient may respond to you. This is why maintaining empathy is so important to nursing practice. The nurse must put themselves in the patient's position and give him or her grace to be angry, frustrated, or even rude, based on the fact that they may be in pain or have just been recently diagnosed with a life-changing diagnosis. Can you still care and serve someone even if it appears to be unappreciated? If you remain empathetic and do not take things personally, you will be an excellent nurse in practice.

Though nursing is different than working in a service industry that depends on tips, the same principles of serving, making the patient (customer) the center of everything that you do and anticipating needs all translate to the essence of what it means to be a highly engaged nurse in practice. Though being a certified nursing assistant is valuable experience to prepare you for nursing, if you have not had this background but were a waiter, waitress, or bartender, the principles you learned from serving others in this context will also benefit and prepare you as a nurse.

7. Is spirituality important to you, and how comfortable are you discussing this with others?

What separates nursing from the medical model that physicians use to diagnose and treat the body is the emphasis of holistic care. Human beings are not only a physical person who require physical care, but also have a soul (emotional care) as well as spirit (spiritual care). When providing care in any setting, the nurse must be sensitive to care for all three aspects of a person's being.

Though spiritual care is expected and within the nurse's scope of practice, I find that most students as well as nurses in practice are uncomfortable with this responsibility. Spiritual care is much more than simply asking the question that is on many admission forms. "Are there any spiritual or cultural needs we can support you with during your stay?" and then determine if they would like a chaplain consult.

Nurses must be willing to be sensitive to the spiritual component of each patient and be willing to support their spiritual needs as needed.

Leading nurse theorist Jean Watson has developed a theory of human caring. She has shown that when the nurse is supportive with the patient's spirituality, these patients have a greater measure of hope, peace, and improved outcomes ("Core Concepts of Jean Watson's Theory of Human Caring/Caring Science," 2010).

I have observed that those most comfortable with spiritual care find their own faith and spiritual traditions personally meaningful and relevant. When it comes to spirituality, you cannot give to others if you do not have something within to give. Just because you may not be a participant of a faith tradition or value the relevance of spirituality, remember that if spirituality or a faith tradition is important to your patient and his/her worldview, it must also be central and important to the nurse!

8. What biases and attitudes may you have toward those of other cultures?

Do you have assumptions about other people based on past experiences? For example, if you have had negative experiences with those of the opposite sex, or those of another religious or ethnic group, it's easy to generalize and transfer those assumptions to those from the same group whom you do not even know. Swanson in her research on caring (1991) identified one practical way that nurses can demonstrate caring to each patient is to "avoid assumptions" or preconceived judgments about them. Once an assumption or judgment of any kind is made, the nurse ceases to be authentically engaged and is unable to demonstrate caring to the patient.

Uncovering cultural bias and attitudes can begin with any classmates from another culture. One nurse educator shared the following example from her program:

I had a group of students who were struggling with a group project. The American-born students were pointing a finger at two foreign-born male students and accusing them of being rude and disrespectful by dominating group work and failing to make eye contact with female students. We did a group conflict exercise and discovered that the group had not taken time to understand each other. They had failed to understand that in some cultures men are dominant and feel disrespected by females who look them in the eye. We found a way to work together by understanding each other and developed mutually acceptable goals. Because these students took time to be open and learn, they ended the bias toward each other and the group project was very successful.

9. Do you possess a strong work ethic?

Nursing is hard work. Being a student can be even harder at times. To get through nursing school successfully you must embrace the hard work required and be willing to do what is needed without taking shortcuts to get by. A strong work ethic and the willingness to work hard were also emphasized as an important virtue of the professional nurse at the beginning of the modern era in the late 1800s. In her text *Nursing Ethics*, Hampton Robb (1900) wrote:

"A pupil (student nurse) should esteem it a piece of good fortune to be put on duty in the heavy wards, where one is always busy, where the work never seems to be done, and where there is so much in the way of nursing going on…Never be afraid to work and to work hard. Work pure and simple is not likely to do you harm…Never seek for the soft spots or the easy places in hospital work (p. 69)."

How did you respond to Hampton Robb's insight? If you said to yourself, "bring it on," you can be assured you are on the right track to become a professional nurse! Ironically, little has changed in the world of nursing more than 100 years later. Depending on the care setting, it is not uncommon for a nurse to be directly responsible for five to ten patients or even more. In many care settings, 12-hour shifts are the norm as well as off shifts and every second or third weekend. Those who embrace this ethic toward work will be well prepared for professional practice.

In addition to being a hard worker, nurses must also be prompt and punctual. Being on time for class and clinical as well as for work is an essential component of professional behavior. If you struggle with this, now is the time to make it a strength and begin to act like the professional that you are and will soon become!

10. Are you inwardly motivated to take responsibility for your own learning?

Nursing is a very difficult major. In order to be successful, students must be willing to apply themselves and make nursing education a priority. They must be inwardly motivated to do so. Learning is a partnership or a collaboration between the student and nursing faculty. Nursing school is much more stressful and difficult than some students expect. Adult learners value participation, discovery, and construction of knowledge through active learning that requires them to apply knowledge. A less effective way of teaching is a passive environment where students attend class, take notes, and then ask the educator, "Just tell me what I need to pass the test."

As a result of this struggle, they want to know what they will be tested on so that they can continue to progress through the program. But for others, this statement represents an unwillingness to do the hard work that is needed to master a difficult major. Maintain this perspective: Nursing education is a partnership between student and faculty. As a student, you have the responsibility to make nursing education a priority and do the hard work that is needed to understand and master what you need to know to be the best possible nurse in practice.

11. Do you feel that your college owes you a degree because you paid for it?

Is education something that is earned, or something that is given to a student because they paid a price to access it? This is an important question that you must honestly answer as it relates to your mental mindset toward nursing education. Some nursing students communicate in no uncertain terms that because they paid their tuition they are owed a passing grade. This is nonsense. Nursing faculty are guardians of professional practice standards to protect the public trust and produce safe entry-level nurses. Regardless of any preconceived notions you may have as a student, faculty do not want to make your life miserable or fail you, but care about helping you! They want you to be well prepared for the challenging role of the nursing professional who must safely care for others.

Any sense of entitlement thinking must be removed upon entering the door of your nursing program if you want to be successful. Remember that learning is a partnership. A healthy educational climate is one where both students and educators are treated with respect. Students show respect for the learning process by owning their part to collaborate with nursing faculty to strengthen and develop their learning. Maintain this mindset to make the most of your nursing education.

12.   Are you naturally inquisitive about how things work?

Do you ask questions about things you don't know so you understand? Do you continue to ask "why" questions such as, "Why is the sky blue?" and then investigate to find the answer? If this comes naturally to you, this curiosity will translate to becoming an excellent nurse in practice. Here's why. One of the important responsibilities of the professional nurse is not just to perform the task but to understand the rationale or why for everything that is done in clinical practice. When the rationale is known, the foundation of critical thinking is established. The nurse is a knowledge worker and must be able to use this knowledge to benefit each patient by understanding the rationale and being clinically curious (Benner, Hughes, & Sutphen, 2008).

Clinical curiosity can improve quality of care when a patient has a problem that you have not seen previously. What is the pathophysiology of this problem and what are the most common complications seen as a result? When this is investigated and understood by the nurse, it lays the foundation of critical thinking and clinical reasoning, which is how a nurse thinks in practice. There are more than 5,000 medications in a nursing drug handbook. When you administer a medication you have not given previously, will you be clinically curious to look it up and identify the mechanism of action and safe dose ranges or will you just assume that everything is just fine because the physician ordered it? Clinical curiosity develops and strengthens your knowledge base and translates to safe patient care.

13.   Do you consider yourself a lifelong learner?

Do you love to learn for learning's sake? Or is learning just about passing a class and getting through the program? To be successful as a student and nurse in practice, you must embrace the role and responsibility of being a lifelong learner and enjoy the ride to maximize your learning. If you are internally motivated and enjoy learning for learning's sake, you will thrive as a nursing student.

In 2014, the Institute of Medicine (IOM) made its position on the value of lifelong learning in nursing education evident. In its report, "The Future of Nursing," issued jointly with The Robert Wood Johnson Foundation, it listed eight recommendations for moving the nursing profession forward. Recommendation six was to the point: Ensure that Nurses Engage in Lifelong Learning.

The IOM's blue-ribbon panel suggested that everyone involved in nursing education, from accrediting bodies to continuing education programs on down, unite to create an atmosphere where lifelong learning helps "gain the competencies needed to provide care for diverse populations across the lifespan ("Lifelong Learning," 2014).

14.   Do you have a natural aptitude for science?

Though nursing has its own body of knowledge or nursing science, the applied sciences of pharmacology, pathophysiology, fluid and electrolytes, and the math skills of dosage calculation are foundational to nursing. You may wonder, "Why are these applied sciences so important?" As a nurse in clinical practice for more than thirty years, I will briefly highlight why these applied sciences, though difficult, must be mastered by nursing students.

Pathophysiology

Most nursing students had pathophysiology as a required prerequisite for nursing. You may have thought that once you completed this difficult class you were done and could look forward to the nursing major. Unfortunately, this is wishful thinking! In order to deeply understand the mechanism of action for medications, accurately interpret lab values, and understand the disease process of the patients you care for, anatomy and physiology (A&P) must be DEEPLY understood so you can use this knowledge and apply this content to the bedside.

For example, understanding the complexities of the inflammatory and immune response is foundational when caring for a patient who has sepsis. Heart failure is another common disease process that requires the nurse to know the physiologic differences between right-sided versus left-sided heart failure. The symptoms unique to each type of heart failure begin to make sense and specific clinical signs of worsening heart failure will be anticipated by the nurse who understands these differences.

Nursing students need to understand the mechanism of action of every medication that is administered, the pathophysiology in the mechanism of action described in nursing drug manuals, and the physiological impact of the drug on the body must be understood. The unique variances of pharmacology and how a drug is metabolized and absorbed depending on the age of the patient (pediatric vs. elderly), chronic medical conditions (liver and/or renal disease) must also be known and considered.

For example, a common cardiac medication that is given for hypertension is atenolol, whose pharmacologic classification is a beta blocker. To understand what a beta blocker such as atenolol is blocking, students must be able to know which nervous system (sympathetic or parasympathetic) beta receptors receive stimulation and the physiologic effects or expected outcomes when these same receptors are blocked. If a patient with acute or chronic renal failure is receiving opiate narcotics for pain control, how would this influence dosage that the nurse would administer and excretion by the body? Knowing that opiate narcotics are excreted primarily by the renal system, this knowledge is relevant and must be considered by the nurse when considering dose to administer as well as adverse effects of over sedation.

Pharmacology/Mechanism of Action

Nurses administer medications every day. They must possess a DEEP UNDERSTANDING of pharmacology. Most students aren't aware that if a nurse administers a medication that is wrong (contraindicated), even though a physician or nurse practitioner has written the order, the nurse is held professionally responsible for this error.

To ensure safe practice, nurses must know and understand why your patients are on the medications that are administered and do all necessary safety checks. This is more easily said than done. You will have multiple patients and medications to pass and will be tempted to take shortcuts. There are more than five thousand medications used in practice and nursing drug manuals are more than a thousand pages in length.

Nursing drug manuals include indications, mechanism of action, pharmacologic classification, time/action profile, contraindications, side effects, interactions, route and dosages, nursing implications, and patient education. If a student has multiple medications to pass, what content areas of the drug manual are the most important?

Though all aspects of a drug manual are important and need to be known, I believe that the MECHANISM OF ACTION is the most important area to master. When the nurse understands how the medication affects the body, understanding this relationship will make the resultant nursing assessments self-evident as well as anticipating the most common side effects. When the mechanism of action is deeply understood, the nurse does not need to consult the drug manual for this content, but will know it based on their applied knowledge.

Fluids & Electrolytes

Fluids and Electrolytes (F&E) are foundational to critical thinking in the clinical setting. This content is challenging because it requires application of chemistry, acid/base knowledge, and physiology. Just as anatomy and physiology is essential to understand the mechanism of action, applied A&P must be integrated into F&E in order for practical application and contextualization to the bedside to be realized.

Laboratory values provide a window to EARLY physiologic status changes that may not be initially evident in vital signs or assessment data collected by the nurse. Examples of this in clinical practice are TRENDS of an elevated serum lactate in any shock state, elevated neutrophils, bands, or WBCs that are typically seen in sepsis, or elevated serum creatinine in acute renal failure or severe dehydration.

For example, in acute renal failure (ARF), would you be able to identify the relationship between ARF and elevation in creatinine, BUN, potassium, and decrease in CO_2 (serum bicarbonate)? Would you be able to anticipate the expected electrolyte derangements most often seen with dehydration caused by severe vomiting and diarrhea? WHY are they present? Students must be able to APPLY knowledge to practice by identifying the most important labs based on the patient's disease and why they are present. When students have this level of understanding, they will be PROACTIVE and anticipate problems early because they will use knowledge and understand the WHY or rationale.

Math/Dosage Calculation

Though computers and calculators have made basic math skills much easier with little thinking required except to input the required data, dosage calculation must be understood and the results correctly validated to ensure safe practice. A simple miscalculation can be deadly! For example, an incorrect calculation of potassium chloride can result in a lethal injection that results in arrhythmias and cardiac arrest (heart stops beating). Dosage calculation is a unique subset of math that you likely did not have in high school.

Actor Dennis Quaid and his wife, Kimberly, had newborn twins who were given 1,000 times the intended dosage of heparin twice by the primary nurse. Fortunately no lasting harm occurred, but a lawsuit was filed as a result. In one five-year period more than 16,000 heparin errors were blamed on incorrect dosing (Ornstein, 2007).

Make it a priority to understand the principles behind setting up a correct formula, correctly calculating, and then administering the correct dose. Another key component of dosage calculation is understanding and memorizing the metric equivalents of micrograms, milligrams, grams, and kilograms. Be sure you know how many micrograms make a milligram, how many milligrams make a gram, and how many milliliters make up a kilogram.

Though a natural aptitude for science and math will make it easier to master this essential content, it is NOT in itself a prerequisite to nursing school success. Go into nursing school with your eyes wide open! If you know that science and math are not your strength, know up front that it will require additional time and energy to strengthen your learning so you can make this and any other weakness strengths by the time you graduate!

15.   What are you willing to give up to make school a priority?

You have 168 hours in each week. No more, no less. There is no way to purchase additional hours in life if you find yourself short. Something has to give. For some students, this dilemma is represented by the amount of hours they work while in nursing school. To be blunt, if you really want to not only pass your program but deeply understand what is being taught so you can apply it at the bedside of each patient you will care for, you need to reboot your priorities and eliminate activities to more effectively manage your time! One of the areas directly under your control is placing clear boundaries in your social life and social media.

Have you ever counted the minutes and hours you spend on Facebook, Twitter, YouTube, or other avenues of social media? I would encourage you to keep a log for a few days. Could this time be better spent studying? What about your social life? Do you feel obligated to maintain the friendships you have while in school in the same manner as you did before? This, too, may be an unrealistic expectation.

Are you willing to make needed short-term sacrifices for long-term gain? This is the mindset that will help you be successful while in nursing school. If you are willing to do what is needed to make nursing school a priority, you will not only make it through the program, but more importantly, you will be the best nurse you can possibly be. Trust me, it will be worth it and your true friends will still be there for you after you graduate!

You may have many competing life priorities. Determine how and where you spend your time and what you can give up. It does not always have to be work. If you are a mom with kids at home, can you assign chores or jobs to the kids for folding laundry, cleaning, cooking, and making lunches? You may need to "lower your standards" for a season. It's okay if your home is not perfect. Again, it is a temporary sacrifice for a long-term gain. You are also role modeling how important college education is to your children and family. Minimize any outside distractions. Say a temporary goodbye or cut back the amount of time you commit to volunteer opportunities in the community or at church. You will come back to those later, but for now, do not feel guilty to put them on hold if needed.

Another important area to consider is how many hours you work each week. Some students must work in excess of 30 hours a week to support their family or have other obligations. I understand. But if possible, work less than 30 hours a week, while no more than 20 hours a week should be a goal. This observation is based on students I have taught who realized too late that their decision to work more than 20 hours a week and be a full-time nursing student was too much. They ended up failing or dropping out before the end of the semester.

One can hear you crying out, "I am the exception, I have been to school before and handled this load." That may be true, but there is one small but significant difference. You did not go through nursing school before. If you are carrying a full-time load, you will need to commit to an additional 20 hours of studying a week in addition to attending class and clinical. You do the math. Something has to give. Do not let it be your nursing education.

16. Do you have strong attention to detail?

If you manufacture a product on the assembly line and fail to pay close attention to the manufacturing process nobody dies. But as a nurse in practice, you must never forget the implications if you fail to pay close attention to the details and miss subtle signs and symptoms of a change in status such as sepsis progressing to septic shock. Your patient could die as a result. The nursing literature has identified this ongoing problem as "failure to rescue." It occurs when the nurse does not recognize early signs of a complication that needlessly progresses and an adverse outcome, including patient death, occurs (Clarke & Aiken, 2003).

Step back and ask yourself, "Do I possess or have a strong attention to detail or do I tend to hurry up and just get the task done?" The most common tasks in nursing include medication administration, vital signs, and a head-to-toe assessment. If these tasks are not combined with critical thinking and strong attention to detail, this can result in an adverse outcome and even patient death.

How strong is your attention to detail when you pass medications? Are you meticulous and committed to not take shortcuts to identify the essential rights of safe administration? Do you routinely check expiration dates of everything that you pass? These little things are really the big things in clinical practice. If you struggle in this area, it is important to identify and recognize this as a weakness, but then work hard to make it a strength before you graduate!

Never forget that mistakes and errors in practice have implications for the patient. In 1999, the Institute of Medicine report estimated that almost 100,000 patients died annually in this country as a result of errors by health care providers. Many changes have been implemented since then to prevent needless death. Though mistakes will still happen because you are human, do your part to minimize the likelihood of errors. Take no shortcuts in school or in practice.

17.   When you make a mistake, do you learn from it, or do you try to cover it up?

You are human. You will make mistakes as a student nurse or in practice. It is inevitable and only a matter of when. What is your initial response to any type of mistake that you make in your life? Do you make it personal and use it as an opportunity to berate yourself for what you have done and cover it up at all costs? Or do you use mistakes as an opportunity for reflection and personal growth? The best and most healthy response is to learn from your mistakes so they don't happen again!

I made a medication error and gave the incorrect dose. No harm was done, but as I reflected on how this could have happened, I realized that I was stressed by multiple patient demands and made a shortcut by not doing the required medication checks to ensure the correct dose. I learned from this mistake and made a commitment to not sacrifice the rights of medication administration regardless of how busy I am. To the best of my knowledge, I have not made a similar mistake since.

If you make a mistake, are you honest and own up to it? Or do you tend to minimize and hide your mistake from others so no one finds out? If so, this character trait will follow you into nursing and you will likely attempt to cover your tracks. This is unacceptable. A lack of disclosure with any type of error or mistake does not just impact you, it also affects the patient and can result in a possible adverse outcome. Be honest with yourself and carefully reflect on how you handle mistakes in your life. Make it a priority to commit to be a person of integrity who consistently does the right thing.

The culture in health care is changing from blaming the individual to looking at the systems that may have contributed to a medication error by the nurse. When nurses honestly report errors made in practice, this data is collected to identify trends that will result in improving patient safety. By self-reporting errors, it is less likely that the nurse will be personally targeted, but will instead contribute to making health care safer for all!

18.   How well do you perform under stress?

Nursing school as well as nursing practice is extremely stressful. There is a large amount of content that must be learned in order to safely care for patients. The passing percentage is higher than most other majors and the stress and anxiety of testing and getting through the program is significant. You will need to have a high tolerance for ongoing stress in school. More importantly, you must be able to perform well with the unexpected stress and fast pace you will experience caring for patients in clinical practice.

For example, you will be trained in basic life support as a required prerequisite to care for patients in the clinical setting. Being trained to do CPR is one thing, but what if you have to use it unexpectedly when you find your patient pale and without a pulse or respiratory effort? Will you still be able to remember what you have been taught and do what is needed to save your patient's life? Though this example is dramatic, this can and will likely happen sooner or later. It is only a matter of when. Less dramatic stress includes the high acuity levels and demands of patients you care for, families that can be difficult, and multiple patient assignments. The nurse must be able to think clearly and handle these stressors and remain attentive to detail to thrive in clinical practice.

19.   How well are you able to multitask?

To handle the ongoing demands and stress of nursing practice, you must be able to multitask or be able to successfully manage and prioritize competing tasks. Recognize the most important thing that needs to be done first and then quickly go to the second, the third and the fourth in quick succession. It is a learned activity. Though the ability to recognize what is most important will be developed with clinical experience, it is important to honestly reflect and determine how well you typically handle the stress of numerous pressing demands that seem to come all at once.

You will experience this reality in nursing school with numerous ongoing demands, assignments, and readings that must be completed. The ability to multitask becomes even more essential once you are in nursing practice. Because you will have larger patient assignments – and with each patient numerous demands – if you can successfully balance two or three platters in nursing school as well as in life, you will be well suited and prepared for nursing practice!

20.   Do you readily recognize your limitations and what you do/don't know?

Have you ever heard the term "intellectual humility"? It is a character trait that is essential for every successful nursing student. You must give yourself grace to be a student learner, that you do not know it all and will even make mistakes. Be in tune and know your limitations. Some nursing students struggle with being less than perfect and will resist any suggestion that they do not know what they really don't know. This is the opposite of humility, which recognizes one's weaknesses. If you can accept yourself as less than perfect but willing to work hard to be the best nurse you can possibly be, you are well on your way to being successful not only in nursing school, but in practice as well.

The "everyone gets a trophy" approach to athletic competition and the consistent and undue praise that students may have received growing up may have had the unintended consequence of creating an over-inflated ego that can impact adult learners by making them prone to being more narcissistic with an inflated sense of self-worth (Walton, 2015). This could affect a nursing student's receptiveness to criticism and constructive feedback.

21.   Are you comfortable asking questions about anything that is unfamiliar to you?

Men have been stereotyped as being resistant to asking questions even when they are hopelessly lost. They would much rather figure it out with their road map than stop and ask for help. If you fail to ask for help, nobody gets hurt, but you will likely be delayed in getting to your destination. In nursing education and especially in the clinical setting, this reluctance to acknowledge what you do not know and ask questions can directly impact patient outcomes and possibly harm your patient.

This is why intellectual humility is such an important trait for nursing students. There is no such thing as a dumb question, only the one you know the answer to! When you are comfortable and willing to acknowledge what you don't know, you will readily ask questions to understand your knowledge deficits and be safe in clinical practice. If you try to fake it, you will likely end up harming your patient. You can never know it all. Each clinical setting has different protocols and procedures that will often need clarification. I am much more fearful of those students and new nurses who never ask questions than those who readily acknowledge their limitations and ask a question to clarify their knowledge.

When I surveyed experienced nurses for the wisdom they would offer to a brand-new nurse for my book *THINK like a Nurse!* the most common response these experienced nurses offered to new nurses was the importance to be willing to ask questions. One experienced nurse's response captures the essence of this topic and says it all:

"A good nurse is always willing to ask questions even if it makes them look stupid. It is better to be willing to appear stupid than be dangerous to your patients" (Rischer, 2013, p. 169).

22. Are you comfortable doing intimate cares and handling body fluids while maintaining privacy and dignity for the patient?

As a nurse you will have access to the most intimate aspects of a person's life and being. You will know things about them from their history that may be unknown to others in their family. Nursing care involves both physical and emotional intimacy. Patients are often incontinent and cannot control their bowel or bladder. Therefore, the nurse provides perineal care for both men and women. How comfortable would you be with this level of patient intimacy and cleaning up while emotionally supporting the patient who may be totally embarrassed that he has lost control of bodily function?

Foley catheters are tubes that are inserted into the urethra to measure urinary output or placed when there is urinary retention. How comfortable would you be cleansing the labia of a woman or the head of a penis and then inserting the catheter?

Though you will be trained to do this procedure in nursing school, are you comfortable performing this level of intimate care on another man or woman? It may take time to be comfortable with intimate care, but this comfort level must be attained because it is a required and expected for clinical practice.

Just as important as being comfortable performing this intimate skill is to remain empathetic and treat the patient with dignity and respect. This is especially relevant when you are working with someone who grew up in another culture and may have concerns about modesty and exposure to a caregiver who is of the opposite sex.

A nurse educator colleague shared her personal story of what it feels like when this dignity and respect is NOT evidenced by the nurse:

While I was a patient in the hospital I had to have a Foley catheter inserted. The nursing instructor came into my room and asked if she could have a student perform the procedure. I said "sure" because I always enjoyed working with students as a nurse. She came back with two students, not just the one, to perform the procedure. Then eight additional students followed to "observe" and formed a semicircle around the end of the bed like they were watching television. They were silent as the instructor walked the student performing the procedure how to do this, until one of the students shouted as they pointed to my bottom area "There it is!" They seemed proud that they could identify the urethra (opening to the bladder) and at that point I felt like a science experiment. I had a towel next to my head and pulled it over my eyes until they all went away as the procedure was completed.

One simple takeaway is to remember that as nurses we are caring for a human being of infinite value and worth; therefore, be sure all that is done while providing care treats them as such!

23.   How well do you handle responsibility?

In the movie "*Spiderman*, it was said, "With great power comes great responsibility." This is also true for the responsibilities that come when working as a nurse. As a practicing nurse, you literally hold the life of another human being in your hands. You are responsible to apply knowledge and identify a possible complication before it needlessly progresses. When you recognize a complication early, you can be a superhero like Spiderman and save a life! Unfortunately, the converse is also true. If you fail to recognize a complication until it is too late, the same patient could experience needless complications and could even die.

This is the incredible responsibility that every nurse must embrace. How well do you handle responsibility in general? Are you willing to own and embrace this responsibility, or does it frighten you? As a student you will be inexperienced and have much to learn. That is expected. You must be willing to be accountable and embrace the responsibility that comes with caring for patients of infinite value and worth.

This is why every student must embrace the desire to be the best nurse you can possibly be. Commit to making this a priority now while you are in school. You must resist the natural tendency to just want to get by. You must dig deep and DESIRE to be the best nurse that you can possibly be. This mindset and attitude needs to begin the first day of nursing school and continue until you retire after many years of clinical practice!

24.   How well do you communicate with others?

Nursing is all about relationships:

- Nurse to patient
- Nurse to family
- Nurse to nurse
- Nurse to physician or primary care providers
- Nurse to other members of the health care team

Enjoying the relationships of others and communicating effectively are personal skills that will predict your success as a nurse. The ability to connect on this person to person level is also perceived as a caring behavior by your patients. Conversely, if you are a loner, enjoy being by yourself, and are more comfortable texting than talking with another person, this could be a challenge that will affect your ability to communicate effectively and relate authentically to your patients.

One practical way to intentionally engage with each patient and relate to them on a person to person level is to take the time to uncover the unique story of your patient's life. Take the time to learn details about the patient's family, children, grandchildren as well as their past occupation or life roles and any unique accomplishments. I have had patients share their unique contributions as an engineer in the space program in the 1960s, battlefield heroics in World War II and the Korean War, and other unique roles that are detailed in history books.

When the patient's story is known, something transformative begins to take place. The nurse begins to see the patient on a personal level that builds and strengthens this person to person therapeutic relationship and trust. Relevant information helps to put the clinical picture together. Remember that our relationship is focused on the patient for therapeutic purposes as well as establishing trust so we can advance the plan of care for their recovery. This level of emotional connectedness requires energy from the nurse that can easily become depleted over time (Self-care is crucial and is discussed further in chapter 2.

Being effective and comfortable communicating with others in a therapeutic manner is a life skill that is relevant to nursing. If the nurse is unable to effectively communicate the plan of care to the patient and family, the patient's ability to be an active participant in the plan of care will be affected. If the nurse is unable to effectively communicate a clinical concern to the oncoming nurse or the primary care provider, this can also directly impact patient care and outcomes.

Incivility and bullying behaviors among nurses and health care providers is endemic. The essence of incivility is a lack of respect for others and an indirect style of communication. If you evaluate your communication style, are you direct or indirect in how you communicate a concern to another person? If another person did something that offended you, would you go directly to that person to address your concern or would you be more likely to discuss your thoughts and feelings about this incident with everyone but the person with whom you had the concern?

Make it a priority to adopt a more direct and respectful style of communication. Commit to never speak negatively of another person in their absence. This includes your feelings regarding other students, nursing faculty, and the nursing program. I have found this to be all too common in nursing school. This is another way that the seeds of incivility are sown.

If you find yourself an unwilling participant in another student's critical rant of another person, do the hard but right thing and stand up for the absent colleague. Encourage the person to go directly to the other and keep it between them and NOT the group. Make a supportive comment such as, "It sounds like you have a problem with this person. It seems you should discuss it with them personally," then wait for a response or walk away.

25.   How well do you handle conflict with others?

How you honestly respond to this question will strongly suggest if you will be part of the problem or part of the solution to bullying and incivility in the nursing profession. If you have conflict and disagree with another person, do you still value and respect their perspective and seek to find common ground? Are you able to step back and view this conflict from the other's perspective and any stress that may have influenced the conflict? Do you have strong conflict resolution skills? This is an important interpersonal/communication skill that is a weakness for many nursing students.

Grover (2005) identified eight skills that are essential for effective communication. These skills include:

- Listening to the other person
- Asking open-ended questions to gain more in-depth information
- Asking closed questions to gain facts
- Clarifying in order to get more details
- Paraphrasing so that meaning can be interpreted
- Using facilitators to encourage continuing dialogue

- Assessing nonverbal communication cues
- Using silence to promote thinking.

Though many of these communication skills are learned from an early age, when facing a challenging or confrontational situation, these fundamental approaches may be forgotten.

If you experience conflict with another person, do you tend to interpret this conflict as an attack on yourself and think negatively of this person and share your critical concerns with others? Though this type of behavior may appear to be normal to some, it is unprofessional and must be called out for what it really is, bullying and disrespectful behavior that has the power to deeply wound and devastate another human being.

The most common overt bullying behaviors in nursing include patterns of fault-finding, intimidation, gossip, put-downs, and nonverbal innuendo such as raising eyebrows or sighing. More subtle bullying behaviors include isolation, exclusion, ignoring/refusing to help, and unfair assignments (Bartholomew, 2006). Other categories of bullying behavior include the resentful nurse who holds grudges and encourages others to join in as well as the cliquish nurse who intentionally excludes others from their "group" (Dellasega, 2009).

Be the needed change in nursing by incorporating an attitude of valuing and respecting one another regardless of any differences. Here are some practical guidelines to live this out in all that you do as a student as well as a nurse in practice:

- VALUE the perspective and expertise of ALL health care team members.
- RESPECT the unique attributes that members bring to a team.
- APPRECIATE the importance of all professional collaboration.
- VALUE TEAMWORK and the relationships within the team.
- VALUE different styles of communication used by patients, families, and health care providers.
- Contribute to resolution of conflict and disagreement ("Pre-Licensure KSAS," 2014).

Results

So how did you do on my quiz? Using the same general passing guidelines in nursing education of 80 percent, if we agreed on 20 or more of my reflections, you may have the aptitude essential to nursing practice and this might be a good fit for your professional career. If you scored 14–19, nursing may be a career you could consider exploring further. Discussion of this with a college career counselor might be helpful. Consider exploring shadowing a nurse for a part of a day or doing an informal informational interview of a nurse to understand more about the profession.

If you scored 13 or less, nursing may not be good fit for you, but discuss this further with a college career counselor. To see for yourself what nursing entails, determine the options available to you in your community to shadow a nurse or volunteer in a health care setting. If you are already enrolled in a nursing program, discuss the areas that are a current weakness with your nursing faculty and collaborate to come up with a plan that will help develop these weaknesses into strengths!

CHAPTER 1 HIGHLIGHTS

- Nursing requires a unique set of aptitudes and skills.
- Each student needs to honestly reflect and determine areas that may be a weakness or a strength.
- The nurse must care as well as possess character.
- The nurse is a knowledge worker who must be able to apply the sciences and all that is taught to the bedside of patient care.
- Nursing school must be a priority and nursing students need to be willing to do whatever is needed in order to maximize learning.
- Practice direct communication and manage conflict by maintaining an attitude of respect, seek common ground, and make a commitment to not speak negatively about others.

Chapter Reflections

1. What was the total score on your quiz?

2. What areas were your personal strengths?

3. What were areas for improvement?

4. What will you do to develop and make any identified weakness your strength by the time you graduate?

The human brain is amazing. It functions 24 hours for 365 days a year. It functions right from the time we were born and only stops when we...TAKE EXAMS!

Chapter 2

How to THRIVE, not Merely Survive, as a Nursing Student

Most of you have taken that next big step and have applied for or are in the nursing program of your choice. What are some additional strategies and information you need in order to successfully complete this challenging and rewarding major? Your goal is not merely to survive, but thrive as a nursing student. It is possible! Let me share some additional thoughts to guide you on the next step of your journey.

Have Realistic Expectations

I have observed that nursing students as a whole are driven, perfectionistic, and used to getting A's in high school or college. You must remind yourself that you are no longer in high school or a less difficult major in college. You are in nursing school. Nursing is typically the most difficult major on most college campuses and is not a program that you can simply attend class and expect to pass. You must spend at least 20 hours a week studying and be highly engaged in your learning.

Even if you were an A student or the valedictorian of your high school class, you may struggle to maintain the grades you have been accustomed to receiving. Accept this reality as your new normal. Most students do not receive an A, but B's are typical. Continue learning and applying yourself to do your best. This is what matters most!

Step back, take a deep breath, and remind yourself that your letter grade or your behavior does not define your value and worth as a person or student. Nor is it a predictor of whether you will be successful as a nurse in practice. I believe that your true identity, value, and worth is defined by God and His unconditional love for you, not by your performance. It is important that you also recognize the incredible intrinsic value and worth of who you are.

Don't Do It Alone

Burnout is higher in nursing than any other health care profession and the level of professional dissatisfaction is four times greater than the average worker (Aiken et al., 2001). Stress in nursing students is higher than medical students and in the general population (Jones & Johnstone, 1997).

The most common sources of stress for nursing students are related to academics and include student workload and problems associated with studying. Fear of unknown situations in the clinical setting, mistakes with patients or handling of technical equipment can also cause stress. These stresses persist throughout the time a student is in nursing education (Pulido-Martos, Augusto-Landa, & Lopez-Zafra, 2011).

In order to counter the inevitable stress of nursing education, maintain social support during your time in school. Student nurses can be reluctant to seek help for stress (Ajzen, 2011) and may even harbor negative attitudes toward those with mental health difficulties (Halter, 2004). These negative attitudes may leave student nurses less willing to seek help for stress should they need it. As a result, they may use avoidance and ignore what they are feeling, which may raise the risk of burnout even further (Gibbons, 2010).

Though nursing students were less likely to seek out formal counseling, social support was the most common approach to cope with the stress in nursing students (Galbraith, Brown, & Clifton, 2014). Make it a priority to seek out support throughout your time in nursing education. Resist the temptation to do it alone and you will be one step ahead. Trust me, the storms will come. It is the wise student who seeks supportive and collaborative relationships with family, friends, and other nursing students!

Peer Support

Social support from student colleagues is important and can benefit students by reducing stress, enhancing learning, and facilitating the socialization into the nursing profession (Hatmaker, Park, & Rethemeyer, 2011). Students who perceive themselves to be all in the same boat and are able to share their unique experiences, reinforce each other's knowledge and can enhance their confidence as a nurse (Ranse & Grealish, 2007). Ironically, the support that student colleagues require can have a negative effect in the clinical setting.

Students can develop a parallel community, which can isolate them from potential supportive relationships in the clinical setting when they congregate and isolate themselves from staff and potential learning opportunities (Roberts, 2009). I have witnessed this as a clinical instructor and it is a common behavior of nursing students. To promote your learning, resist this temptation to lean too heavily on other students in the clinical setting and seek support from your assigned nursing staff as much as possible.

Learning Resilience

Though high levels of stress are inevitable in nursing education, this stress can be used to promote resilience in each nursing student. Resilience is the ability to not only survive adversity but learn and grow from the experience. (McAllister & Lowe, 2011). Resilience will help you find meaning and cope more effectively with the stressors you will inevitably face in the clinical setting (Stephens, 2013).

Nursing programs are rigorous and require determination and resolve in order to complete the program. Baldacchino and Galea (2012) found that in addition to pure desire to complete a nursing program, students require high levels of hardiness (students who remain emotionally strong during stress) in order meet the comprehensive demands of the program. Students also need self-confidence to realize that they can meet the expectations of nursing education (Schmukle & Egloff, 2008; Griswold, 2014).

As a novice nursing student, you will experience many "firsts" that can cause high levels of anxiety and stress. These "firsts" include the intimate care of both male and female patients, death and dying, exposure to communicable diseases, and incivility and bullying in both academia and in the clinical setting. These experiences have been linked to high attrition rates in nursing education (Thomas & Burk, 2009).

If you are a young adult, you are particularly vulnerable to the negative effects of stress due immature coping abilities and lack of experience in dealing with conflict (Stephens, 2013). Resilience is one of the key components that will help you not just to survive, but thrive in nursing education and over the years of clinical practice. The importance of self-care and finding supportive relationships will help you develop this resilience in nursing school as well as in clinical practice.

The Importance of Self-Efficacy

The very stress and rigor of nursing education can also help you build self-efficacy. Self-efficacy is your belief and ability to rise up and successfully overcome adversity that impacts your life (Bandura, 1994). Your ability to develop self-efficacy can predict how well you will overcome the difficulties in nursing education, academic performance, ability to successfully complete your program, clinical performance, and even your emotional and mental health (Taylor & Reyes, 2012).

Conversely, students who were not able to overcome challenges can undermine the development of self-efficacy. Developing resilience through persevering and overcoming hurdles and difficulties while in nursing school may play an important role in persevering through the challenges inherent in the nursing profession (Taylor & Reyes, 2012).

The Power of Empowerment

When you experience difficulties in your life, do you tend to play the victim? Or do you respond with resolve and take control of those aspects of the situation as you are able? It has been shown that your ability to be resilient and overcome difficulties in nursing education will be directly related to the degree of your feelings of empowerment. Empowerment is the ability of an individual who believes in her or his own abilities and does not focus on deficiencies. Those who feel empowered are more likely to succeed in school as well as in clinical practice (Simoni et al., 2004).

Why You Must Possess Passion

What is it that separates those that are successful in everything they do and those who are not? Is it intelligence, education, or social status? No. The most important characteristic of your success will be your passion. You must have a burning desire to be the best and overcome any obstacles that may be in front of you. If you have this burning passion, even if you are average or ordinary in your abilities you can and will achieve and accomplish great things! This is why nurturing and cultivating passion is so important for you as a student or as a nurse in practice (Maxwell, 1999).

Passion is the first step to accomplishing your goals. Your desire determines your destiny. Those who live extraordinary lives have great desire. A small fire creates little heat. The larger and stronger your fire, the greater your desire and the greater your potential will be to achieve great things as a nurse in practice (Maxwell, 1999).

Passion also increases your willpower. There is no substitute for passion. It is the fuel for your will. If you want to be a nurse bad enough you will find the willpower to achieve it. The only way to have this kind of desire is to develop a burning passion that must be in you. Passion makes the impossible possible. If you have a burning fire in your heart this will lift everything in your life (Maxwell, 1999).

This is why passionate educators and nurses are the best in practice. Passion is also contagious. If you possess this fiery passion you will impact those around you and be a leader by your example.

What Is Your Temperature?

Do you possess this fiery passion to be the best nurse you can possibly be? Are you overwhelmed with stress and just wanting to survive each day? To increase your passion, the following are some practical strategies to see this realized in your life (Maxwell, 1999):

- **Take your temperature.** How passionate are you really about nursing and nursing education? Does it show? Ask those around you including students and family about your level of desire and if it is hot, cold, or waning.
- **Return to your first love.** Too many students allow the tyranny of the urgent and stress of nursing school or practice to get them off track and steal their joy and passion. Look back to when you were just starting out as a student or as a nurse in practice. Try to recapture this enthusiasm. Then evaluate your current passion in light of those former desires.
- **Associate with people of passion.** Birds of a feather really do flock together. If you've lost your passion and desire, you need to get around some firelighters! Because passion is contagious, make it a priority to have friends and colleagues who will infect you with passion instead of stealing your joy with their negativity.

Take Care of Yourself!

Nurses have one of the highest rates of burnout among all health care professionals. This can be attributed in part to the tendency to put the needs of others ahead of their own, as well as the ongoing physical and emotional strain of caring for patients who are sick, dying, or demanding. When these forces are combined with the prevalence of extended (12-hour) shifts, high acuity/high stress settings such as oncology, med/surg, ED, and critical care as well as increasing patient workloads and staffing challenges, the end result is physical and emotional exhaustion that can begin a slow flameout that can eventually lead to burnout (Alexander, 2012).

Burnout has been described as the progressive loss of the initial idealism, passion, energy, and purpose to enter the profession (Edelwich & Brodsky, 1980). Burnout can also be defined as the loss of human caring or the separation of caregiving and caring (Benner & Wrubel, 1989). Students are not immune to this all-too-common reality. High levels of stress and ongoing demands in nursing education can contribute to the early progression of burnout that typically manifests as mental and physical exhaustion.

Value of Self-Care

To maintain a healthy balance and to prevent burnout in practice, nursing students must recognize the value of self-care. This must start while you are a student! Though school will consume you with new challenges and additional learning, do NOT let nursing education become your life! Fight to overcome the "tyranny of the urgent" or the tendency to allow your life to be dictated by the pressing "urgent" aspects of nursing school. Do not neglect those things that are really more important (faith, family, relationships) simply because they do not demand your immediate attention.

Pursue and fight for balance by establishing "margin" in your life. Margin is the space between your current demands and your limit to handle them (Swenson, 2004). Those blank spaces on the sides of each page of a book have a purpose, as do margins or blank spaces in your daily life. If you continually push yourself to the point of your load limit, you will soon find out that this cannot be sustained for the long haul of nursing education.

The perpetual "gerbil wheel" you feel in school with its incessant, ongoing demands requires you to be fully aware of the need to renew your body, mind, and spirit. If your "tank" of personal renewal is empty or dangerously low, this will directly affect your ability to be fully engaged and caring in practice.

The essence of The Serenity Prayer is relevant to prevent burnout and encourages self-care. The Serenity Prayer emphasizes the importance of accepting what cannot be changed, courage to change those things that are within your control, and wisdom to know the difference (Niebuhr, 1942). Most of the stresses that you will experience are NOT easily changed or within your direct control. You must learn to accept those things, but recognize that you have the power to directly control and change your RESPONSE to stress.

Following are specific strategies to empower you to make change and adjustments in school as well as in practice. It is important to note that as a result of high levels of stress while in nursing school, students are at a higher risk of developing physical and even mental illness. Managing stress effectively is not an option as a student or nurse in practice!

Personal Lifestyle Strategies

- **Obtain adequate sleep.** The magic number is SEVEN hours of sleep minimum every night. Adequate amounts of sleep are the easiest way to prevent emotional and physical exhaustion.
- **Eat healthy.** The common saying "Garbage in, garbage out" certainly has relevance here!
- **Engage in regular physical activity.** Thirty minutes of sustained activity three to five times a week reduces stress. For those who have exercise aversion, a brisk walk is just as effective. Look up the pathophysiology of endorphins and the secondary benefits this provides as well!
- **Identify what is MOST important in life and make time for it.** I readily identify with students who are highly driven and task/goal oriented and who struggle to achieve balance. Though successfully completing nursing education is important, spouses, children, and friendships require QUANTITY time, not just quality, to thrive and survive the rigors of nursing school and practice.
- **Nurture your spirituality.** In addition to cultivating your spiritual life for balance and purpose in life, spirituality has relevance to patient care as a nurse. In order to provide meaningful spiritual care in the clinical setting, you must personally cultivate this in your own life.
- **Participate in outside interests.** It's tempting to keep the pedal to the metal and make nursing school your life. Although it is important to be committed and serious about your education, you must also remember the importance of BALANCE.
- **Recognize your limitations.** Don't push yourself to the brink of exhaustion to pursue perfection as a student.

Professional/Educational Lifestyle Strategies

- **Set realistic goals.** Recognize the difficulty of the nursing major, and readjust your GPA goal to reflect this reality and "new normal."
- **Seek support from colleagues or other students.** The relevance of this principle was validated over 2,500 years ago in the book of Ecclesiastes in the Old Testament: "Two are better than

one... For if they fall, the one will lift up his fellow: but woe to him that is alone when he falleth; for he hath not another to help him up" (Ecclesiastes 4:9–10).

- **Grieve well.** You should never remain oblivious or indifferent to the pain and suffering of patients you will encounter in practice. Remain empathetic, but realize the need for support when grief or painful feelings need to be addressed.
- **Take breaks as needed.** Make time for rest, hobbies, relationships, faith, and any other interests that are important to you. Nursing students tend to be highly driven, and need to be reminded that what comes naturally may not benefit them in practice. I have found the book *Margin: Restoring Emotional, Physical, Financial, and Time Reserves to Overloaded Lives* a helpful book in this ongoing battle for balance!

My Story

Though I did not experience burnout as a student, it did happen to me as a nurse in the ED. I share my story as a word to the wise. Learn from my experience, especially as you graduate and work in the clinical setting.

When I first started in the ED, it was a dream come true. From the adrenalin rush that came with caring for critically ill patients, to the wide range of clinical presentations, it was a stimulating environment for me. I became more proficient in clinical skills and critical thinking as I drew from my prior years of experience in critical care. I was engaged and truly cared about what happened to each patient I saw and cared for. I enjoyed what I was doing so much I began to pick up overtime on a regular basis because it was readily available. I became more physically and emotionally tired, but I did not realize that I was beginning to DRIFT.

Slowly but gradually over time, I began not to care. What I once enjoyed, was now just a job and putting in my time. Patients became burdens. I had critical patients and some of them died as a result of their injuries or illness. I did not truly care. When I began to reflect and saw how far I had fallen from my original motivation to care for others, I knew I had to do something dramatic to recapture my heart. I left the ED and renewed my passion for caring in an entirely different environment in acute care. In addition to a change of scenery, I also needed REST, which led to RESToration.

I have experienced the wisdom of Benner and Wrubel, who wrote:

"It is a peculiarly modern mistake to think that caring is the cause of the burnout and that the cure is to protect oneself from caring to prevent the 'disease' called burnout. Rather, the loss of caring is the sickness, and the return of caring is the recovery" (1989, p. 473).

There is no reason to remain highly stressed in a setting that may contribute to burnout when there are so many opportunities to change your practice environment. With the wide variety of acute care units in any hospital, and clinical practice environments in the community, change is readily possible and must be pursued. The ability to further your education and pursue advanced practice roles can ensure that you will remain caring and engaged throughout your career. But introspection and reflection are also needed before making any needed changes. The "if I were somewhere else I would be happier" line of thinking may only bring current baggage to a new practice setting. It may be a temporary fix that does not get to the root of contributing factors.

Breaking Free from the Tyranny of the Urgent

The trap that many students fall into while in nursing school is that what is most important in life (taking time to cultivate relationships) does NOT insist on being done immediately. But the URGENT things or never-ending tasks of nursing school demand our immediate attention and action. Without realizing it, we become slaves to the TYRANNY of the URGENT. By choosing the urgent, we can begin to neglect what is most important in our life.

In the classic article "Tyranny of the Urgent" (1967), Charles Hummel insightfully stated that there is a constant tension in our life between the URGENT and the IMPORTANT.

Filter your day by identifying what is "nice to do" and what is "need to do." The urgent tasks that continually press are NICE to do, but the most important things in your life are the NEED to do and must become your priority. As I have gotten older, I have observed that the URGENT tasks will always be present in one form or another, but the things that are most IMPORTANT may not.

Our five children have left our home and we now have an empty nest. In the past two years, one of my closest friends suddenly died of a massive myocardial infarction, and another has stage IV small cell lung cancer. The old Joni Mitchell song got it right, "You Don't Know What You Got 'Til It's Gone." What about you? What is most important to you? Do you consistently make time for it in your busy schedule? I would encourage you to make this a priority and schedule time for it, before it's too late.

CHAPTER 2 HIGHLIGHTS

- Have realistic expectations of your academic performance. This is imperative to manage the inherent stress present in nursing school.
- Solicit the support of other students and friends to help cope with the inherent stress of being a nursing student.
- Resilience, self-efficacy, and empowerment are all strategies that can help you overcome the difficulties present in nursing education and can even personally benefit you as you successfully overcome struggles.
- Maintain a healthy balance between all competing demands of your time. Take time just for yourself and do not allow the "tyranny of the urgent" to dictate your daily schedule.

Additional Resources

- Book: *The Resilient Nurse: Empowering Your Practice* (2011) by Margaret McAllister and John Lowe
- Book: *Margin: Restoring Emotional, Physical, Financial, and Time Reserves to Overloaded Lives* (2004) by Richard Swenson
- Article: Tyranny of the Urgent by Charles Hummel

Chapter Reflections

1. Do you have unrealistic expectations for yourself as a student learner that need to be adjusted?

2. Do you tend to base your personal value and worth on your letter grade or perceived success as a student?

3. What do you need to do differently to make self-care a priority or provide a healthy balance in your current schedule?

4. What are the urgent things in your schedule that keep you from taking care of the most important?

5. What could you do differently to put first things first?

> *There is a story behind every patient. There is a reason why they're the way they are. Remember that before you decide to judge that person.*

Part II

GET READY...

Preparing for Practice

Now that you have determined that nursing is a good fit and you are going to persevere to be the best nurse possible, it is time to thoroughly prepare and understand what is required to be a successful nurse.

Building the "Living House"

Nursing is not just a job but a profession. A practice-based profession has three apprenticeships. The three professional apprenticeships that embody nursing practice include:

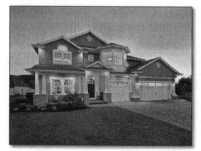

1. **How to act.** Ethical standards that guide practice. Develop the dispositions and ethical actions the profession values and represents.
2. **What you must know.** Knowledge, science, and theory of the profession.
3. **How you must think.** Clinical reasoning and knowledge required for practice (Benner, Sutphen, Leonard & Day, 2010).

As I reflected on these three apprenticeships using my lens as a nurse and nurse educator, I began to see how these three apprenticeships parallel the primary structural components of a home that include the foundation, walls, and roof. To visualize the development from student to practicing nurse, I will use the metaphor of building a house.

This is not just any house or a static structure, but a unique, vibrant, "living" house. Building this "living" house requires the active and intentional engagement of the nurse educator as well as the student. Both must fulfill their responsibility to see this structure take shape to be the best it can possibly be.

How to Act

To be strong and last over time, this "living" house must have a firm and stable foundation. The ethical apprenticeship or the art of nursing is this foundation for every student. Caring behaviors, nurse engagement, and professionalism in practice must be present or your nursing practice will be on an unsteady foundation before it even begins.

If the student's "living house" is established on a shaky foundation because they lack caring, compassion, or professionalism in practice, it will soon come crashing down like a house built on the sand. But if this "living" house is built on a rock-solid foundation of caring, compassion, nurse engagement, and professional behaviors, it will withstand any storm and last a lifetime in the profession. Every student must be prepared to experience a multitude of storms in professional practice, especially in the first year!

In chapter 3, I discuss why the ART remains the "heART" of nursing. The art of nursing includes caring, compassion, nurse engagement, and providing spiritual care. If these foundational aspects of your practice are a current weakness, they must be strengthened, or your ability to authentically engage with your patient, avoid burnout, and even critically think will be impacted.

What does it mean to be a health care professional? This is discussed in chapter 4. The personal character of the nurse that includes a self-motivating desire to be the best nurse possible is essential to practice. Practical ways to demonstrate professionalism while a student as well as identifying and avoiding the destructive and unprofessional behavior of incivility and bullying are discussed.

What You Must Know

Once the foundation is strongly established, it is time to build. The apprenticeship of knowledge, theory, and the science of the profession comprise the walls of the "living" house of professional practice. This includes a DEEP understanding of the applied sciences of nursing and how they relate to the bedside: pharmacology, fluid and electrolytes, and anatomy and physiology.

In addition to behaving the right way, the nurse must also know the right things. Chapter 5 discusses the importance of pharmacology and why the mechanism of action must be understood. Though fluids and electrolytes is difficult content, it is foundational to interpreting and understanding lab values. In chapter 6, the most important labs to the nurse are identified. What to do with an abnormal lab and how to create a plan of care around a relevant abnormal lab value are discussed.

Chapter 7 addresses the most important concepts or principles related to professional practice. This includes the preeminence of safety in all that is done as well as knowing your ABC's (airway, breathing, and circulation priorities) and how to use this knowledge in clinical practice.

Chapter 3
Why the "Art" of Nursing Is Foundational to Practice

"The spirit in which she does her work makes all the difference. Invested as she should with the dignity of her profession and the cloak of love for suffering humanity, she can ennoble anything her hand may be called upon to do, and for work done in this spirit there will ever come to her a recompense far outweighing that of silver and gold."
–Isabel Hampton Robb, 1900
Founder of the American Nurses Association, *American Journal of Nursing*,
and National League for Nursing

"Caring practices are central to nursing. What it is to nurse cannot be separated from what it is to care for and about others."
–Christine A. Tanner, PhD, RN, FAAN

The quiz at the beginning of this book had numerous questions that represented the importance of caring, compassion, empathy, and spiritual care. These questions included:

- Do you easily identify with the feelings of others?
- Do you enjoy and find fulfillment in serving others?
- Is spirituality important to you and how comfortable are you discussing this with others?
- Are you aware of your own internal biases and attitudes toward those of other cultures?
- How well do you relate to others and communicate effectively?
- What kind of character do you possess?

Collectively, these foundational values comprise what is commonly known as the "art" of nursing. The provision of holistic care that not only addresses and cares for the physical needs, but also the emotional, and spiritual needs of patients is a distinctive of professional nursing practice.

To lay the foundation of the "art" of nursing, the essential building blocks are comprised of:

- Caring and compassion
- Empathy
- Engagement
- Spiritual care
- Presence

- Use of touch
- Professionalism (this will be discussed in chapter 4)

The ability to bring these aspects of practice to the bedside is not optional and needs to be developed as you progress through nursing education. I will share practical strategies that I have found successful in my work with students to see the "art" strengthened in your practice as well!

Before I address the specific components that comprise the art of nursing, it is important to first define nursing and how it is distinct and separate from medical practice as well as the historical context of nursing. When this context is properly understood, it will become readily apparent why the "art" really is the heart of nursing and remains foundational to nursing practice.

What Is Nursing?

Though nursing is currently closely associated with medical practice, nursing and medicine are two distinct professions with two different histories as well as worldviews in how they originated. A worldview is the ideas and beliefs through which an individual, group or culture interprets the world and is akin to a lens through which you view things. Western medicine, beginning with Hippocrates, developed from the Greek body–mind dualism worldview that viewed man as composed of a mind and body (Bullough & Bullough, 1987). The mind and the physical body were regarded as two separate and distinct entities. Medicine traditionally focuses on the scientific dimensions of the human body, relegating spiritual and psychosocial concerns of patients to those who are experts in religion and psychology (Shelly & Miller, 2006).

In contrast, nursing grew out of a Christian or biblical worldview (Berman, Snyder, & Frandsen, 2016) that viewed human beings as an integrated whole of physical body, soul, and spirit. Nursing is defined as both an art and a science (Berman, Snyder, & Frandsen, 2016) that emphasizes care for the whole person. Numerous nurse leaders have identified the essence of what it means to care for others using in part this holistic emphasis.

- "Nursing is a ministry of compassionate care for the whole person…which aims to foster optimum health and bring comfort in suffering and death for anyone in need" (Shelly & Miller, 2006, p. 17–18).
- The nurse assists the individual who is sick or well in the performance of those activities that he would perform if he had the necessary strength, will, or knowledge and to do this in such a way that will help him gain independence as rapidly as possible (Henderson, 1991).
- "At its most basic level nursing is a human, caring, relational profession" (Watson, 1995, p. 67).

History of Nursing
Early Christian Church
Though caring for the sick occurred in numerous cultural settings, including India, Rome, and Greece in the BC era, from the first century AD to the late Middle Ages, caring for the sick was primarily a ministry of the Christian church performed by lay deacons and deaconesses and later through convents and monastic orders (Berman, Snyder, & Frandsen, 2016).

There has always been a strong link between nursing and religious orders (Wilkinson & Treas, 2011). Showing compassion and caring for the sick was founded on the teachings and example of Jesus, who demonstrated high regard for human life through His model of service and sacrifice. He stressed the importance of love for God and one's neighbor. His example of healing and giving personal attention to the sick and being present and willing to touch the "untouchable" has strongly influenced nursing and the value given to caring for the sick (Pavey, 1952). The first organized group of nurses was established in response to His teachings and example (Dolan, Fitzpatrick, & Krohn Herrmann, 1983).

Phoebe, a deaconess in the first century church whom the apostle Paul refers to by name in his letter to the Roman church (Romans 16:1) was a nurse who took care of both men and women (DeWit, 2009). While pagan religions seldom offered help to the sick and dying, the early Christians were willing to nurse those in need of care regardless of their religion (Blainey, 2011). The Christian emphasis on compassion and caring for others gave rise to the development of systematic nursing and hospitals after the end of the persecution of the early church in the third century AD (Knight, 2012).

Early Middle Ages

In the Byzantine (eastern Roman) Empire beginning in 325 AD, construction of a hospital began in every cathedral town. Some hospitals maintained libraries and training programs, and doctors compiled their medical and pharmacological studies in manuscripts. Byzantine hospital staff included a chief physician, nurses (deaconesses), and orderlies. Thus, in-patient medical care and what would be considered a hospital today, was an outgrowth of Christian mercy and Byzantine innovation (McClellan & Dorn, 2006). To care for the sick was often self-sacrificing in this era, because exposure to diseases could be incurable and result in death for caregivers (Wilkinson & Treas, 2011).

Middle Ages

During the Middle Ages, nursing and caring for the sick was centered in monasteries. By the twelfth century, Constantinople had two well-organized hospitals, staffed by doctors who were both male and female. Facilities included systematic treatment procedures and specialized wards for various diseases.

1600's to1800's

The Renaissance through the eighteenth century was literally the Dark Age in the history of nursing. Catholic religious orders were disbanded and suppressed in Protestant Europe. As a result, hospitals and the care provided deteriorated. By the nineteenth century, with the exception of a few nursing orders of nuns, nursing was disorganized and corrupt. Author Charles Dickens portrayed the worst of nursing in this era in the character of Sairey Gamp, a self-serving alcoholic nurse in his novel *Martin Chuzzlewit.* Dickens also addressed the substandard care that was provided by alcoholics, prostitutes, and women who were uncaring and immoral (Shelly & Miller, 2006).

In the mid-1800's, a German Lutheran pastor, Theodor Fleidner, responded to the pressing needs of the poor and sick in his community, and his church began to care for these people. Over time, this ministry grew into the Kaiserwerth Institute and became a large organization that included a hospital and training programs. When Florence Nightingale felt God calling her to future service, she began her studies at the Kaiserwerth Institute and then Catholic hospitals in Paris (Shelly & Miller, 2006).

Nursing Today

Some fundamental textbooks of nursing include little to none of the history of our profession that puts caring, compassion, and calling in needed perspective. If a person is unaware of this legacy, they will not realize what is needed to live out the foundational values that are unique to nursing. Many nurse educators are concerned about the lack of emphasis on caring in the curriculum as well as the primary motivation of some students who are attracted to the economic benefits. One nurse educator writes:

> I'm seeing an increasing number of students who are not entering nursing for the same reasons you and I did. They don't have a caring attitude. They have a goal and that goal is to get a job that pays a decent wage. What impact will that have on the professional organization and the profession (Stocker, 1995).

Once in practice, some new nurses become focused on the numerous financial and other benefits that come with the job. A slow fade can take place that can impact any new nurse regardless of their motivation. A nurse can drift from being patient-centered to self-centered by focusing on what he or she can get from being a participant in the profession rather than serving others and improving patient outcomes by providing compassionate care. This is another reason why motivation to become a nurse matters.

Observant nurse educators who interact with nursing students in a wide range of academic settings can see that the altruistic motivation to care for others has been replaced in some by a stronger appeal of how much money they will make as a nurse. Because of instability and resultant layoffs during economic decline in other industries, the realization that nursing pays well, is stable and recession-proof has been the deciding factor for some students to enter nursing today.

Calling vs. Profession

It is interesting to note that it was Nightingale's influence and example that set the stage for an ongoing struggle between those who view nursing as a profession (secular), and those who understood nursing as a calling. The professional nurse serves primarily for financial reimbursement and though concerned for the physical welfare of the patient, is not concerned with their eternal future. Nurses who have a sense of calling or religious motivation serve and care for others out of love for humanity. They recognize the spiritual significance of caring and the eternal rewards for caring for the sick as well as the eternal future of the patient (Shelly & Miller, 2006).

The tension between these two intrinsic motivations was present over 100 years ago as influential nurse leaders were outspoken and against the idea of nursing as a religious calling and wanted to remove religious motivation for serving, caring, and demonstrating compassion as a nurse. Other nurse leaders insisted that the intimacy inherent in nursing practice required religious goodness, discipline, and obedience (Shelly & Miller, 2006). In her 1924 nursing ethics text, Charlotte Aikens acknowledged that religion is "the relation which an individual fixes between his soul and his God" as the basis for nursing ethics (Aikens, 1924, p. 51–52).

The tension between the secular and religious influences in nursing was ongoing in part due to the deaconess hospitals that established their schools of nursing based on the Nightingale system. Hospital-based diploma programs saw no conflict between service and professionalism. As baccalaureate nursing education grew in prominence in the 1950s and beyond, the academic and secular university culture emphasized the scholarly aspects of nursing education instead of religious service (Shelly & Miller, 2006).

Caring and Compassion

Caring has traditionally been viewed as the essence of nursing practice and the most important characteristic of a nurse (Leininger, 1988). Caring is also a distinct, dominant, central, and unifying focus for nursing practice (Leininger, 1991).

Caring theorist Jean Watson describes caring as a heart-centered encounter with another person. This takes place when two people come together in a human-to-human transaction/interaction that is meaningful, authentic, intentional, honors the person, and share a human experience that expands each person's worldview and spirit ("Core Concepts of Jean Watson's Theory of Human Caring/Caring Science," 2010).

Caring as a recognized core value in nursing is not new. It was emphasized at the beginning of the modern era by influential nurse educator Isabel Hampton Robb, who later went on to found the American Nurses Association, the *American Journal of Nursing*, and what would later become the National League for Nursing. In 1900, she wrote the following in her textbook *Nursing Ethics:*

> *"The spirit in which she does her work makes all the difference. Invested as she should with the dignity of her profession and the cloak of love for suffering humanity, she can ennoble anything her hand may be called upon to do, and for work done in this spirit there will ever come to her a recompense far outweighing that of silver and gold"* (Hampton Robb, 1900, p. 36).

While Hampton Robb stated in the language of her day that nurses should provide care by embracing *"the dignity of her profession and the cloak of love for suffering humanity,"* it is important to recognize that this must NOT be treated as an abstract philosophical platitude. This ethic must not only be embraced, but also seen by nursing students as a philosophical truth that must also be lived out (Benner, 2013). Each patient is a valued person with whom nurses share a common humanity.

Though the importance of caring to nursing practice can be taught in the curriculum, what cannot be taught is a heart motivation to serve others as a caregiver. Faculty can help develop caring behaviors in students through their role modeling and caring attitude (Labrague, McEnroe-Petitte, Papathanasiou, Edet, & Arulappan, 2015). If you lack empathetic caring, your practice will reflect this and your practice will be devoid of life and be primarily technical in its emphasis. But if you are truly caring and engaged in the story of each patient you care for, you will relate person to person and bring hope, life, and joy through your engaging and caring presence!

Defining Caring and Compassion

Caring and compassion are essential components of the foundation that must be established in your practice. How do you define caring in the context of nursing?

CARING DEFINED
The ability to recognize the value and worth of those you care for and that the patient and their experience MATTER to you (Benner & Wrubel, 1989).

This definition beautifully captures the essence of applied caring to practice.

Compassion literally means to "suffer with" another. This is a feeling of deep empathy and sorrow for someone who is stricken by misfortune, accompanied by a strong desire to alleviate the suffering. You must actively demonstrate this ethic in the clinical setting for every patient you care for. Though the emphasis in nursing education is knowledge acquisition and skill development, this in itself is not enough; every student must CARE and have COMPASSION for others.

Patricia Benner also affirms that caring is central to nursing practice. *"Nursing can never be reduced to mere technique…the nature of the caring relationship is central to most nursing interventions"* (Benner & Wrubel, 1989, p. 4). *"The nurse is both a knowledge worker and one who cares…knowledge is dangerous if it is divorced from caring"* (p. 400).

Caring is an essential component of expert practice that has the power to not only impact the patient but enriches the nurse in the process (Benner & Wrubel, 1988). This is the unique legacy of the nursing profession throughout history, including the modern era ushered in by Nightingale.

Lessons from the Good Samaritan

Another foundational internal motivator is empathy, which desires to relieve the suffering of another and meet the other as a fellow human being. Helping people during periods of vulnerability and distress is the essence of what it means to be "good" as a nurse in practice (Benner, Hooper-Kyriakidis, & Stannard, 2011). As a nursing student, do you have eyes to see that every patient you care for is your "neighbor" for whom you are called to have mercy and compassion? This timeless truth is found in the parable of the Good Samaritan taught by Jesus and has been an influential example for nurses to emulate since (Walsh, 1929).

A religious leader of the Jews asked Jesus, *"Who is my neighbor?"* Jesus shared a brief story of a man who was severely beaten, left for dead, and was lying on the side of a road. Two religious leaders saw the man, but ignored his plight. They even walked on the opposite side of the road. But the Samaritan, when he saw the man, was moved with compassion. He responded by taking action to alleviate his suffering and took him to a place to be cared for. Jesus then asked this religious leader a question that is relevant to all who provide care for those in need today. *"Which of these three…was neighbor unto him that fell among the thieves?"* The religious leader replied, *"He that shewed mercy on him."* Jesus then replied, *"Go, and do thou likewise"* (Luke 10: 29–37).

Influential nurse educator and scholar Patricia Benner validates this truth as relevant to nursing today:

> *"As nurses, we have been given the ministry and tradition of compassionately caring for strangers, of loving our neighbors as ourselves. We do not have to have great will power to do this, or even great determination and motivation. We do need knowledge and skilled know-how, but we need to be open to see every patient as an opportunity to demonstrate this compassion to those we do not yet know"* (Benner, 2012, p. XX).

Hampton Robb (1900) also recognized the value of this ethic when she wrote that the nurse will receive a *"recompense far outweighing that of silver and gold"* through compassionate care for others.

Though I try to make this principle a part of my practice, I am inconsistent and often allow the "tyranny of the urgent" to distract me from this ideal. I had a recent clinical example that made it clear how important this ethic is to nursing practice and illustrates how the "little" things done in providing care are really the "big" things that your patients and family will not soon forget.

Little Things that Make a Difference

I had a typical busy shift in the ED with numerous demands. I was pulled in all too many directions at the same time. One of my patients was a healthy middle-aged man who had numerous vague respiratory complaints the past week including shortness of breath. The physician ordered a chest X-ray and numerous tumors were found in both lung fields. Because a full workup is not done in the ED, the physician explained that it was likely cancer with a poor prognosis, but he required hospital admission to complete a full workup. I went into the room 15 minutes later and found the patient with tears in his eyes, He realized that his world would never be the same. I did not know what to say, except that I was so sorry, and then had to leave because the admitting physician had just arrived.

I then called report to the receiving nurse, and transport came to take the patient to the floor. I wanted to share some encouraging thoughts that were on my heart before he left the ED, but when I went to his room, he was gone. Though he was a stranger, his experience really did matter to me. Though it would have been easy to forget it and move on to deal with the next crisis in the ED, I could not shake the need to visit him before I left at the end of my shift. I punched out and went to his room on the oncology floor. He lit up when he saw me as I entered. I briefly shared what was on my heart. With tears in his eyes, he said something I will never forget. "Your decision to come and see me is special, and it makes me feel special because you care."

Benefits of Caring

Nursing literature and research has conclusively shown that the patients of a caring, engaged nurse have better outcomes (Swanson, 1999). Caring gives the nurse a heightened sense of awareness and guides the evaluation of nursing interventions by recognizing subtle changes in the patient's condition. In this context of caring, the nurse pays close attention to the patient's body language, facial expressions, tone of voice and interprets the significance of what is communicated (Benner & Wrubel, 1989).

In one study, the degree of critical thinking and the emotions of caring and emotional engagement by students had a positive clinical relationship. The higher the degree of caring measured in students showed an improved disposition to critical thinking. This study recommended emphasizing caring behaviors in the curriculum to improve the adoption of critical thinking in nursing students (Pai, Eng, & Ko, 2013).

Caring behaviors also create healing environments that positively influence and improve patient outcomes. The benefits patients receive when they experience caring by the nurse include enhanced healing, decreased length of stay, increased well-being and physical comfort. Caring influences nurse engagement, which helps the nurse notice the effectiveness of interventions and subtle signs of patient improvement or deterioration (Benner & Wrubel, 1988). Practicing in a caring manner also benefits the nurse and enhances the nurse's well-being, both personally and professionally. The nurse feels more connected both to his/her patients and colleagues and is more satisfied with bedside care (Swanson, 1999).

Patients can readily detect a nurse's nonverbal communication that contradicts caring behaviors. You must learn to recognize the influence and significance of eye contact, body language, and tone of voice with every patient you encounter and how these nonverbal actions communicate caring and contribute to a patient's well-being (Benner & Wrubel, 1989). Some patients lose hope and a sense of connection to others as a result of their illness and feel that they do not matter.

When the nurse demonstrates that the patient matters to him/her, this has the power to reintegrate the patient with his/her world and can be seen as the integrative power of caring. Being approachable and available is central to effective nursing care and essential ingredient to patient recovery (Orlick & Benner, 1988). When the head and heart are integrated and fully engaged in practice, the nurse clearly communicates in both verbal and nonverbal communication that each person matters and is more likely to recognize EARLY changes that may signify a change in status.

Caring as "Covenant"

Characteristics of a covenant relationship include bonds of responsibility and faithfulness, without expectation of a return for service. Though the use of covenant is described to define the marriage relationship and God's relationship with man, another perspective that is relevant to nursing is to view the nurse–patient relationship as a sacred covenant (O'Brien, 2006). How will you respond when the patient or family are difficult and do not value the unique contributions that you provide as a nurse? Will you walk away, or will a sense of responsibility and faithfulness keep you engaged and present in the sometimes difficult situations that are present in health care?

This is especially important for nurses who practice in the emergency department. Patient waits can be long, stress is high, and many patients are in pain and demand that their needs be met now. This can create a volatile cocktail that causes some nurses to disengage and become cynical. But if the nurse can maintain a sense of covenant in the nurse–patient relationship, this can guide engagement and presence that is required for all patients, not just those who are appreciative and kind!

Patient-Centered Care

Your nursing program may use Quality and Safety Education for Nurses (QSEN) as a framework of four competencies to structure safe patient care. QSEN emphasizes the practical values that are needed to guide the provision of holistic patient care.

Patient-centered care is the first competency of the Quality and Safety Education for Nurses (QSEN) that situates in this framework the value of caring and compassion. QSEN defines caring and compassion by its recognition that patient-centered care happens when the nurse *"recognizes the patient or designee as the source of control and full partner in providing compassionate and coordinated care based on respect for patient's preferences, values, and needs"* ("Pre-Licensure KSAS," n.d).

The underlying attitudes that are required by the nurse to provide patient-centered care according to QSEN include seeing health care situations through the patient's eyes, respect, encouraging individual expression of what the patient needs, and valuing active partnership with the patient and family in all aspects of care ("Pre-Licensure KSAS," 2014).

Caring for Families

Holistic, compassionate care must also be extended to and include the family of the patient. They are an extension of the patient and their needs must also be considered. Families also need information, reassurance, guidance, and care. For patients with large families, make it a priority to identify the primary family spokesperson so that all health-related information goes to this person and prevents the nurse from receiving numerous phone calls for updates.

When the nurse begins to understand how the patient's current illness has impacted his life and family, she or he acquires a lens to see from the patient's point of view. This is the core to empathetic caring and patient-centered care. This allows the nurse to not just react, but INTERPRET the current situation (Benner & Wrubel, 1989). For example, if the nurse goes into the patient's room and he states angrily, "Can't you just leave me alone! I am so tired of being messed with!" knowing he was recently diagnosed with stage IV pancreatic cancer and has three months to live will provide contextual interpretation to the nurse, who can remain engaged and present in his care instead of reacting to this outburst and taking it personally.

The importance of including the family in providing care is also emphasized throughout the QSEN competencies. Under the competency of Patient-centered Care, it is expected that the nurse will involve the family and identify their preferences and values, remove barriers to the presence of families, elicit expectations of the patient and family regarding pain relief, value active partnership with patient and family surrogates, examine how safety can be improved through the active involvement of patient and families, describe strategies to empower patients or families, and finally, assess levels of communication skill in encounters with patients and families ("Pre-Licensure KSAS," 2014).

How to Handle Difficult Families

You must have realistic expectations as you enter the clinical setting as a new student or nurse. Though you may have a heart overflowing with love and compassion for others, this love will not always be reciprocated by those you care for or the families of patients.

Working in the emergency department, I often see patients and families who are not feeling well and as a result are not at their best. The following are some simple strategies that I have incorporated into my practice to manage these situations with grace and not allow their response to define and influence me in a personal way:

- **Remember that families and patients are under duress and stress**. They need your support, not your judgmental attitude. Practical ways to support families include taking the time to update them in a non-hurried manner with what they need to know at their level of understanding, conveying availability by making it clear they can call anytime for an update, speaking in a gentle, respectful tone of voice, and involving them as much as possible in the care of the patient.

- **Clearly communicate the plan of care.** When families have no idea what is going on and what is going to happen next, it can create significant stress for them in the clinical setting. The nurse who routinely explains and updates all that is taking place has the power to defuse that stress and improve family well-being.

- **A gentle answer turns away wrath**. Though the family or patient may be obviously angry and upset and speaking in an angry voice, resist the temptation to fight fire with fire. Speak in a restrained, respectful tone of voice. This response can quickly defuse an escalating situation.

- **Assume the best, not the worst of others.** When the nurse is able to empathize with the stress and difficulties the family is experiencing, this will encourage empathy and understanding. Assume that this is NOT the way they always relate to others, but is likely the exception because of high levels of stress.

- **Maintain a firm boundary of respect at all times.** The patient or family may be angry or frustrated, but this does NOT give them the right to cross lines by being verbally abusive or personally demeaning toward the nurse or any member of the health care team. If this line of respect is crossed, it must be addressed by making it clear that it is unacceptable and will not be tolerated. If the patient or family continues to escalate when respectful boundaries are communicated, do not hesitate to call security or the house supervisor, depending on your facility, to defuse the situation.

Empathy

To practically demonstrate empathy to your patient, make it a priority to UNDERSTAND the plight and experience of those in your care (Scott, 2009). In the clinical setting, it is imperative that you are able to readily place yourself in the patient's shoes and attempt to identify and understand all that the patient is encountering and experiencing from their perspective. In one three-year research study, Sweeney (2012) identified that 96 percent of patients had fears and anxieties about being in the health care setting.

The following empathetic caring strategies were derived from Sweeney's research and patient reflections that nurses can use to demonstrate sensitivity to the patient's needs and provide empathetic care.

Entering the Room for the First Time:
- Always knock before entering the patient's room. Remember, it's their personal space.
- Tell the patient your name, school where you are a student, and why you are there.
- Ask the patient how they want to be addressed. Be sure to avoid calling the patient "Honey," "Sweetheart," or "Darling."
- Show honor and respect. Address your patient by "Mr.", "Mrs." or "Ms" during your first encounter and then allow the patient to express their preference regarding how they want to be addressed; by their first name, nickname.
- Before leaving the room, ask if there is anything else the patient needs.
- When you leave the patient's room, always offer to shut the door. Give them the choice.

Beginning of the Clinical Day:
- Do not immediately start taking vital signs and doing tasks. Instead, remove the stethoscope from your shoulders, sit at their bedside, and ask them how they are doing today. Engage person to person, not nurse to patient.
- Start your shift by asking your patient about their greatest fear or concern they may have.
- Have your patient identify their greatest hope and goals.
- Encourage the patient to share his or her story. This can involve the number of children, grandchildren, or their interests or hobbies.
- Know what is most important about your patient and give him or her the opportunity to talk about it.

While Providing Care
- Honor and respect patients' privacy and keep them appropriately covered at all times.
- Offer a soapy washcloth to cleanse their hands before eating.
- Keep the patient's room clean. A clean room is a healing environment.
- Anticipate the needs of your patient. This includes the need for water or pain medications.

- Offer a back rub, wash hair, or give a shave to your male patients. They will appreciate this extra effort!

General

- If your patient is from a different culture, ask relevant questions to increase your cultural sensitivity and show that you care.
- Never share your problems with your patient. It's always about them, not you.
- Never tell a patient how tired or busy you are.
- Encourage your patients by letting them know what they are doing well.

Final Takeaways

- Take care and treat each patient as you would a beloved family member.
- Treat your patient the way that you would want to be cared for.
- Be completely engaged and maintain your focus on the patient at all times in the clinical setting.
- Remind yourself that you have been called to do the most important work in the world as a nurse!

These patient-centered observations reinforce the importance of the art of nursing. Be sure to incorporate these practical strategies next time you are in the clinical setting and see for yourself what a difference empathetic caring can make!

Compassion Fatigue

It is important to recognize that each nurse is vulnerable to developing the potential boomerang of compassion fatigue. Although patient care is rewarding, it can come at a cost. Repeated exposure to life-altering or life-threatening illness or the aftermath of critical illness puts nurses at high risk for compassion fatigue. Compassion fatigue is a subset of burnout unique to nurses (Figley, 1995).

Another component of compassion fatigue is traumatic stress, which results from feelings of distress and pain from the patient that causes feelings of despair for the nurse. Empathetic caring that identifies with the patient's experience is the essence of understanding traumatic stress that adversely impact nurses over time (Sacco, Ciurzynski, Harvey, & Ingersoll, 2015).

Compassion satisfaction is the other weight on this teeter-totter that can balance and even negate the stress that can lead to compassion fatigue. Compassion satisfaction is simply the positive feelings the nurse experiences from helping others and is the sum of the positive feelings a nurse derives from helping others. The balance between the levels of compassion satisfaction and compassion fatigue can be defined as the professional quality of life. The higher the feelings of compassion satisfaction, the higher the positive work–life balance (Stamm, 2002). The converse is also true. If the work environment and patient care experiences are consistently highly stressful with little compassion satisfaction, this will more likely lead to compassion fatigue.

In addition to the practical self-care strategies that were discussed in chapter 2, a healthy work environment that has appropriate staffing, team collaboration, and healthy and effective communication can directly influence the degree of compassion satisfaction or compassion fatigue a nurse experiences in practice (Sacco, Ciurzynski, Harvey, & Ingersoll, 2015).

Nurse Engagement

Skillful nurse engagement complements caring and compassion and is basic to nursing practice and care. The nurse must remain clinically curious and responsive to the patient's story and situation. When distracted and not engaged, the nurse will be unable to invest the energy needed to recognize relevant and urgent clinical signs that may require intervention. When nurses are not engaged with the patient and their clinical problem, patient outcomes will suffer (Benner, Hooper-Kyriakidis, & Stannard, 2011).

The importance of nurse engagement was also identified in Sweeney's (2012) research on empathy. Patients made it clear that they wanted a nurse who was completely engaged in the clinical setting and focused entirely on the patient and their needs.

To be engaged in practice also implies that the patient is your priority, focus, and motivation for all that you do as a nurse. Use the following questions to evaluate if you are living this out in your practice:

- Do you volunteer and offer to help your colleagues whenever you have a chance?
- Do you consistently ask your patient what they need?
- Do you avoid activities that distract you from patient needs such as unit gossip and surfing the web (Scott, 2009)?

Remember to leave personal distractions and feelings of anxiety at the door once you enter the clinical environment. This is especially important for first-year students who are new to the clinical setting. If a patient can sense that the student nurse is stressed or anxious, he or she will NOT feel cared for (Swanson, 1991). Personal, family, and any other stressors or problems will affect the quality of care and nurse engagement needed for practice. Though difficult to fight through at times, students must learn to focus on the patient to whom they are assigned. Students must understand the need to hide their anxieties and become a good actor or actress in order to communicate caring to their patients!

Listening

One practical way to engage is to actively listen to your patient. It is important to listen to not only what your patient is saying, but to investigate the meaning of what they are communicating, and to make needed adjustments to patient care based on what you discover. As you listen, pay attention and accurately interpret the nonverbal messages that your patient may be communicating (Scott, 2009). For example, if you ask your patient if he is having pain, and he is obviously tense and appears uncomfortable but says he is just fine, do not hesitate to communicate what you are observing and that he appears tense and uncomfortable.

Remember to listen twice as long as much as you speak. Active listening communicates caring, which allows you to further engage with the patient and their story. I have noted in practice that when I make that caring connection with my patient and family, they tend to be much more gracious and understanding if I get busy and am unable to address a need or concern immediately. They are on my side because trust was established.

Caring Made Practical
Two Questions to Ask Yourself Each Clinical

As a new nursing student, you will be focused on what needs to be done for your patient. As a result, you will be TASK oriented (Benner, 1984). When I taught fundamental clinical, some students seemed to forget at times that there is a person in the bed; they were preoccupied with obtaining vital signs, head to toe assessment, and passing medications! To integrate caring behaviors and make them intentional in your practice, I have created two open-ended questions that I use with my students in the clinical setting that cause them to reflect and consider the relevance of empathy, caring, compassion, and nurse engagement in the context of each patient under their care.

1. *What is the patient likely experiencing/feeling right now in this situation?*
   This question emphasizes empathy, which is the ability to imagine and put oneself in another's place with the intention to understand what another is feeling or experiencing. Empathy is a synonym of compassion and represents another perspective to situate the necessity of compassion to nursing practice.

2. *What can I do to engage myself with this patient's experience and show that they matter to me as a person?*
   This question begins with an emphasis on nurse engagement and what can be practically done to communicate empathy. The last half of this question is derived from Patricia Benner, who defines the essence of caring as a nurse is that you recognize the value and worth of those you care for and that the patient and their experience matter to you (Benner & Wrubel, 1989).

My students expected me to ask these questions each clinical day. Even if I was not able to ask them personally, they were prepared to answer them. This simple strategy kept caring on their radar regardless of how task-oriented they tend to be as a novice nurse. I encourage you to do the same. By reflecting on these questions and choosing to intentionally engage with each patient, their personal story, clinical situation, family dynamics, and culture/ethnic traditions, you will be well on your way to tailoring and providing the best possible holistic care for your patients!

Can Caring Be Taught?

Are caring behaviors in nursing students innate, or can caring be taught? One of the characteristics of a novice nurse is an emphasis on tasks, but he/she may have difficulty in establishing priorities and recognizing what is relevant due to the lack of clinical experience (Benner, 1984). Nursing is both a science and an art. The art of nursing, including the teaching of caring theories, has historically received less emphasis in nursing curriculum than the science of nursing (Leininger, 1988).

Caring is a behavior that can be taught and learned (Cronin & Harrison, 1988). Tanner (1990) recognized that caring is learned by students when they experience caring practices between faculty and students. Tanner (1990) warned that the language of health care institutions is dehumanizing and detached. It is imperative that students are helped to retain their caring practices in these settings and have them continuously nurtured and cultivated. How can nurse educators accomplish this objective? Nursing practice is grounded in theory. One nursing theory that I have found practical and relevant to provide a framework for understanding and integrating caring behaviors into nursing practice is Swanson's Middle Range Theory of Caring (1991).

Swanson's Middle Range Theory of Caring

I was introduced to Kristen Swanson's caring theory during my graduate studies in nursing education. Swanson based her theory on the foundational caring theory work of Jean Watson and Patricia Benner. Swanson validated their observations by building her caring processes through qualitative research in a perinatal context. Mothers who had a critically ill infant in the NICU or had experienced the death of their baby through miscarriage or stillbirth were asked what the nurse did to show that they cared. Swanson identified five qualitative themes that the mother perceived as caring behaviors from nurses (Swanson, 1991). I have found these themes of caring apply to any patient-care setting despite the specialty practice settings from which they were derived.

Swanson's Caring Processes and Their Definitions:

1. **Maintaining Belief (Esteem)**
   - Sustaining faith in the other's capacity to get through an event/transition and face a future with meaning
2. **Knowing (Empathetic Understanding)**
   - Striving to understand an event as it has meaning in the life of the other
3. **Being With (Emotionally Present)**
   - Being emotionally present to the other
4. **Doing For (Enact For)**
   - Doing for the other as he/she would do for oneself
5. **Enabling (Empowering)**
   - Facilitating the other's passage through life transitions and face a future with meaning (Swanson, 1991)

In addition to each theme, Swanson also identified three to five caring interventions for each theme that described what the nurse did to practically demonstrate caring. For example "conveying availability" is one of the caring interventions from the "Being With" theme. When the nurse "conveys availability" to a patient, this demonstrates caring (Swanson, 1991). In the article "Caring Made Visible" Swanson further explains her caring theory so that it can be easily understood.

Convey Availability

A practical application of this caring theory for students to integrate into their practice is to communicate to their patient that the nurse is available to them. So instead of saying to your patient, "Here is the call light," the student can convey availability by stating, "Here is the call light; do not hesitate to call me. I am available if you need me." Both statements involve making the call light available to your patient, but the latter does it in a way that will be interpreted as a caring behavior.

Avoid Assumptions

Another relevant caring intervention is "avoiding assumptions" from the "Knowing" theme. "Avoiding assumptions" stresses the importance of the nurse to not rely upon another nurse's judgments about the patient, but to make her own assessments by approaching the patient with a "clean slate" (Swanson,

1991). A common example of this in practice is when a nurse gives a "loaded" report filled with judgments about the patient and the kind of shift the next nurse will have.

It is imperative to make your own assumptions based on your interaction with the patient. When a nurse makes a preconceived judgment, he/she ceases to be able to demonstrate caring. I have experienced this reality firsthand when I practice in the ED, where it is very easy to make judgments/assumptions with the unpleasant experiences I may have had with a certain patient who may be identified as a "frequent flier."

Holistic and Spiritual Care

Professional nursing has its roots in the early Christian church and Roman Catholic religious orders. The provision of nursing care included both physical as well as spiritual comfort. As a founder of the modern era, much of Florence Nightingale's nursing knowledge and skill came out of her own religious heritage that included training at the Lutheran Deaconesses Institute at Kaiserwerth, Germany (Wilt & Smucker, 2001). Nightingale recognized the value of spirituality to nursing that would be present in the way the nurse has an inner belief and commitment that link a nurse's work and personal life (Attewell, 2012).

The emphasis of spirituality and healthcare has been diminished as scientific knowledge and medical technology have currently taken precedence. Nursing education has emphasized the scientific and medical model. In this vacuum, spirituality is easily devalued as human life is reduced to biological processes. But things are beginning to change. Both medicine and nursing are beginning to realize that health and healing involve much more than physiologic processes. Science and technology alone are not able to fully answer the deeper questions of purpose, meaning, and value of human life.

Today, we have come full circle in nursing in recognizing the importance of spiritual care as a key component of holistic care. Human beings are also spiritual beings. Spirituality and the provision of spiritual care can be a difficult concept to grasp because one is trying to put that which is unseen and invisible into words.

The spiritual dimension is beyond us yet somehow within the physical and material world. We usually cannot see or touch it, but when we experience the spiritual, it becomes very real. Ironically, we are much more likely to experience the spiritual in times of great joy or great sadness (Wilt & Smucker, 2001). The recognition of a transcendent reality and the feeling that a spiritual reality that one can have communion with exists is the most important aspect of a person's spiritual nature (Hardy, 1979).

Holistic Care

Holism teaches that each individual is more than the sum of his or her parts. Each person is multidimensional and has its own unique characteristics that cannot be separated from the whole. This philosophy and worldview has been foundational to nursing going back over 2,000 years and reinforced as central to nursing practice by Nightingale and current nursing theorists and leaders today. As a result, professional nurses are taught to embrace holistic care in practice by caring for all aspects of each patient's being.

This bio-psycho-social-spiritual model of patient care is also supported and endorsed by the American Holistic Nurses' Association that recognizes that all disorders of health also influence psychological and spiritual health and well-being. Healing interventions then also impact these same domains of a person's being.

High patient acuity levels, decreased length of stay, and heavy patient assignments make it difficult to take time to explore the spiritual needs of patients. The "tyranny of the urgent" is a daily reality for nurses as the pressing urgent demands of physical care result in a neglect of what may be just as important, the emotional and spiritual needs of those you care for.

By providing compassionate care, the nurse directly impacts both the patient's physical and emotional needs. Holistic care also involves supporting spirituality as defined by the patient. For some students, spiritual care may conjure up images and expectations of religious practices or prayer and going way out of their comfort zone. Though spiritual care may include prayer, it is much more.

The essence of spiritual care is caring and serving the whole person: the physical, emotional, social, and spiritual aspects of their being (Murphy & Walker, 2013). It is important to view spiritual care as a thread to naturally weave into the tapestry of care that you provide for each patient (Wilt & Smucker, 2001).

Religion vs. Spirituality

Religion is a set of beliefs, texts, and other practices that a community shares in its pursuit of relationship with God or that which is transcendent. Spirituality is a broader concept than religion and specific beliefs and practices. Spirituality is the recognition of a dimension of life that is invisible, yet within us and beyond the material world that provides a sense of connectedness to the universe (Wilt & Smucker, 2001).

It includes your concept of the sacred and the development of your personal value system. It represents the individual pursuit and search for meaning and purpose in life. "Why am I here?" "What is my purpose?" "Why did God allow ____ to happen?" are common questions that each of us have asked at some point in our life that reflect the relevance of spirituality. You may care for patients in crisis because of life-altering medical conditions. Questions of a religious or spiritual nature may be internalized or openly expressed by the patient and need to be discerned and explored.

Spiritual Needs

The physical needs that each of us require for life are obvious: food, water, and oxygen. But each of us also have universal spiritual needs.

These universal spiritual needs include the following:

- Meaning and purpose in life
- Faith or trust in someone or something beyond ourselves
- Hope
- Love
- Forgiveness (Bensley, 1991; Fish & Shelly, 1983; Highland & Carson, 1983)

Meaning and Purpose in Life

Trying to make sense of the world we live in, especially in a time of crisis, is a natural human response (Frankyl, 1978). Meaning provides one with a basic understanding of life and our place in it. We may look for understanding through our lived experiences, our relationships with others, or our faith community. Meaning also provides a stable structure in the midst of a storm and can bring a sense of control when chaos appears to be present. Each of us needs to feel that life is worth living and having an ultimate purpose or goal in life regardless of circumstances (Wilt & Smucker, 2001).

Faith

Many associate faith with religious beliefs and practices. This is one aspect of faith that must be considered and addressed, but faith can also include a moral philosophy or ethical teachings. Faith can be defined as a deep conviction of those things that are not seen as well as the assurance of things hoped for. Though having a sincere and strong conviction of God is present in many faith traditions, this concept can vary because some faith traditions such as Judaism, Christianity, and Islam emphasize God's transcendent nature, while Hinduism emphasizes God's presence in all creation and oneness with the human soul.

Other faith traditions such as Buddhism do not even include the concept of God but are based on ethical teachings. Some people may not have faith in a supreme being, but may put their faith and trust in people, natural laws, or their own philosophy of life. Regardless, faith is an important concept that one's mental and psychological health depend on in order to draw from in a time of need. The source of faith for your patient is something that you, the nurse, may need to explore in order to provide meaningful spiritual care.

Hope

Hope is related to meaning and purpose but its emphasis is on having a future hope or expectation. In both Protestant and Roman Catholic churches, the Apostles' Creed summarizes their faith traditions. The Apostles' Creed ends with the belief in "the forgiveness of sins, the resurrection of the body, and life everlasting." Those who are Muslim have a belief in the resurrection of the dead and that good deeds will be rewarded with entry into heaven. If a patient has this hope grounded in their faith, they may be more likely to face suffering, adversity, and even death with confidence and peace.

Love

Unconditional love is one's greatest spiritual need. Every one of us needs to experience this love or there is something missing in our lived experience. When we are able to experience love from God as well as others, we feel valuable and worthwhile, cared for, with a renewed purpose to live. Recognize that others around you, including your patients, need the care and love of others. This is what distinguished the good Samaritan from the religious leaders who saw a wounded man in the ditch. The good Samaritan was moved with compassion to do what was needed to care for the needs of the other.

Forgiveness

Many religions address forgiveness as an important principle and provide ways to receive forgiveness as well as the need to forgive others. Forgiveness has the power to restore broken relationships between God and others. Research also shows a connection between forgiveness and physical and emotional health. If one is unable or unwilling to forgive others, this resentment produces negative emotions that generate stress hormones that take a physical toll. Harboring unforgiveness continues to separate and isolate one from others and the social support that one needs in life.

Spiritual Care

Identifying spiritual needs and providing spiritual care are an important part of nursing assessment. The principles in this section will help you recognize the importance of spiritual care to your patients' health, healing and well-being. Make it a priority to embrace this responsibility to provide spiritual care based on their needs.

The nurse must recognize when a concern requires the attention of a professional counselor or chaplain. Many of the same principles that guide chaplaincy are part of the nurse's scope of practice. This includes providing/offering hope, support at the end of life, and maintaining presence to reduce anxiety and stress.

Because HOPE and MEANING are key components of spirituality, spiritual care can be simply defined as helping a patient to find/make MEANING out of his/her experience and find HOPE. Practical interventions that students can use include listening, encouraging the expression of feelings, compassionate presence, open-ended questions, instilling hope, and prayer (Murphy & Walker, 2013).

A practical, holistic approach to providing spiritual care in nursing recaptures the perspective that all that is done for the patient by the nurse can be an act of spiritual care. Instead of compartmentalizing patient care as "nursing interventions" and spiritual care as something you will do when you have the time, everything that is done for the patient can become a demonstration of spiritual care. For example, taking a set of vital signs becomes an opportunity for presence and spiritual assessment. You can further intentionalize spiritual care by thinking with every interaction, *"What are this patient's needs, fears, anxieties, or questions?"* Every interaction is filled with meaning as the student engages the "entire" patient (Murphy & Walker, 2013).

Though spiritual care is a responsibility that is clearly within the nurse's scope of practice, I find that most students and many nurses in practice are uncomfortable with this duty. Contributing factors to this discomfort for some may include the dominant physical/medical model in health care, secular-humanistic worldview of educational and health care institutions, and a lack of emphasis on spiritual care in nursing education. In one survey, 87 percent of nursing programs do not have specific content on how to practically incorporate spiritual care in practice (Murphy & Walker, 2013)!

I have observed that those most comfortable with spiritual care find their own faith and spiritual traditions personally meaningful and relevant. When it comes to spirituality, you cannot give to others if you do not have something within to give. But regardless of where patients are in their faith journeys, I encourage you to nurture and develop your own spirituality so that you can holistically support and care for your patients. You may not be a participant of any faith tradition or may be an atheist or agnostic, but you must recognize that if spirituality or a faith tradition is important to the patient, it must also be central and important to you!

The Art of Spiritual Care

Nursing has been compared to a fine art that requires the nurse to provide physical as well as spiritual care with creativity, sensitivity, and intelligence. Nursing must not be reduced to a mechanistic step-by-step approach. Though certain aspects of the tasks of nursing do not change from patient to patient, the nurse must remember that each patient is distinct and has unique holistic needs. The essence of spiritual care is to use awareness, intuition, and sensitivity to know when to speak, when to listen, when and how to touch a patient, and when to ask if prayer would be helpful (Wilt & Smucker, 2001).

The nurse must relate to the patient on a person to person level through the skillful use of observational listening, therapeutic communication, empathy, and intuition. If you have a living, personal faith to draw upon, you may integrate this in your nursing practice by asking God to guide and lead you throughout your day and what to specifically say or do with specific patients (Wilt & Smucker, 2001). This can also include silently praying for you and your patients throughout your provision of care.

Although nursing education is grounded in the sciences, you must also incorporate your unique self and personality into your art. Use your authentic self as an artist, like a painter with a brush and palette of paints (Rhodes, 1990). What you bring as an "artist" to each patient interaction is unique as each patient. It is this ongoing giving and receiving of what the nurse and patient bring to each encounter that makes nursing an art (Wilt & Smucker, 2001).

Hildegard Peplau, a highly regarded nursing leader and theorist on interpersonal relations, recognized the power of the use of self to help patients make needed change. She believed that spiritual care was the purest form of the art of nursing because it required the nurse to go beyond routine care and to be present as a concerned, caring, compassionate person as well as a competent nurse (Peplau, 1988).

Just as it takes time to develop proficiency with any new skill as a nurse, you will also develop proficiency in providing meaningful spiritual care to your patients over time. To obtain this proficiency will require practice. Make it a priority to integrate spiritual care in practical ways each clinical experience. Develop a therapeutic relationship with your patient, using active listening, empathy, and presence. Each of these actions will provide spiritual comfort, because caring in any form will also touch the patient's spirit. Since caring and compassion are the heart of spiritual care, you can minister to the spirit and provide spiritual care in every encounter with your patients when this is part of your practice (Wilt & Smucker, 2001).

Use Nursing Process

The nursing process is not just for your patient's pressing physical needs, but can also help you effectively administer spiritual care through this systematic approach. Although the traditional steps of assessment, diagnosis, implementation, and evaluation may be more difficult when compared to physical care, I will highlight briefly each aspect of the nursing process relevant to spiritual care to make this tangible and readily grasped so you can incorporate it into your practice. For more on this topic, *Nursing the Spirit* by Dorothy Wilt and Carol Smucker is an excellent resource.

Assessment

The use of spiritual assessment will identify your patient's current level of spiritual well-being and long-term needs so that these needs can be addressed. Because matters of the spirit are more nuanced and not as tangible as physical needs, the nurse must look at the present situation and nonverbal communication or statements of losing hope that may indicate a spiritual concern or crisis. The following questions (Wilt & Smucker, 2001) are organized based on the five universal spiritual needs addressed earlier and can be naturally woven into your conversation with your patient if you sense through intuition or obvious need that you need to go there and address a possible spiritual need.

Meaning and Purpose
- What gives your life purpose?
- What keeps you going in life?
- What meaning do you give to your current situation?
- How has this illness affected the way you view life?

Faith
- Are you connected with a faith community?
- How has your health problem affected your spiritual beliefs?

- What is your source of strength?
- What can I do to support your faith?
- How do your beliefs help you cope with suffering and illness?

Hope

- What is your source of strength or support?
- Do you believe in a power greater than yourself?
- What gives you hope?
- Where have you found strength in the past?

Love

- Who do you receive love and support from?
- Describe a time when you received unconditional love from God or another person?
- Are you lonely?

Forgiveness

- From whom do you receive forgiveness?
- Do you feel like God has abandoned you or is punishing you?
- Are you angry with God?
- Do you have any unfinished business?
- Is there something you need to confess? (Wilt & Smucker, 2001, p. 55–56)

One easy to remember acronym to implement a spiritual assessment with your patient is S-P-I-R-I-T.

S-P-I-R-I-T Acronym for Spiritual Assessment
S-Senses: Use all your senses to gather data about your patient's beliefs, practices, and needs.   **P-Presence:** Be present and available to your patient.   **I-Intuition:** Tune in and listen to that still, small voice.   **R-Respect:** Communicate respect for your patient's spiritual beliefs and practices by being nonjudgmental.   **I-Interpretation:** Accurately interpret the data you have collected. Validate your assessment with your patient or family.   **T-Trust:** Develop a trusting, therapeutic relationship with your patient.   Wilt & Smucker, 2001, p. 52

Diagnosis/Priority

Once you have completed an assessment by using spiritual assessment questions that are relevant to your patient, you can make a diagnosis or determine the nursing priority by understanding and interpreting what has been collected. The NANDA-I (International) nursing diagnostic statement that addresses a need for spiritual intervention is spiritual distress. The essence of spiritual distress is that the spirit of your patient is clearly troubled and deteriorating.

Spiritual distress is present when your patient begins to openly question the purpose and meaning of life or existence of God (Smucker, 1996). In this scenario, the nursing goal would be to help the patient find meaning, hope, and rediscover his/her purpose in life. Nursing interventions to address spiritual distress include providing compassionate care, active listening to concerns, and making referrals to chaplaincy.

Implementing

Remember that the nurse is not meant to serve as a chaplain. The primary role of the nurse includes facilitating and connecting the patient and/or family with spiritual support such as chaplaincy or the patient's pastor/priest/imam. In one study, the interventions that patients found most meaningful when they needed spiritual care was when the nurse helped to enable transcendence of the present situation so they could see the bigger picture, provide hope, and establish an authentic connection with the caregiver (Conco, 1995). When patients feel cared for, their spirit has been touched. That is why caring and compassion are so important to nursing practice and was addressed at length earlier in the chapter.

Evaluating

If a patient experiences spiritual distress, the nurse can help the patient find meaning, hope, and rediscover his/her purpose in life to a certain degree. Though successful resolution of spiritual distress will likely involve pastoral or chaplaincy support, the nurse is on the front lines. When a patient is in crisis and you are "it," you must be prepared to do the best you can. Let me share some examples from my practice and show you how the provision of spiritual care can present in the context of bedside care in an acute care setting.

Spiritual Care Made Practical

Spiritual care can be done in a short period of time depending on the circumstances. Let me share a real-life example from my practice in the ED to show how this can be possible. Some details have been changed to protect patient confidentiality.

One of my patients, a middle-aged Hispanic woman, presented with a chief complaint of vaginal bleeding at 12 weeks gestation. She had an ultrasound that was unable to locate a fetal heartbeat or intra-uterine pregnancy. She unfortunately had a miscarriage. For this woman, this was an especially devastating event because it was not her first miscarriage, but her fourteenth without bringing a pregnancy successfully to term. She was so hopeful that this would have been the one that would result in a child she would someday hold in her arms. The primary care provider saw the patient, informed her of the ultrasound results, and promptly left the room and wrote orders to discharge the patient to home.

I came into the room a few minutes later with the discharge paperwork. She was still sobbing and in obvious distress. I had two choices. I could quickly give her the paperwork and send her home so we could see the next patient in a very busy ED, or I could acknowledge her pain, show that she mattered to me, and offer her hope in some small tangible way. I chose the latter.

I pulled up a chair, sat down beside her in silence for several seconds. I then said, "I am so sorry." But I didn't just say it; I truly meant it because her experience and the loss of her fourteenth baby really did matter to me. I remembered that she made a reference earlier that her church was praying for her. There was no chaplain. There are going to be times in practice when all you can do is pray, and this seemed to be one of those times. I asked if I could pray for her before she left. She quickly agreed, and I did so.

Afterward she opened her eyes, wiped away a tear, looked a bit more relaxed and said, "Thank you so much! You have no idea how much this meant to me!" I then went through her discharge instructions and she left the ED. This nursing intervention took only a couple of minutes but made a difference as she felt holistically cared for. Every nurse has the ability to make a lasting difference by caring not only for the physical needs, but those of the spirit as well.

Pay close attention to what is in a patient's room. If there is a Bible, Koran, or other material of a spiritual nature, if/when appropriate, engage the patient regarding their faith and current illness. For example, I recently cared for a patient who had a Bible in his room. I asked, "Do you have a favorite passage, and if so would you like me to read it to you?" He wanted me to read the Twenty-Third Psalm: "The Lord is my shepherd; I shall not want..." He closed his eyes and appeared relaxed as I read this to him. He thanked me afterwards and asked if I would pray for him. After a short prayer he fell asleep. This took only a couple of minutes, but it clearly ministered and cared for his spirit.

If you have a faith tradition that recognizes the value and the power of prayer, do not hesitate to integrate this into your nursing practice. Pray for yourself before you come into work (see appendix D). Pray for your patients as you provide care. Be sensitive to your patient's spiritual needs. If you sense that they are in need of prayer and would be open to this intervention, offer to pray for them. I have found that most patients are thankful of this gesture and appreciate it when the nurse is willing to go there.

Patient Presentations

Not every patient will have a clinical presentation that will require the nurse to provide spiritual care. In my experience, it is the exception, not the norm. But there a specific clinical situations that often have a high correlation to a potential crisis of the spirit that the nurse must have on his/her radar and be willing to "go there" as needed.

These scenarios include:

- Patients who have been recently diagnosed with a life-altering or terminal illness such as cancer
- Patients who are transitioning to hospice care
- Patients who are facing decisions regarding withdrawal of aggressive interventions such as dialysis
- Patients who are facing major surgery
- Patients who have lost hope
- Patients who are depressed
- Patients who are anxious

Application Case Study: Anxiety or Spiritual Distress?

I have created a unique series of case studies titled "Clinical Dilemmas" that address the unique nursing dilemmas that are most common in clinical practice and require the "art" of nursing to address and resolve. By capturing the salient themes of a scenario that situates a patient in spiritual distress, apply what you have learned by using this case study to apply this important content to practice. This case study is found in its entirety with a blank student version and fully developed answer key in the attachment in the eBook .

Power of Presence

It is the LITTLE things that the nurse does that are in reality the BIG things that make a lasting difference. One example of this axiom is the power of nurse presence. Most students are unaware that their physical presence, while providing care, can meet the emotional and even spiritual needs of each patient in their care.

But what does it mean to be "present"? To be present means that the nurse is AVAILABLE and ACCESSIBLE and this is clearly communicated to the patient. Presence can also be defined as "being with" and "being there" for the purpose of meeting their needs in a time of need. Other ways to define or explain presence include caring, nurturance, empathy, physical closeness, and physical touch (Rex–Smith, 2007).

Being present also implies a spiritual presence, to be attuned with the situation in such a way that it becomes spiritually transcendent when you quiet your mind to hear, see, and feel not only your current thoughts and feelings, but those of your patient (Dossey, 1995). When truly present, the nurse experiences what the patient is feeling (Faas, 2004). This is also the essence of empathy applied to practice.

To practically integrate the power of presence while providing patient care, be open to this unique person you are about to meet. As you introduce yourself, establish eye contact, let go of any assumptions, specific concerns or all the tasks that you need to complete. Instead let the patient tell you his/her story. Allow the patient to lead you on their journey. Remember that you are a companion with your patient on their current journey (Wilt & Smucker, 2001).

Presence is a nursing intervention that can be used in situations where there is nothing more that can be done but BE THERE by being supportive, physically close, offering a touch, or sitting in silence (Rex–Smith, 2007). Sitting quietly in times of need can communicate so much more than any words, even if it is for just a moment. This was what I did when I sat briefly and was "present" to the woman who had just suffered a miscarriage.

In contrast, a "non-present" nurse would be aloof, outside the situation, or preoccupied with other thoughts though physically present (Benner & Wrubel, 1989). This is the tension students will experience as novice nurses who are focused on the "tasks" to be done. They may not be able to recognize the importance to be "present" in a way that communicates caring. As a novice nursing student, you must give yourself grace to grow and develop as a new nurse, knowing that you will initially be focused on the tasks that need to be completed. As you develop greater proficiency and progress, you will be able to be grow in the ability to be more intentionally present to your patients.

Presence is also a nursing intervention recognized by the Nursing Interventions Classifications (NIC). Specific NIC presence interventions include:
- Demonstrate accepting attitude.
- Verbally communicate empathy or understanding of the patient's experience.
- Establish patient trust.
- Listen to the patient's concern.
- Touch the patient to express concern as appropriate.
- Remain physically present without expecting interactional responses (Cavendish et al., 2003).

Power of Touch

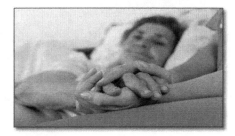

Touch is a fundamental human need and an appropriate intervention that nurses should integrate into their practice. Touch is a positive way to influence the patient's physical environment. It uses nature to influence the patient's well-being. This understanding of touch is consistent with the holistic nursing theories advocated by Florence Nightingale (Bush, 2001). During times of stress, patients have an increased need for reassuring touch. Simply placing a caregiver's hand on top of a dying patient's head reduced isolation and fear of death (Kubler-Ross, 1970).

Though older adults, especially those with dementia in long-term care settings are receptive and value touch, they are touch-deprived and less likely to receive touch from nurses and other care providers. In addition to communicating caring, touch can also decrease anxiety, lower heart rate and blood pressure, and reduce cardiac dysrhythmias (Weiss, 1990).

The elderly are most comfortable with the touch of a hand on their arm. Massage is another effective form of touch that has been shown to improve relaxation, relieve tension and anxiety, decreased pain medication, and improved sleep patterns in those who are terminally ill (Carnahan, 1988), but I have seen these same positive results of touch and massage in patients regardless of their diagnosis and need for care.

Another aspect of human touch that needs to be considered is that caring and acceptance can also be communicated through physical touch, especially by those in our culture who are considered "untouchable." An example of the power of physical touch to bring healing and acceptance is powerfully demonstrated in the life and ministry of Jesus. He was approached by a leper who desired healing. In the context of this man's lived experience, he was "untouchable" and had never experienced the warmth and acceptance of human touch since he became a leper.

Instead, he heard daily the loud cries of "Unclean! Unclean!" as people moved out of their way to avoid his presence if he left the leper colony. Recognizing not only his need to be healed, but also his deep unmet emotional need of acceptance that only human touch could communicate, the very FIRST thing that Jesus did before He brought needed healing, was to reach out and TOUCH the man who was "untouchable" and "unclean" (Matthew 8:1–4). Jesus also demonstrated the power of presence by not running away, but willing to approach and be present to the leper.

What can nurses learn from this example? Who is "untouchable" and "unclean" today in health care? What about those with HIV/AIDS, the homeless, or the increasing prevalence of patients who are in various forms of contact precautions that require the nurse to wear a gown and gloves every time they enter the room? What do you think the patient over time feels in this lived experience? Recognize the power of touch and be sensitive to the needs of those in contact precautions as well as anyone else whose illness has a similar stigma and is considered "untouchable" or "unclean" by cultural norms today. The use of your personal touch can powerfully communicate caring and acceptance.

The following true story from one nurse's practice graphically illustrates the power of touch and how it made a difference to this patient.

One Nurse's Story

I went in to meet my patient on the night shift and in report I had been told she had HIV. I went in for my first round of assessments and extended my hand to warmly introduce myself and said, "Hi, I'm Kathy and I'll be your nurse tonight." She stopped and looked at me incredulously and said, "Do you know my diagnosis?"

Thinking I was missing something, and likely hoping she meant something else, I looked at my clipboard and said the admitting diagnosis to her. She said, "No, do you know my diagnosis?" I looked at her and knew exactly what she meant. I said, "Yes, you also have HIV." Then she said, "Yes, I have been here a week and you are the first person here

> *to touch me" (my handshake).*
>
> *This opened a flood gate of emotions and we had many conversations that night. I learned that she was being discriminated against at work and her ex-husband (who had an affair and gave her HIV) had passed away. She was trying to re-establish contact with a family member so they could take care of her kids when she died. All of this started with the offer and touch of a handshake to a patient with HIV.*

I have observed that many new nurses, once in practice, are in the habit of wearing gloves any time they touch their patient with a routine nursing assessment when no blood or bodily fluids are evident or present. There is no substitute for direct human contact. I would encourage you to use gloves only when necessary and maintain the human touch in your clinical practice as much as possible. Your patients as well as your physical assessment will be better off as a result!

Becoming Culturally Competent

As our nation becomes more ethnically and culturally diverse it is imperative for all nurses to work toward becoming culturally competent. Cultural competence can be defined as a "lifelong process of examining values and beliefs and developing an inclusive approach to practice with active intercultural engagement. This definition reflects a broad description of culture that includes, but is not limited to age, gender, race, ethnicity, religion, sexual orientation, socioeconomic status, and physical or mental abilities" ("Nurturing Cultural Competence in Nursing," 2010, p. 6). As new immigrants join our culture, it can be challenging to keep up with various cultures. This is an ongoing aspect of professional development and lifelong learning nurses need to embrace.

Since religious worldviews provide a window to the prevailing values and ethnic norms of any cultural group, knowledge and understanding of the most dominant religions of ethnic groups in your community are essential and will facilitate cultural sensitivity. But remember that there will always be exceptions, so be careful not to make assumptions!

For example, the religious identity of most who are from Somalia will be Muslim, most Hispanics will be Roman Catholic, those from Ethiopia may be Christian, Orthodox, or Muslim, and those from India are most likely to be Hindu, but Islam, Christianity, and the Sikh religions are also practiced by some.

Becoming knowledgeable about another cultural group and integrating this knowledge into your practice is the essence of becoming culturally competent. It means respecting each patient's cultural diversity and examining how their beliefs may affect their health care. When nursing care does not intersect with the patient's worldview or belief set, compliance with the proposed treatment plan will be less likely (Ward, 2012).

America is a nation comprised of immigrants from all around the world. Many of these immigrants will require health care and will be patients in your clinical setting. What does the nurse need to know to demonstrate respect and provide culturally competent and sensitive care based on their patients' unique culture and worldview? It isn't enough to know others have different religious beliefs. It is imperative to get beneath the surface and explore your attitudes and any assumptions you may have toward the most common ethnic groups in your community.

Use the professional behavior of reflection to determine if you have any internal bias or prejudice toward any of these cultural groups. Address this head on and be aware that any bias impacts your ability to engage and care. Learn as much as you can about the dominant ethnic and cultural groups in your community that you will likely encounter in the clinical setting. This knowledge will help develop understanding and higher levels of engagement for the wide diversity of humanity in your care.

One way to grow is to develop cross-cultural friendships with others. Reach out and expand your friendship circles. Learn to enjoy and appreciate others and their culture and live out an ethos that truly "celebrates" diversity.

This principle also applies if you are an international student. Reach out to American students and form friendships that will help you better understand and become culturally sensitive to American culture. This will also help you care more effectively for American patients by recognizing cultural attitudes that are similar to yours as well as different and to incorporate this knowledge into your practice.

Practical Strategies to Build a Bridge

Regardless of the color of our skin, the language that we speak, or the way that we dress, we share a common humanity and oneness with each other. Despite what may be obvious differences, never forget that you have much in common with those from other cultures. In order to build a bridge with those from other countries, here are some simple strategies to not only build a bridge to provide needed care, but in the process will clearly communicate that you care!

- **Identify the most common ethnic/cultural groups in your community.** For example, where I practice at a large inner-city metropolitan hospital in Minneapolis, Minnesota, the most prevalent cultural groups are from Somalia and Mexico.
- **Memorize several greetings and phrases for each ethnic group.** Communicating even the simplest greetings will put a smile on the patient and family members when they see you reach out in their native language. This simple gesture practically communicates that you care.
- **Become knowledgeable of the role the patient's family plays in the healing process.** For example, it might be customary for the patient's family to stay with the patient whereas in other cultures, the family might refrain from visiting (Ward, 2012).
- **Refrain from stereotypes.** Be careful about making assumptions based on other patients that share the same ethnicity. Stereotyping is a judgment that will impact your ability to engage and demonstrate caring. Remain open-minded (Ward, 2012).
- **Assess for understanding.** If the patient is not fluent in English, health care terminology can be difficult to understand. Assessing for comprehension is crucial. Make sure you have an interpreter with you if there is a language barrier present (Ward, 2012).
- **Ask about alternative practices to healing.** It is important to understand the alternative healthcare practices that are customary for the patient from this culture. If there are no contraindications, the nurse may be able to integrate this into the plan of care (Ward, 2012). The book *The Spirit Catches You and You Fall Down: A Hmong Child, Her American Doctors, and the Collision of Two Cultures* is an excellent presentation of the dynamics present when two cultures collide in the health care arena.

- Nursing is both an art and science because of its unique emphasis of holism that emphasizes care for the physical, emotional, and spiritual needs of patients.
- Caring for the sick did not begin with Florence Nightingale in the 1800's, but has its origins in the first century AD, as a ministry of the early Christian church.
- Caring and compassion are foundational to nursing practice and are the most important attitudes of the nurse.
- The essence of caring as a nurse is the ability to recognize the value and worth of those you care for and that the patient and their experience matter to you.
- Caring disposition not only improves patient outcomes by improving nurse engagement but also benefits the nurse by decreasing stress and resultant burnout in clinical practice.
- Spiritual needs that are universal include finding meaning and purpose in life, faith, hope, love, and forgiveness.
- Spiritual care is within the nurse's scope of practice and can be implemented by using nursing process and questions that incorporate the themes of universal spiritual needs.
- By using nurse presence as well as appropriate use of touch, the nurse can communicate caring as well as care for the emotional and spiritual needs of patients.
- Make it a priority to become culturally sensitive regarding the largest ethnic groups in your community. Utilize practical strategies to build a bridge between cultures that communicate caring.

Additional Resources

- Case Studies: Clinical Dilemmas: Case Studies that Cultivate Caring, Civility and Clinical Reasoning: http://www.keithrn.com/home/store/
- Book: *Nursing the Spirit: The Art and Science of Applying Spiritual Care* (2001) by Dorothy Wilt and Carol Smucker
- Book: *Spiritual Care: A Guide for Caregivers* (2000) by Judith Allen Shelly
- Book: *The Nurse with an Alabaster Jar* (2006) by Mary Elizabeth O'Brien
- Book: *Spirituality In Nursing: Standing on Holy Ground* (2013) by Mary Elizabeth O'Brien
- Book: *The Spirit Catches You and You Fall Down: A Hmong Child, Her American Doctors, and the Collision of Two Cultures* (2012) by Anne Fadiman

Chapter Reflections

1. What caring behaviors do you utilize in the clinical setting?

2. Are you easily "moved with compassion" with each patient you care for?

3. What barriers do you encounter that prevent you from seeing your patient as "your neighbor" in the clinical setting?

4. What can you do to address these barriers as you progress through your program?

5. Is religion and/or spirituality important to you? If so, how can you integrate care for the spirit of each patient in your care?

6. How can you practically incorporate physical touch or nurse presence while you provide care?

7. What are the dominant ethnic groups in your community that you need to become culturally sensitive to?

8. What do you need to know in order to provide culturally sensitive care?

Your goal as a nurse:
Have a heart that never hardens, a temper that never tires, and a touch that never hurts!

Chapter 4
How to Act Like a Professional

"Let us all have the benefits of the opinion that some high resolve or pure motive actuated us. Are we proud to be Nurses? to be called Nurse?"
–Florence Nightingale, 1883, Probationer address, St. Thomas Hospital

"Professional, personal, and professional identity act as one as a nurse. When individuals become members of a profession they become identified with the profession. Their membership in it cannot be separated from their personal identity. I am a nurse is a statement that enumerates who I am, not just what I do."
–Timothy Porter O'Grady, DM, EdD, ScD(h), APRN, FAAN

The quiz at the beginning of this book had numerous questions that represented the importance of professional dispositions and attitudes toward nursing practice. Each of these questions reveal an important aspect of what it means to be a member of a profession vs. just having a job. These questions included the following:

- How do you see nursing? Is it a job or a profession?
- Do you possess a strong work ethic?
- Do you consider yourself a life-long learner?
- Do you have strong attention to detail?
- When you make a mistake, do you learn from it, or do you try to cover it up?
- How well do you perform under stress?
- How well do you handle responsibility?
- How well do you relate to others and communicate effectively?
- How well do you handle conflict with others?

How did you do on these questions that relate to the professional behaviors of nursing practice? This is relevant and must be reflected upon by each student because, from my vantage point, there is a crisis of professionalism in nursing today. We are health care professionals, but our behavior often betrays this truth with the prevalence of incivility, bullying, and disrespectful behavior that is well-documented as a problem in our profession.

In one study, nurse managers reported a current increase in inferior work ethic, poor attendance, and an attitude of entitlement in new nurses entering the profession ("Managers Note Less Professionalism among Nurses," 2013). Unfortunately, many of these behaviors were evident while these same students were in school. Because incivility and entitlement have become normalized in popular culture, many students may be unaware that they are being unprofessional. Because of the presence of bullying and incivility in nursing education, students may also see this unprofessional behavior role modeled by nursing faculty.

But despite these challenges, I am confident that things can change. The essence of professionalism in practice is that it is not so much something that you do as it is something that you are. It is a way of life that is demonstrated by your character, your high standards of excellence, and your desire to be the best possible nurse you can be and to settle for nothing less.

What values would you emphasize as the essence of professionalism for nursing? One study answered that question and determined that the following qualities should be emphasized in nursing education:

- Strong interpersonal relationship/communication skills
- Appearance
- Time management
- Being ethical
- Strong work ethic ("Managers Note Less Professionalism among Nurses," 2013).

A strong work ethic and the willingness to work hard is a practical value that is timeless and was also emphasized as an important virtue of the professional nurse at the beginning of the modern era. In *Nursing Ethics*, Hampton Robb (1900) wrote the following:

"A pupil (student nurse) *should esteem it a piece of good fortune to be put on duty in the heavy wards, where one is always busy, where the work never seems to be done, and where there is so much in the way of nursing going on...Never be afraid to work and to work hard. Work pure and simple is not likely to do you harm...Never seek for the soft spots or the easy places in hospital work"* (p. 69).

Professional behaviors are also part of the American Nurses Association (ANA) Code of Ethics. Section 1.5, Relationships with colleagues and others, states:

"The principle of respect for persons extends to all individuals with whom the nurse interacts. The nurse maintains compassionate and caring relationships with colleagues and others with a commitment to the fair treatment of individuals, to integrity-preserving compromise, and to resolving conflict" ("Code of Ethics for Nurses with Interpretive Statements," 2001).

The foundational professional behaviors that students need to demonstrate before graduation can be boiled down to CARING, COMPASSION, and RESPECT. These core values are also a part of our code of ethics! Are you aware of the ANA code of ethics and the values it calls each nurse to embody? These same principles that we are called to demonstrate toward our patients must also be shown to other students and nursing faculty.

Character Matters

Character matters. Florence Nightingale, the founder of the modern era of the nursing profession, recognized the importance of personal character and virtue to those who would aspire to become a nurse. Nurses at the time of Nightingale had little to no training. Women who were caregivers included alcoholics and prostitutes who routinely came to work drunk, and immoral conduct was not uncommon on the wards where patients received care.

Nightingale identified the following character traits as central to nursing (Woodham-Smith, 1951). Though written more than 150 years ago, they remain relevant today. Honestly reflect on the questions with each essential character trait below and see if these values are well established in you.

- **Truthfulness/honesty.** Do you consistently tell the truth regardless of the consequences or only when it's convenient? Are you willing to cheat on an exam to get a passing grade?
- **Obedience.** Do you find it easy to follow the directions of those in authority over you?
- **Punctuality.** Are you on time for class and clinical learning? How about your current job or appointments?
- **Sympathy.** Are you able to identify easily with the pain and suffering of others or are you distant and aloof?
- **Humility.** Do you readily recognize your limitations as a student learner? Are you comfortable asking questions to validate your knowledge base?

Building on Nightingale's legacy, the American Nurses Association has identified the following values and character traits as essential to the professional nurse (American Nurses Association, 2015):

- **Integrity.** What are you like when nobody is watching? Are you the same or different?
- **Accountability.** Are you willing to allow others to hold you accountable for areas that may be a weakness for you?
- **Credibility.** Are you known to those close to you as being honest and trustworthy?
- **Advocacy.** Are you willing to take a stand for what you believe is right even if others may not agree with you?
- **Compassion.** Do you identify with the sufferings of others in such a way that you "suffer together" with them? This is the essence of what it means to be compassionate.
- **Respect.** Do you see others as having infinite value and worth regardless of their socioeconomic status or ethnicity? Do you have a high regard for the value and sanctity of every human being?

Moral Courage

The professional nurse must embrace the responsibility of being a patient advocate by willing to do what is best for the patient, even if it comes at a personal or professional cost to the nurse. The ethical principle of *primum non nocere*, "above all do no harm," is foundational to medical as well as nursing ethical practice. Nightingale recognized the relationship between the character of the nurse and living out this ethical principle. A concise definition of moral courage is standing up to do the right thing by acting on moral values when faced with known risks to self through speaking up.

What if the physician insists that the dose of the medication ordered is correct and insists that you administer it, despite your reservations? What if you smell alcohol on the breath of the physician who is rounding on patients or on a nurse colleague who shows up for work? What would you be willing to say or do?

In one study where nurses were asked to respond to a scenario in which a surgeon or a nurse colleague appeared to have alcohol on their breath, moral courage was influenced by the education of the care provider. A nurse with an associate or baccalaureate degree was more likely to do something and confirm the suspicion with another health care provider. Perioperative nurses in urban hospitals were significantly more likely to stop the procedure with the physician than nurses in a rural hospital setting.

When there was a culture of reprisal and retaliation, nurses were much less likely to address the concern but when the fear of reprisal was low, the nurse would be more willing to address the problem (Dinndorf-Hogenson, 2015).

I want to encourage you as a student or new nurse to successfully pass the mirror test after every clinical day. This means that you can look yourself in the mirror and know that you not only did the very best you could do, but you did the right thing and did not compromise your values and moral character in order to do what was easy and expedient.

Treatment Dilemmas

Treatment dilemmas may arise when a physician advocates for full medical treatment or the family demands treatment while the patient is unsure or unwilling to undergo aggressive medical treatment. What if a patient with stage IV metastatic cancer wants to go straight to hospice/palliative care and not go through the rigors of chemotherapy or radiation treatment? Nurses are the ones who are troubled morally by non-beneficial treatment if it is implemented and continues. How would you handle this dilemma once in practice?

Some principles to guide ethical and moral decision making in practice include initiating open communication among all members of the care team in the context of a family conference or among the health care team alone. If the nurse is still morally troubled by a course of treatment that is not consistent with the wishes of the patient but caters to the demands of the family, a medical ethics consult would be the next logical step. Most hospitals have a team that typically includes a chaplain, physician, nurse, and other members of the health care team who are unbiased. This team looks objectively at the concerns that are brought forward and suggests steps to successfully resolve the issue.

Excellence Matters

Excellence means that you have a strong desire to excel and be the best that you can possibly be. Excellence is inwardly motivated and is present because you cannot imagine doing anything less than your very best. If you are content to be average and just good enough to get by, you sell yourself short and will not live up to the potential that you could be as a person and nurse (Grossman & Valiga, 2013). Do not accept the status quo, but push yourself to do what is needed and sacrifice to be the best nurse you can possibly be.

What about you? Do you have an attitude of excellence as a nursing student who will soon be a practicing nurse? Or do you consistently do what is needed and the bare minimum just to get by? One example of this get-by attitude that I have heard more than once from my students when I am presenting a lecture is, "Tell me what I need to know to pass the test." Determine right now that you will not be that student! Giving your all and nothing short of your best is your goal if you want to excel in nursing school as well as a nurse in practice.

Excellence is also a choice and a habit. It does not just happen by chance or by accident. It is always the result of sincere effort and strong intention. I want to encourage you to make the pursuit of excellence incorporated into not just your studies as a student but in everything you do (Grossman & Valiga, 2013).

Vince Lombardi, the former coach of the Green Bay Packers said, "The quality of a person's life is in direct proportion to his or her commitment to excellence, regardless of the chosen field of endeavor."

The implications of pursuing excellence impact not just the quality of nurse you will become but all aspects of your life!

For the health care professional, excellence needs to be a way of life. Excellence begets excellence, for ourselves and for those we work with. Studies have shown that when nurses work on units where excellent nursing is the norm, nurses strive to continually reach the level of excellence they see in their nurse colleagues. But the converse is also true. When nurses practice on a unit where the standard of care is poor or merely average, the other nurses are satisfied with merely maintaining the status quo and doing just enough to get by as well. The quality of nursing practice tends to descend to this lowest common denominator instead (Grossman & Valiga, 2013).

Just because bad behavior may be evident in your clinical setting and may reduce your practice to the lowest common denominator, this will not only impact the patient's you care for but also your license. The excuse that "everyone else does it" is not a legal defense in court or before the board of nursing!

Historical Examples of Excellence to Emulate

Though difficult at times to live up to and pursue, excellence and the moral character traits can be lived out and need to be "in you" at some level. Several years ago, Gatorade® had a popular ad campaign centered on Michael Jordan, who was at that time, a basketball star for the Chicago Bulls. Do not underestimate the power of a relevant lived-out example to role model. Though popular culture has numerous examples of individuals who do not provide positive role models of life and character, I have chosen three individuals from three different historical time periods who capture the essence of the foundational values of our profession who compassionately and sacrificially served and cared for others that can provide an opportunity for students to imprint and learn from their example.

St. Camillus de Lellis

St. Camillus de Lellis (1550–1614) was a male caregiver from the Middle Ages. St. Camillus entered a Franciscan monastery after he recognized that he was not living a life worthy of God and desired to turn his life around. While needing hospital care for a chronic infection, he was concerned about the lack of compassion by caregivers he saw in practice and vowed to be different. As he cared for others, he recognized that good nursing depended on loving humanity, and he believed nursing would be better if it was not influenced by being paid for services provided (O'Lynn, 2012).

He made it his primary goal to gather men who would care for others, who were motivated by love for humanity and would let the wages take care of themselves. As he looked about the streets of Rome, he realized that it was the sick outside the hospital who needed care. He set up the first hospice service in the roughest part of Rome and began to focus his ministry on caring for the dying and providing comfort. His order was known as the Brothers of the Happy Death, since they brought compassion and comfort to those who were dying.

Some of the caregivers of his order became ill and died of the plague. The remaining men in his order continued to sacrificially serve and care for others. This order was formally titled the Congregation of the Servants of the Sick (the Camellians) and still exist today, providing health care in 35 countries. His example of caring, service, and sacrifice embodies the spirit of the nursing profession and remains relevant today. This order had

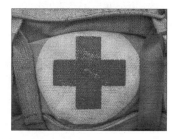

a unique symbol that identified their order of male caregivers; the RED CROSS that remains the universal symbol of health care today (O'Lynn, 2012)!

Florence Nightingale

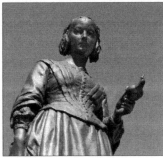

At the age of 17, Florence Nightingale felt that God had spoken to her and called her to service. Nightingale (1820–1910) was influenced by a belief in God that motivated her to transform health care and the nursing profession (McDonald, 1999). Her heart to serve and obey God through her life is evident in this passage from her diary at the age of thirty, *"Today I am 30, the age Christ began His mission...now Lord, let me only think of Thy will, what Thou willest me to do, O Lord, Thy will, Thy will"* (Widerquist, 1992, p. 51).

As a young woman who sensed God leading her to devote herself to works of charity in hospitals, she recognized the need for health care training. However, her parents were wealthy and respectable, and caring for the sick in England was not practiced by respectable women. Nurses in this era routinely came to work drunk, and immoral conduct was present even on the wards.

Therefore, she left England and obtained her health care training at the moral and respectable Lutheran Deaconesses in Germany. She willingly chose to sacrificially serve during the Crimean War, caring for the wounded, making rounds as the "lady with the lamp," and educating nurses. Florence demonstrated God's care for humanity when she wrote:

> *"I have not a moment. The whole Army is coming into the hospitals. The task will be gigantic. Alas how will it all end? We are in the hands of God. Pray for us. We have at the moment five thousand sick and wounded. My only comfort is, God sees it, God knows it, God loves us"* (Dossey, 1999, p. 121).

She implemented numerous reforms to lower the 73 percent mortality rate from diseases alone and wrote a one-thousand-page report of statistics she compiled during this time. Nightingale established her schools of nursing after the war based on her "evidence-based practice" (Lewis Coakley, 1990). Despite poor health later in life, Nightingale continued to devote herself to nursing research, using her gifts and passion as a statistician. As the first nurse educator and researcher of the modern era, her legacy includes the value and importance of applied research to practice and how it can lead to better patient outcomes (Berman & Snyder, 2011). Nightingale's life clearly demonstrates that faith, service, and nursing can and do complement one another in practice.

Agnes Gonxa Bojaxhu

Though not a trained professional nurse, one caregiver who is worth emulating is Agnes Gonxa Bojaxhu (1910–1997). Never heard of her? I am sure you have if I use her more commonly-known name of Mother Teresa!

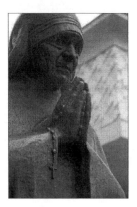

Like Florence Nightingale, Agnes responded to the call of God on her life to serve others. At the age of 18, she joined an Irish community of nuns with missions located in India. While teaching at the high school in Calcutta, she received further clarity of the call of Jesus to serve him in the poorest of the poor and received permission to start a school for the children of the slums. She then started her own order, The Missionaries of Charity (active in 133 countries), whose primary task was to love and care for persons nobody valued, the sick and dying homeless poor ("Mother Teresa – Biographical," 1979). Her primary mission was not about the work, it was all done for Jesus. She sacrificially served in this capacity until her death at the age of 87.

Out of her heart of love for God and love for others, the following quotes capture the essence of the example of her life. Regardless of your faith tradition, these principles have relevance and embody the essence of compassionate caregiving by striving to be "like" Mother Teresa:

- *"Do ordinary things with extraordinary love."*
- *"It is not how much we do, but how much love we put into that action."*
- *"Let us touch the dying...and let us not be ashamed or slow to do the humble work"* ("Her own words", n.d.).

Vocation vs. Occupation

Each of these caregivers from the past has a common thread of vocation as the primary motivation to care for others. Vocation can be defined as doing all that is possible and whatever is necessary for the good of the patient. Others, including Nightingale, have spiritualized vocation by referring to it as a divine "calling."

In the first nursing textbook of the modern era, *Notes on Nursing*, Nightingale (1859) writes, *"Every nurse...must have a respect for her own calling, because God's precious gift of life is often placed literally in her hands"* (p. 71). Nightingale also affirmed this sense of calling in a probationer (new graduate) address at St. Thomas Hospital in 1883, *"We nurses should remember to help out suffering fellow creatures in our calling...let us make our calling sure"* (Attewell, 2012, p. 75).

Christine Tanner (2004) affirms that nursing is a calling that requires each nursing student to recognize the importance of renewing their body, mind, and spirit. Nursing as vocation remains relevant today and can guide students to care deeply for their patients. This vision of nursing makes values, faith, and the patient the primary motivation to care for others. Financial compensation then becomes a secondary motivator to be a caregiver (O'Lynn, 2012).

Developing a Personal Mission Statement

Purpose

What do the business you work for, the college you attend, and nursing programs all have in common? They all most likely have a mission statement. A mission statement used to guide the actions of an organization, spell out its overall goal, provide a path, and guide decision making. For example, the health care organization I work for has the following mission statement, "We serve our communities by providing excellent care as we prevent illness, restore health and provide comfort to all who entrust us with their care"("Our Mission," 2014). This statement concisely captures its purpose (provide excellent care) as well as the outcome of this purpose (restore health and provide comfort).

What's Your Mission?

If a mission statement is essential for an organization, what about a personal mission statement to concisely capture the purpose and goals that you want to see realized for yourself as a student nurse? At the beginning of this book I encouraged you to reflect upon why you want to become a nurse. Now it is time to take the essence of your motivation and put it into writing. This will provide a literal stake in the ground so you remain grounded in your purpose of becoming a nurse. Because of the hard work and stress that most students experience, you will at times wonder if it is worth it and can easily lose your perspective.

Principles to incorporate in a personal mission statement can include the following:
- Vision to be the best
- What is your motivation to serve?
- What do you want to accomplish?
- What is your overriding goal?
- What values will you embody?

Student Examples

I recognized the value of this exercise and had my entire class develop and write out their own personal mission statement that would define them as a student nurse as well as a nurse in practice. I encouraged them to write down their personal mission statement and put it in a place such as their smart phone or notebook where they would be able to see it and review it often. I have included a few of their examples to guide you as you develop your own:

- *"To be a knowledgeable and compassionate professional nurse that truly makes a difference in patients' lives through providing holistic nursing care."*
- *"To integrate critical thinking knowledge and the nursing process to serve people in a Christ-like manner."*
- *"To be a competent and lifelong learning nurse while providing empathetic and compassionate care, maintaining honesty and integrity, and being respectful of all cultures and individual choices."*
- *"To never lose sight of my passion and drive to become a nurse. I will work with an open heart to give the best care possible to every patient I come in contact with. I will remain educated, honest, and professional for the duration of my career as well as in life."*
- *"To provide unwavering care for each individual to the best of my ability and to incorporate optimal skill, compassion, and character into every situation I am involved in."*

Unprofessional Behavior

Though I have held up a high standard of what professional behavior looks like in practice, the time has come to reveal and expose what bad behavior looks like in the nursing profession. Do you talk negatively about other students, faculty, or the nursing program to others, but NOT to the person you have an issue with? If so, this is indirect communication and is unprofessional behavior that does not befit a student entering the nursing profession.

Do you believe that your college owes you a degree because you paid for it? This, too, is an unprofessional attitude of entitlement. Coming late to class or texting during lecture are also uncivil actions and disrespectful to nursing faculty. While you are a nursing student, make it a priority to embrace the highest level of professional behavior in word and deed!

Incivility Defined: Student to Faculty

Entitlement and incivility have become increasingly pervasive in American society and contribute to incivility in nursing education (Clark & Springer, 2010). Unfortunately, students may reflect these attitudes as they enter nursing education. Student "entitlement" is exhibited by those who expect high grades for modest amounts of work, assume a "consumer" mentality toward education, refuse to accept responsibility and make excuses for their failures.

The most common student incivility behaviors are:

- Disruptive behaviors in class/clinical that include
  - ✓ Rude comments, engaging in side conversations, dominating class
  - ✓ Cell phone, texting, inappropriate computer use in class
  - ✓ Late to class and leaving early
  - ✓ Sleeping in class (Clark & Springer, 2010)
- Anger or excuses for poor performance
- Inadequate preparation (Clark, 2008)
- Pressuring faculty until they get what they want (Clark, 2008)
- Bad-mouthing other students, faculty, and the nursing program (Clark, 2008)

Contributing Factors

What other factors influence incivility in nursing students? Could the highly competitive and academically rigorous culture of nursing education itself be a contributing factor to student incivility? In one qualitative study, the themes that students identified that contributed to incivility included burnout from demanding workloads and competition in a high-stakes academic environment (Clark, 2008).

Incivility Defined: Faculty to Student

Students are not the only ones who can be uncivil and disrespectful in nursing education. Nursing faculty also can be responsible for this unprofessional behavior. What is it that influences nursing faculty to demonstrate incivility toward their students? Faculty identified STRESS as the primary problem. Ironically, many nurse educators are also burned out from their demanding workloads. Other causes of faculty stress include high faculty turnover, lack of qualified educators, role stress, and incivility from all sides: students, other faculty, and administration (Clark, 2008). Though faculty may not be aware of perceived uncivil behaviors toward students, any verbal/nonverbal communication that students perceive as disrespect, abruptness, or rudeness must be guarded against by faculty.

According to Henderson (2009), bullying is "verbal abuse and maltreatment between nurses" and is a problem in health care settings and in nursing education. Henderson reported there are various forms of bullying within the nursing hierarchy, ranging from intimidation to verbal abuse. Bullying that occurs from one in a position of power (faculty or administrator) to someone without power (student) is referred to as vertical bullying (Bartholomew, 2007).

Vertical bullying is under-reported and is one of the nonacademic reasons for withdrawal from nursing schools. Students have experienced incivility by instructors, which made the learning environment difficult and, at times, hostile (Sengstock, 2008). The results of a study by Cooper et al., (2009) revealed that nursing students repeatedly encountered multiple bullying behaviors by faculty and nurses during their clinical rotations. This is problematic because students who have negative experiences in both the classroom and clinical areas of hospitals will often decide that they do not want to be a part of a profession or organization that does not value them, and withdraw from nursing programs (Bartholomew, 2007).

The most common uncivil and disrespectful behaviors by nursing faculty towards students are:

- Exerting position and control over students (Clark, 2008)
- Setting unrealistic student expectations (Clark, 2008)
- Assuming a "know-it-all" attitude (Clark, 2008)
- Being rigid, unapproachable, or rejecting students' opinions (Clark, 2011)
- Devaluing students' prior life experiences that can include work and academic experiences (Clark, 2008)
- Ineffective educators who cannot manage the classroom (Clark, 2008)
- Making condescending remarks or put-downs to students (Clark, 2011)
- Showing favoritism to certain students (Clark, 2008)
- Refusing or reluctant to answer questions (Clark, 2011)

There are two common denominators that both students and faculty have regarding the contributing factors to incivility: STRESS and DISRESPECT. Students are stressed by juggling many roles as provider/parent and student, as well as financial pressures and too little time. Faculty are stressed by multiple work demands, heavy workload, problematic students, and lack of faculty and needed support (Clark & Springer, 2010).

The lack of respect by both faculty and students creates a poisonous, downward spiral. If faculty are rigid, set unrealistic expectations, and do not allow open dialogue, students will inevitably respond with anger and lack of respect toward faculty. A cycle of incivility is set in motion. But it doesn't have to be this way; respect begets respect. If both faculty and students respectfully and openly communicate and engage with one another, a culture of civility can be nurtured instead (Clark, 2008).

The "Dance"

Clark likened incivility in academia to a "dance"; one leads and the other follows. It is important NOT to point fingers and say this is a student or a faculty problem. In reality, uncivil behavior does not exist in a vacuum, but both student and faculty are partners and interdependent in this "dance" (Clark, 2008). When both student and faculty engage, communicate, and seek resolution of conflict before it digresses to incivility, a culture of respect and the "dance" of civility are present.

But if opportunities to promote engagement by both faculty and student are missed, the root of disrespect is established and a "dance" of incivility is perpetuated. Once this dance has begun, regardless of who may be responsible for initiating it, incivility can escalate and become a blame game with no end in sight (Clark, 2008).

Pursue Civility

To create a healthy academic culture, there must be a healthy relationship between faculty and students. The principles that apply to healthy personal relationships are relevant and apply in academia. This includes the foundation of open/honest communication, working together, and establishing boundaries that are clearly defined and enforced.

Civility can become normative as a culture of respect is cultivated in academia. The following are practical steps from the literature (Clark & Springer, 2010) that educators can implement to make civility possible:

Educator Responsibilities of Civility:

- Model caring and respect in all that you do so your students can see what true professionalism looks like in practice!
- Provide opportunities to dialogue with students in open formats, such as a town hall meeting. This can provide needed dialogue and understanding.
- Establish clearly written policies or place expectations in student codes of conduct that address consequences of incivility. Enforce them consistently.
- Listen carefully; give students positive feedback.
- Incorporate time management/stress reduction/self-care in the curriculum.

Student Responsibilities of Civility

- Be prepared, respectful, and engaged in your learning (Clark, 2011).
- Do not speak in a negative, derogatory manner openly about other STUDENTS, FACULTY, or the nursing PROGRAM.
- Abide consistently by the standards of student conduct of your institution.
- Communicate your needs, and what you need/expect from faculty (Clark, 2011).
- Work toward a common goal of civility and respect (Clark, 2011).

Incivility in the Clinical Setting

Just like nurses in practice, nursing students are also at high risk to experience incivility and bullying in the clinical setting from other staff nurses and even patients and their families (Jackson et al., 2011). In one study 95 percent of students experienced hostile and bullying behaviors (Randle, 2003). When students experience these hostile behaviors, it adversely and negatively impacts student learning and well-being. Bullying behaviors that nursing students experience in the clinical setting include:

- Feeling ignored or unwelcome (Hoel, Giga, & Davidson, 2007)
- Undervalued (Pearcey & Elliott, 2004)
- Invisible (Vallant & Neville, 2006)
- Verbal abuse (Ferns & Meerabeau, 2009)
- Unfair treatment (Thomas & Burk, 2009)

The effect of a hostile environment as perceived by nursing students in the clinical portion of their program is evident in a report from the Joint Commission on Accreditation of Healthcare Organizations (2008), which showed that as negativity increased in hospitals, so did errors by nurses and nursing students. A positive environment in which students can develop a sense of self as a nurse and increase their self-esteem must be developed (Videbeck, 2007). Creating a nurturing clinical environment can promote a student's decision to remain in the nursing program (Griswold, 2014).

Student Responses to Incivility

Students and new nurses tend to feel powerless in the clinical setting (Boychuk Duchscher, 2009) and find it difficult to advocate for themselves when they experience any of these unprofessional behaviors. When students experience these hostile and disrespectful behaviors, they are not prepared to manage this conflict. As a result, they most often use avoidance and do not address it directly (Pines et al., 2011). I will discuss cognitive rehearsal, which is an empowerment strategy that prepares any student or new nurse with a direct and respectful response when incivility or bullying behaviors are directed toward you, later in this chapter.

Incivility as a Nurse in the Practice Setting

The prevalence of incivility that is often referred to as "nurses eating their young," is a current and ongoing dilemma in the nursing profession where the young and less experienced are often the targets of victimization.

If you have worked in health care or have had clinical in the practice setting, you have likely observed or experienced the disrespectful behavior of bullying or incivility. Would it surprise you that health care occupations such as nursing have the highest rates of bullying (Johnson & Rea, 2009)? Surveys have shown that 93 percent of nurses have witnessed bullying and 85 percent reported that they were victims of bullying (Coursey, Rodriguez, Dieckmann, & Austin, 2013).

Sixty-four percent of nurses cited this as the primary reason for leaving their current job (Stagg, Sheridan, Jones, & Gabel Speroni, 2011). New nurses as well as men (Dellasega, 2009) are more likely to experience incivility most often from other more experienced or senior nurses (Griffin, 2004).

Incivility is defined as a disregard for others that creates an atmosphere of disrespect, conflict, and stress that results in rude speech that can progress to more threatening situations (Clark, 2013). The most common overt bullying behaviors in nursing include patterns of faultfinding, intimidation, gossip, put-downs, and nonverbal innuendo such as raising eyebrows or sighing. More subtle bullying behaviors include isolation, exclusion, ignoring/refusing to help, and unfair assignments (Bartholomew, 2006). Other categories of bullying behavior include the resentful nurse who holds grudges and encourages others to join in as well as the cliquish nurse who intentionally excludes others from the "group" (Dellasega, 2009).

Other specific examples from the literature most commonly seen in the clinical setting include:

- Having information withheld so it affects your performance
- Having your views and opinions ignored
- Being personally ignored or excluded
- Micromanaging your work
- Persistent criticism of your work and effort
- Having insulting/offensive remarks made about you
- Repeated reminders of your errors and mistakes
- Having false allegations or accusations made against you (Johnson & Rea, 2009)

The most common examples of incivility I experienced in clinical practice consisted of being marginalized and isolated by nurses who were unwilling to help. If I asked for help, they would sigh and make it clear that I was asking too much from them. During report, some nurses appeared disinterested, distracted, and asked numerous questions not even relevant to the patient's priority problem. When I didn't have this nonessential information, the nurse would look at me in a demeaning manner that clearly communicated disrespect.

I have witnessed new nurses break down and begin to cry when I asked before report how they were doing. One nurse described the need to prove herself, feeling belittled if she asked a question because the nurse would respond, "You don't know that?" in a demeaning tone of voice. New nurses routinely overheard gossip about them or others and did not feel safe asking questions of certain nurses. Those who excel in the clinical setting are often marginalized or demeaned for their excellence. In some practice settings there seems to be a prevailing culture of keeping everyone average. If a nurse chooses to exceed and excel, he or she may pay a very high price from colleagues.

Root Causes

Why is incivility endemic in nursing and nursing education? One perspective from the literature is that incivility is RELATIONAL aggression, which is a feminine form of aggressive behavior. In comparison, men most often resort to PHYSICAL aggression when faced with conflict. But because women comprise the majority of nurses, incivility as relational aggression is endemic and common throughout the nursing profession (Dellasega, 2009).

Just as relational aggression among young women is normalized in adolescence ("mean girls"), this accepted norm becomes a self-fulfilling prophecy of what to expect in a profession where women are the majority. This may explain in part why there is an acceptance or tolerance of incivility in nursing. This pattern continues unchallenged because nurses do not challenge the status quo but put up with it to avoid conflict at all costs (Szutenbach, 2013).

One new nurse shared with me her experience with incivility and the emotional pain she experienced in this open letter:

One New Nurse's Pain
"I started on the unit with a fresh and positive attitude directly out of school. I thought I had found my dream job. However, I quickly learned that there was something incredibly dysfunctional about this unit. I had heard of 'horizontal violence' in nursing school, but I never expected that it would happen to me regularly in my own career and on my own unit. I have found this unit to be one of the most hostile, cold, unprofessional, passive-aggressive, inappropriate, and dysfunctional nursing units I have ever worked on. I find the unit to operate under a 'good old boys' mentality, where new staff fall victim to senior staff until they have 'proved themselves' or 'done their time' like they had to do. *I can honestly say that I cried every shift I worked for the first 6 months, and the only reason I stopped crying was not because it got any better, but because I had to change my expectations about the unit and accept my reality. I cannot put into words what it feels like to have nurses laugh in your face and belittle you when you ask a clinical question, roll their eyes and walk out on your report before it is finished, to literally have a back turned on you when trying to discuss a concern, or to be scolded or yelled at in front of your other colleagues until you are apologizing profusely with tears streaming down your cheeks. At this time I am not interested in making things any more difficult for myself. I would just like to get off of the unit before I lose my passion for nursing altogether."*

Consequences

This open letter validates the devastating consequences of a hostile work environment by creating feelings of inadequacy in a new nurse. Incivility is like putting gas on a fire. Feelings of failure, decreased self-esteem, self-doubt, anger, depression, burnout, and even post-traumatic stress disorder (PTSD) are common (Bartholomew, 2006). This often leads to decreased morale, low job satisfaction, increased absenteeism, and ultimately leaving the unit or even nursing entirely (Murray, 2008). Thirty percent of new nurses leave their first job after the first year when bullying is personally experienced (Johnson & Rea, 2009). Incivility in the clinical setting is an assault on human dignity and self-worth, and the effects can be devastating, debilitating, and enduring (Clark, 2013).

Does this toxic environment affect patient care? Absolutely! The Joint Commission has taken the position that incivility is a safety issue and has issued a standard to that effect. It has been shown that a unit that has a prevalence of incivility can lead to increased medical errors, adverse patient outcomes, and lower rates of nurse retention. By creating an environment that does not make it safe to ask questions, incivility poses a serious threat to patient safety and overall quality of care (Tillman Harris, 2011).

Be the Needed Change!

The article "Teaching Cognitive Rehearsal as a Shield for Lateral Violence: An Intervention for Newly Licensed Nurses" is a must-read for every student or new nurse. It defines professional behaviors as well as the most common uncivil behaviors. But more importantly, "cognitive rehearsal" teaches nurses to have a prepared plan to respond respectfully when specific uncivil behaviors are directed toward them. Because incivility thrives in an environment of passivity, incivility can often be stopped in its tracks when it is directly addressed in an assertive, direct, and respectful way (Griffin, 2004).

In one study where nurses were empowered by this strategy, 100 percent of the nurses reported that when the perpetrator was confronted, the bullying behavior stopped (Coursey, Rodriguez, Dieckmann, & Austin, 2013). This is obviously an effective strategy that must be implemented when any nurse experiences incivility.

For example, if a nurse has a pattern of raising eyebrows or sighs when asked for help, the empowered nurse has practiced and is prepared to respond in the following manner, "I sense (I see from your facial expression) that there may be something you wanted to say to me. Please speak directly to me" (Griffin, 2004).

Make a difference in your clinical setting if incivility is present! Be a leader and embrace the responsibility to be a role model:
- Demonstrate respect for all colleagues.
- Embrace and value the diversity of others.
- Form meaningful relationships with your colleagues.
- Never criticize another colleague publicly.
- If another team member is being slandered by gossip, stand up and speak out for the absent colleague when they are not present.
- Work as a team.
- Accept your share of the workload. (Griffin, 2004)

You Don't Have to Take it!

The song "We're Not Gonna Take It" by Twisted Sister became an anthem for the disenfranchised in the 1980's. In the same way, if you are the recipient of incivility in clinical practice, you don't have to take it! If you experience incivility in practice or see it used against others and have respectfully addressed the perpetrator with no change in behavior, you have done all that you can. Now is the time to communicate your experience to your nurse manager. To effectively communicate your concerns, you must thoroughly document what you have observed or experienced with dates and times.

Once adequate documentation has been collected, communicate these concerns to your nurse manager or human resources department (HR). In some cases, nurse management is part of the problem by allowing incivility to continue unchallenged or they may be the perpetrator of these unprofessional behaviors. In these circumstances, HR should be involved first.

Most institutions now have policies regarding a healthy work environment free of hostility or the lateral violence that incivility represents. Therefore, appropriate discipline can be initiated by management to hold those who perpetrate incivility accountable for their actions. Unfortunately, some HR departments are ill-prepared to deal with these situations. Employees have asserted that the HR department is simply another version of the "good old boys network." If this is the case, it is important to have other resources such as Workplace Bullying Institute (www.workplacebullying.org), or seek legal advice.

I have observed from my own experience that patient care units are like families. Some units are healthy and functional with a team orientation, while others are clearly dysfunctional with no sense of team and in need of intervention. Incivility is a toxic behavior that tends to be contagious and affects everyone on that unit. Being a new nurse can feel like being in middle school again. You will want to do whatever it takes to fit in and be a part of the new group, even if it means being passive or indifferent to incivility around you. By being passive and doing nothing, you are actually part of the problem. Instead, hold yourself to the highest standards of professionalism in practice and be the change that is so desperately needed in nursing today!

In 2015, the Professional Issues Panel on Incivility, Bullying, and Workplace Violence convened to develop a new ANA position statement. The key points of this position statement include:

- The nursing profession will not tolerate violence of any kind from any source
- RNs and employers must collaborate to create a culture of respect
- Evidence-based strategies that prevent and mitigate incivility, bullying, and workplace violence promote RN health, safety, and wellness and optimal outcomes in health care
- The statement is relevant for all health care professionals and stakeholders ("Incivility, Bullying, and Workplace Violence," 2015).

Application Case Study: Nurse-to-Student Incivility

Since incivility is endemic in nursing, the likelihood that you will witness or experience it in your first year of practice is high. Prepare to be the needed change by practicing! I have created a unique series of case studies titled "Clinical Dilemmas" that address the unique nursing dilemmas that are most common in clinical practice.

This clinical dilemma case study on nurse-to-student incivility will capture the essence of identifying incivility and how to directly and respectfully address incivility as a student or nurse in practice. By capturing the salient themes of this scenario, apply what you have learned from this chapter by using the following case study to apply this important content. This case study is found in its entirety with a blank student version and fully developed answer key in the attachment in the eBook.

Principles of Respectful and Effective Communication

To complete this discussion on incivility, it is important to realize that so much hinges on our words and how we communicate with one another. We must strive to be QUICK to listen and SLOW to speak! The importance of wise words in communication was recognized by Buddha, author Mark Twain, Gandhi, and King Solomon.

"To have much learning, to be skillful in handicraft, well-trained in discipline, and to be of good speech, this is the greatest blessing."

–Buddha

"The right word may be effective, but no word was ever as effective as a rightly timed pause."

–Mark Twain

"Keep your thoughts positive because your thoughts become your words.
Keep your words positive because your words become your behavior.
Keep your behavior positive because your behavior become your habits.
Keep your habits positive because your habits become your values.
Keep your values positive because your values become your destiny."

–Gandhi

Solomon, the wisest man of ancient history, wrote the following words of wisdom in Proverbs that, if put into practice, will also work to recapture civility in nursing:

Our Words Have Power
- Life and death are in the power of the tongue. Use your words to bring healing, NOT to crush and to destroy the spirit of others (Proverbs 12:18).
- *"Kind words heal and help; cutting words wound and maim"* (Proverbs 15:4).

The Source of Our Words Is Important
- Be sure that what we speak does not provoke strife, but is based in truth, and that it is spoken in love.
- *"It's a mark of good character to avert quarrels, but fools love to pick fights"* (Proverbs 20:3).

We Must Learn to Listen
- Listen carefully to what is communicated. That is the only way you will learn and grow from constructive feedback.
- *"The ear that listens to life-giving reproof will dwell among the wise"* (Proverbs 15:31).

THINK before You Speak
- Becoming slow to anger is the beginning of wisdom (Proverbs 16:32).

- *"The start of a quarrel is like a leak in a dam, so stop it before it bursts (Proverbs 17:14).*

Speak Less
- Too much talking tends to digress in time to gossip. Let our words be few, and only what is needed.
- *"But whoever restrains his lips is prudent"* (Proverbs 10:19).

Our Tone Matters
- *"A soft answer turns away wrath, but a harsh word stirs up anger"* (Proverbs 15:1)

Practical Professionalism

What follows are practical professional behaviors that, from my perspective, comprise the essence of what nursing students should internalize. They should be established by the time they complete nursing education. This list is not meant to be exhaustive. This summary of professional behaviors is derived from my own observations in practice as well as from those who have been my mentors and what I have seen lived out in their practice.

1. Ask questions!
- Remember that you are a student learner! Your body of knowledge is always growing and questions that you have are an outgrowth of your learning and clarification that you require to grow as a student learner. Many nursing faculty use questions as a way to assess what you know and do not know. Do not become defensive when you do not know the answer, but determine to find the correct response.
- Intellectual humility is an important principle that you must maintain throughout your career, especially as a new nurse. Recognize your limitations and what you don't know, never fake it, but always ask questions of your colleagues to be safe and provide the best possible care for your patients.

2. Reflect on your practice
- Reflect on what went well/poorly and make adjustments to prevent similar problems in the future.
- Reflection will guide students to learn from their mistakes, receive constructive feedback, and grow as a result.

3. Prompt and prepared
- Be on time for clinical, prepare for care in the time allotted, and be ready to receive report on time at the beginning of clinical.
- Complete treatments, medications in the time frame they are ordered.
- Complete all clinical documentation in a timely manner.
- Have all aspects of care completed at the end of shift and be present in post conference before it begins.

4. *Hold yourself to high standards*

- Desire to be the best nurse you can be!
- Resist the natural tendency to do only what is needed to "get by."

5. *Clinically curious*

- Ask questions and desire to know the WHY of what you do not know or understand.
- Use appropriate resources to accurately obtain the information you need to promote your own learning.

6. *Embrace the responsibility*

- You are holding the life of another in your hands. Never take this responsibility lightly!
- Take initiative, ownership, and responsibility for the care of your patients, but do not hesitate to ask for help or collaborate with your colleagues as needed!

7. *Caring*

- Be truly engaged and empathetic toward those you care for and demonstrate this by your caring presence.
- Reflect on what you can do to practically demonstrate empathy and show that every patient and family member matters to you.

8. *ZERO tolerance for incivility*

- Do NOT talk negatively about any student or faculty to others.
- Be respectful and direct in all communication with students and faculty. Make a commitment to go to any student or faculty member you have a concern about.
- Stand up for the absent colleague if students are gossiping about another. Encourage the person to go directly to the other person and keep it between them and NOT the group.

9. *Be a TEAM player*

Though your patient assignment is your responsibility, it takes a team to ensure that the needs of each patient on the unit are met, especially when it is a busy shift. Even at the beginning of the modern era of nursing, Nightingale recognized the importance of teamwork by communicating to new graduate nurses that in providing care, *"We are all one Nurse"* (Attewell, 2012, p. 76). Adopt a mindset of being a team player by role modeling this professional behavior consistently in the following ways:

- Answer call lights regardless if they are your patients or not.
- Offer to help your colleagues whenever you have a chance.
- Be a uniter in all you say and do, not a divider.

- The nurse is a health care professional who must demonstrate by their lived example what this looks like in practice.
- Character traits that are essential to professional practice include honesty, humility, integrity, compassion, and respect.
- The nurse must have an internal motivation to consistently pursue excellence and be the best that he/she can possibly be.
- Historical examples of caring and excellence that today's nurse can emulate include St. Camillus de Lellis, Florence Nightingale, and Mother Teresa.
- Developing a mission statement that defines your personal purpose as a nurse can help you maintain a vision of excellence and perspective.
- Though incivility and bullying behavior are common nonprofessional behaviors in nursing, they can be eliminated by maintaining an attitude of respect for others.
- Practical professional behaviors include the willingness to ask questions, reflect on your practice, remain clinically curious, have zero tolerance for incivility, and be a team player.

Additional Resources

- Book: Illuminating Florence: Finding Nightingale's Legacy in Your Practice (2012) by Alex Attewell
- Book: *The Joy in Loving: A Guide to Daily Living* by Mother Teresa
- Book: *Ending Nurse-to-Nurse Hostility: Why Nurses Eat Their Young and Each Other (2nd ed.)* (2014) by Kathleen Bartholomew
- Book: *When Nurses Hurt Nurses: Overcoming the Cycle of Nurse Bullying* (2011) by Cheryl Dellasega
- Book: *Creating & Sustaining Civility in Nursing Education* (2013) by Cynthia Clark
- Website: Civility Matters: Creating and Sustaining Communities of Civility website of Cynthia Clark

Chapter Reflections

1. What character traits essential to nursing are your greatest strengths?

2. Are there any character traits you need to develop to be more integrated as a professional nurse? If so, what will you do to develop them?

3. What historical example resonated most with you? Do you have any current role models of a professional nurse? What would you like to incorporate from their example into your practice?

4. Is your decision to become a nurse motivated by a "calling"?

5. How will you directly address incivility you experience or witness?

6. What practical professional behaviors are a strength for you?

7. What practical professional behaviors are current weaknesses? What will you do to make them strengths?

8. Write out your personal mission statement that will guide you as a nurse.

> *New students and nurses on the unit are friends, not food!*

Chapter 5

Pharmacology Content You NEED to Know

"What has been gained by knowledge is too easily forgotten.
Look for the ideal, but put it into the actual."
–Florence Nightingale (Sick Nursing & Health Nursing, 1893)

The walls of the "hard" sciences require hard work and countless hours of study to master, not merely memorize. Though memorization may help you pass a test, it will not prepare you to solve problems or use knowledge to make a correct clinical judgment. That is why the walls of the applied sciences of nursing that include pharmacology, anatomy and physiology, and fluids and electrolytes must be deeply UNDERSTOOD.

That is why the following questions from the quiz at the beginning of the book have relevance:

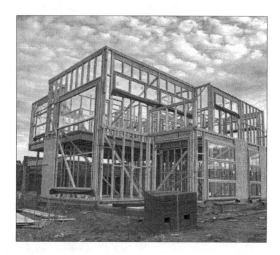

- Are you inwardly motivated to take responsibility for your own learning?
- Do you feel that your college owes you a degree because you paid for it?
- Are you naturally inquisitive about how things work?
- Do you have a natural aptitude for science?
- What are you willing to give up to make school a priority?

The applied sciences must be deeply understood and APPLIED to the bedside because they lay the foundation for the critical and clinical thinking that is expected and required of the professional nurse. Students must be able to take what is learned and USE that knowledge in practice (Eraut, 1994). It is essential for the nurse to also have a strong understanding of the applied sciences that is also relevant to medicine in order to be a better nurse.

This includes the need for nurses to have a basic understanding of physician treatment and interventions with an emphasis of the rationale, understanding of the medical approach to illness and current research on treatments, and a deep knowledge of the applied sciences that include anatomy and physiology, pharmacology, and pathophysiology.

If a nurse understands the essence of physician practice and WHY specific medications and treatments are used to treat illness, the nurse's practice will improve because he/she will see and understand the big picture of both domains of practice. This will develop needed critical thinking so the nurse is able to USE and APPLY knowledge from BOTH domains of practice.

In order to deeply understand the mechanism of action of most medications, anatomy and physiology (A&P) must be DEEPLY understood to make this connection possible. For example, to understand what a beta blocker is blocking, students must be able to know which nervous system beta receptors receive stimulation and the physiologic effects or expected outcomes when these same receptors are blocked. In the same manner, fluids and electrolytes (F&E) must be DEEPLY understood to recognize the significance and relevance of abnormal electrolyte lab values.

Nursing Pharmacology

Once in nursing practice, you will likely pass medications every day. Therefore, it is essential that you possess a DEEP UNDERSTANDING of pharmacology. This is more easily said than done. Currently, there are more than five thousand medications used in practice and most nursing drug manuals are well over one thousand pages in length. Nursing drug manuals have content areas of indications, mechanism of action, pharmacologic classification, time/action profile, contraindications, side effects, interactions, route and dosages, nursing implications, and patient education. If a student has multiple medications to pass, what should she or he be able to state and understand before the medications are considered safe to administer? What content areas of the drug manual are the most important?

Mechanism of Action=NEED to Know!

Anatomy and Physiology (A&P) is a prerequisite for most nursing programs. This class is typically taught with little to no contextualization to nursing practice. Essential content and concepts such as preload, afterload, Starling's law, and the classic formula CO=SVxHR have no clear clinical contextual hook for pre-nursing students to understand how relevant or important this is to bedside practice.

For example, as a clinical faculty assessing a student's safety to pass atenolol, most of my students were able to identify the pharmacologic classification of atenolol as a beta blocker. But when I asked, "What is a beta blocker blocking?" most students had no response or were unable to answer the question correctly. As a student, recognize the importance of understanding the mechanism of action so you can be safe in practice and strengthen your ability to think critically.

This formula of cardiac output is known to all nursing students:

$$CO=SVxHR$$

Cardiac Output (CO) = Stroke Volume (SV) x Heart Rate (HR)

But do you understand this formula DEEPLY so you could describe in your own words how preload, afterload, and contractility influence cardiac output? Can you take it to the next level of application and state how each of these determinates of cardiac output are specifically impacted by each major pharmacologic classification of cardiac medications?

In order to develop a DEEP understanding of the mechanism of action of diuretics, nitrates, beta blockers, calcium channel blockers, and ACE inhibitors, the pathophysiology situated in the mechanism of action must be UNDERSTOOD as well as the implications of the action to cardiac output. This level of applied understanding should be the bar that is expected for the advanced student.

To see why understanding pharmacology is essential to safe clinical practice, let's use the common cardiac medications of atenolol and amiodarone and see why both mechanism of action and its impact on determinants of cardiac output are relevant to nursing practice.

Atenolol

This is the mechanism of action for atenolol as stated from Micromedex, an online data base used by many hospitals:

> *"Atenolol is a synthetic beta (1)-selective adrenoreceptor blocking agent without membrane stabilizing or intrinsic sympathomimetic activities. It inhibits beta (2)-adrenoreceptors primarily found in bronchial and vascular musculature at higher doses"* ("Atenolol," 2014).

In order to understand the physiologic impact of atenolol, students must be able to recognize the differences between beta 1 and beta 2 adrenergic receptors, and the physiologic effects of this beta blockage to the heart and lungs.

Based on the formula CO=SVxHR, would you be able to readily identify how the mechanism of action impacts the following determinants of cardiac output for atenolol?

- Preload (no effect)
- Afterload (directly impacts by lowering systolic BP)
- Contractility (directly impacts by decreasing contractility)
- Workload of the heart (directly impacts by lowering workload due to reduction of afterload and lowering heart rate)

Amiodarone

This is the mechanism of action for amiodarone as stated from Micromedex:

> *"Amiodarone is an antiarrhythmic drug with predominant class III effects of lengthening cardiac action potential and blocking myocardial potassium channels leading to slowed conduction and prolonged refractoriness"* ("Amiodarone," 2014).

In order for a student to safely administer amiodarone, she or he must understand the cardiac electrophysiology concepts of action potential, refractory period, and slowed conduction, and how these physiologic effects will directly affect heart rate and rhythm. Based on the formula CO=SVxHR, would you be able to translate this mechanism of action and how it impacts the following determinants of cardiac output when administering amiodarone?

- Preload (no effect)
- Afterload (little to no effect though in practice it can lower BP)
- Contractility (no effect)
- Workload of the heart (directly impacts by lowering workload by reducing the HR)

My students struggled with this depth of understanding of cardiac medications. To translate this essential content so it could be deeply understood, I created a handout, "Comprehending Cardiac Medications," that is the content at the end of this chapter.

Five Foundational Pharmacology Questions

I used my lens of clinical practice to determine the sequential and logistical questions that I reflect upon to safely administer medications. From this perspective, I have created the following "foundational five" questions that must be verbalized and understood for medications administered in the clinical setting. The use of these questions in your practice will strengthen your knowledge and mastery of pharmacology. I also used these five questions with my students in the clinical setting when the most important or commonly used medications are being administered to develop a DEEP understanding of knowledge with the medications that are most important. If a student is passing a medication that is not commonly used, I keep it simple, and do not go to this depth of validation, but focus on the indication and safe dose range.

Five Foundational Pharmacologic Questions
1. What is the pharmacologic class? What is it for?
2. Why is your patient receiving it?
3. What is the expected patient response based on the mechanism of action?
4. What assessments do you need to know before you administer and follow up?
5. Is this a safe dose? Is the dose range low–mid–high?

1. What is the pharmacologic class? What is it for?

You must be able to identify the pharmacologic class for the most common medications used in practice. This benefits you by simplifying medication knowledge. Though there are thousands of individual medications used in practice, there are far fewer classifications or families. For example, when a student recognizes that any generic medication ending in "lol" belongs to the beta blocker pharmacologic class, the mechanism of action, side effects, and nursing assessments needed before or after administration are all the same for several medications in this family of beta blockers.

Most medications have one primary indication and this must be known. This knowledge allows you to identify the clinical relationship of the medical problem each medication treats. If there is more than one indication for the medication, this must also be identified so you are able to answer the next question!

2. Why is your patient receiving it?

Because many medications have more than one indication, you must be able to identify the indication that applies to your patient. Atenolol is an excellent example. Though it is most commonly given to control hypertension, it also is used to control the heart rate in patients with atrial fibrillation or decrease the workload of the heart in patients with heart failure.

3. What is the expected patient response based on the mechanism of action?

Though I have addressed this earlier, you must make it a priority to understand how the mechanism of action will affect your patient. To help students develop this essential critical/clinical thinking skill, I have had my students state in their OWN words the mechanism of action and not be allowed to "parrot" it word for word from their nursing drug manual or Micromedex.

Make sure you DEEPLY understand the mechanism of action by asking simple questions such as:

- *"What is a calcium channel blocker blocking?"*
- *"What is an ACE inhibitor inhibiting?"*
- *"What is a beta blocker blocking?"*

Then you will know how much you really know and understand!

4. What assessments do you need to know before you administer and follow up?

This is an essential clinical relationship that should become readily apparent when the mechanism of action is DEEPLY understood. An excellent example of this is when you are able to recognize that not all cardiac medications require an assessment of the heart rate and blood pressure. Knowing that the primary physiologic effect of an ACE inhibitor is to cause vasodilation, the heart rate does not need to be assessed in order to safely administer the drug.

5. Is this a safe dose? Is the dose range low–mid–high?

Identifying a safe dose of a medication is an essential assessment that must be verbalized, but is best suited for fundamental level students. If you are an advanced student, build on this basic knowledge by not only determining that it is a safe dose, but use your knowledge of dose ranges to determine if it is a low, mid, or high-range dose. This will develop an awareness of the clinical relationship of dosage and severity of the underlying problem.

Putting the Puzzle Together

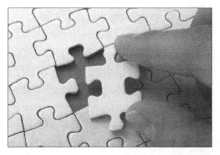

Do you enjoy putting puzzles together? If so, nursing is a good fit for you because patient care and clinical practice is like assembling a puzzle through recognizing and identifying clinical relationships and recognizing patterns. Though there are many pieces of clinical data that may not be readily apparent, most pieces do have a relationship and fit together. I will go into additional detail on this important concept in the next chapter.

But in the context of pharmacology, there are two important clinical relationships that, when recognized and identified, will improve your critical and clinical thinking and help you put the clinical puzzle together as you provide care for your patients.

Pharmacology Relationship #1

What is the clinical RELATIONSHIP between the mechanism of action and the nursing assessments required to be "safe to administer"?

When the nurse UNDERSTANDS the pathophysiology of the mechanism of action and how it impacts the body, essential nursing assessments logically follow. The value of this relationship is readily apparent in the discussion of mechanism of action. When a beta blocker such as atenolol is administered, the need to assess the heart rate and blood pressure are quickly identified.

Pharmacology Relationship #2

The clinical RELATIONSHIP between the dosage of the medication and recognizing if the dose range is low, mid, or high.

This relationship will suggest the likely severity of the underlying problem that the medication treats. The higher the dose range, the more resistive or severe the underlying illness likely has become. For example, when a student identifies and applies these clinical relationships to practice when administering atenolol 100 mg orally, knowing that atenolol 100 mg is in the high dose range, the clinical relationship of the degree of hypertension is identified as likely severe or resistant to treatment.

Portable Nursing Textbooks

You can't know it all – especially when it comes to the sheer volume of medications used in clinical practice! Though you will know many medications well, there are literally thousands of medications you do not know. If you need to administer a medication you are not familiar with and have multiple patients with pressing needs, will you sacrifice safety and wing it? Will you maintain the highest standards of safety even if nobody is watching and determining if you are "safe to give"?

To be consistently safe in practice, I strongly recommend that if your institution allows cell phones in the clinical area and you have a smart phone, make an investment in a nursing drug reference manual that you can carry with you at all times in the clinical setting. Your institution may provide pharmacology software that can assist you with your assessment of dosages and compatibility. If so, please take the time to look up the medication you are questioning. One minute of research may save you hours later in paperwork and the courtroom.

My personal favorite application of informatics technology is *Davis's Drug Guide for Nurses*. It is well worth the current $49.95 download for a number of reasons. It can be stored on your device's memory so it does not have to be on or connected to the Internet. Having this resource is the equivalent of having more than five thousand medication cards at your disposal in seconds!

If you want to have additional resources on your mobile device, Skyscape has an excellent selection of more than two hundred downloads so you can build your own nursing informatics library! I have found the Skyscape platform to be the easiest to navigate. It is recommended to have all of your electronic resources on the same platform. This is another advantage to using Skyscape. I have found *Davis's Comprehensive Handbook of Laboratory and Diagnostic Tests with Nursing Implications* an excellent companion to a drug guide to promote and build your knowledge of lab values. Having quick accessibility while at the patient's chart is PRICELESS!

Diseases and Disorders: A Nursing Therapeutics Manual will help you develop needed critical thinking by understanding the pathophysiology of your patient's primary problem. An additional benefit to having these three resources on your electronic device is the ability to develop the basic nurse thinking skill of identifying CLINICAL RELATIONSHIPS. Skyscape has the ability to SmartLink™, which is a tool that enables you to cross-reference all of your Skyscape resources, quickly and easily.

Let's assume you have these three resources discussed above on your electronic device. You access the topic of heart failure on *Diseases and Disorders*. When you use SmartLink™, the drugs that are used to manage heart failure and the laboratory values specific to heart failure are identified and can be easily accessed on the other resources. This will promote your learning and help you put the clinical puzzle together.

Some of the benefits to having accessible nursing resources include:

Accessibility

- When you need medication or other clinical information fast, do you have time to retrieve and look it up in a hard copy nursing drug or lab manual? This can take minutes compared to seconds with the same resource on your smartphone.
- Using free online resources through your employer, such as Micromedex, may be an option, though an excellent resource, it can be content-heavy. It is geared for physicians and pharmacists, while a nursing drug guide is concise and "just right" for what a nurse needs to know.
- You can purchase a belt clip holster to carry your smartphone with you at all times (if your institution allows).

Nursing Emphasis vs. Physician Emphasis

- Though Micromedex or Epocrates are free downloads for your smartphone, they are geared for physician practice and do not have essential content that nurses require. Though you can get the basics of drug action, side effects, dosages, etc. from these free resources, if you have to give an IV push of metoprolol (Lopressor) 5 mg (or any IV drug), you won't be able to ascertain how quickly you can administer it, and the onset-peak-duration of this drug. Do you need to monitor the patient's blood pressure during administration? You will rarely find it in Micromedex or Epocrates; therefore, a NURSING drug reference is essential to safe practice.
- If you want to get started with a drug reference guide at no cost, I have found that that the abbreviated content found in the application Micromedex is more relevant and richer in detail than Epocrates. Some of the IV med push times are identified under the "Administration" tab of Micromedex, but not consistently.

Usage

- Would you come to clinical without your stethoscope? Accessible nursing references are just as essential and should be a part of your clinical tools that accompany you into practice.

Need-to-Know Medications

From my clinical context of acute care, I have compiled the following list of forty-five medications that I administer consistently in this setting. Use this list as a starting point to acquire deep learning of those medications that are most commonly used. Add or subtract from this list depending on the clinical setting you have clinical or practice in.

Antihypertensives	Respiratory	Non-opioid Analgesics
B-blockers: Atenolol/Metoprolol	Albuterol	Ketorolac
ACE-I: Captopril/Lisinopril	fluticasone/salmeterol (Advair	Acetaminophen
Ca-channel blockers: Diltiazem	Diskus)	Ibuprofen
Antiarrhythmic	**GI**	**Opioid Analgesics**
Amiodarone	*H2 blocker:*	Hydromorphone
Digoxin	Ranitidine/Famotidine	Morphine
	PPI-Pantoprazole/Omeprazole	Percocet/Vicodin (trade name)
Diuretics	Ondansetron/Metoclopramide	
Loop: Furosemide	Docusate/Senna	**Antianxiety**
Thiazide: HCTZ		Lorazepam/Diazepam
K+ sparing: Spironolactone	**Diabetic**	
	All insulins	**Anti-Infectives**
Lipid lowering	Humalog/Novolog	Ciprofloxacin
Statins (all)	Regular/NPH	Vancomycin
	Lente	Metronidazole
Anticoagulants	Glyburide/Metformin	Cefazolin
Warfarin		piperacillin/tazobactam
Heparin/Enoxaparin	**Misc.**	
	Potassium chloride	
	Levothyroxine	
	Prednisone/Methylprednisolone	

To simplify the process of medication knowledge acquisition and develop mastery of the most common medications used in your clinical setting, I created a blank template, "Medications That Must Be Mastered." It is in appendix E and it can be reproduced. It incorporates in a single page worksheet the "foundational five" questions to DEEPEN student knowledge:

1. What is the pharmacologic class? What is it for?
2. Why is your patient receiving it?
3. What is the expected patient response based on the mechanism of action?
4. What assessments do you need to know before you administer and follow up?
5. Is this a safe dose? Is the dose range low–mid–high?

Make it a goal to internalize the essence of these "foundational five" questions of the most commonly used medications by the end of the clinical rotation so that they can be stated from memory. This knowledge can then be readily carried over into your next clinical experience with another 10 to 15 medications to master. This knowledge will also prepare you for the NCLEX licensure examination.

I have created another handout, **"Most Commonly Used Categories of Medications,"** found in the appendix. It identifies the most commonly used categories of medications, individual medications in that category, most common side effects, and essential nursing interventions. This will help you see the big picture of pharmacology because medications are listed by both categories such as anti-hypertensives but also in their respective pharmacologic classification. Once the mechanism of action, side effects, and nursing responsibilities are known for one drug in a pharm class, this knowledge can be translated to other medications in the same family.

Comprehending Cardiac Medications

My students struggled with integrating knowledge from pathophysiology with the mechanism of action of the most common cardiac medications. To help them make the connection, I created a handout for my students, "Comprehending Cardiac Medications." I am confident that it will help strengthen and deepen your learning of this essential content as well.

Foundational Formula for Clinical Practice

$$CO = SV \times HR$$

Cardiac Output (CO) = Stroke Volume (SV) x Heart Rate (HR)

Pathophysiology Definitions

Cardiac Output

The amount of blood the heart pumps through the circulatory system in a minute. The amount of blood put out by the left ventricle of the heart in one contraction is called the stroke volume. The stroke volume and the heart rate determine the cardiac output. A normal adult has a cardiac output of 4.7 liters (5 quarts) of blood per minute (normal range 4–8 liters/minute).

Stroke Volume

Stroke volume (SV) is the volume of blood pumped from one ventricle of the heart with each beat. The term "stroke volume" can apply to each of the two ventricles of the heart, although it usually refers to the left ventricle. The stroke volumes for each ventricle are generally equal, both approximately 70 mL in most adults.

- Stroke volume is influenced by the amount of blood that returns to right atrium from venous circulation (RIGHT SIDE) and left atrium (LEFT SIDE) from pulmonary veins.
    - Higher SV increases workload of the heart…typically due to too much VOLUME.
    - Tachycardia INCREASES cardiac oxygen demands, workload, and DECREASES stroke volume because there is less time for the ventricles to fill.
    - Goal of medication therapy with any cardiac patient is to DECREASE cardiac workload through manipulating SV, HR, preload, afterload, and contractility.

Preload

Preload is the filling pressure of the right ventricle (RV) and left ventricle (LV). It is influenced by how full the body's tank is and amount of venous return. Higher venous return (fluid volume overload) will result in higher SV. Fluid volume deficit will result in lower SV. If monitored with a central venous line, normal values are 2–6 mm/Hg. This is also the same as a central venous pressure (CVP).

- Pressure/stretch in ventricles end diastole just before contraction.

- In a healthy heart, as you increase preload, you will increase stroke volume, which will increase force of contraction (Starling's Law).
- This continues only up to a certain point, then further stretching may actually decrease contractility. This is what happens with patients with chronic heart failure.
- Drugs that cause venous dilation (nitrates) DECREASE preload.
- Diuretics that eliminate excess fluid volume DECREASE preload.

Starling's Law of the Heart

- If preload is increased, a greater quantity of blood is ejected during systole due to increased stretch of the myocardium and larger amount of circulating blood volume present.
- But only up to a maximal point. Greatest force of contraction is when the muscle fibers are stretched 2 ½ times their normal length.
- Overstretch of cardiac muscle is like an overstretched rubber band; it will DECREASE cardiac contractility and efficiency over time. This is why an enlarged heart due to heart failure is NOT a good thing!

Afterload

- Force of resistance that the LV must generate to open aortic valve.
- Correlates w/SBP–How much pressure is needed to push blood out of the LV, and into systemic arterial circulation.
- Influenced by resistance of blood vessels in the body. Are the arteries dilated or constricted? If arterial vasodilation is present, afterload is DECREASED and workload of the heart is DECREASED. If arterial vasoconstriction is present, afterload is INCREASED and workload of the heart is INCREASED.
- Arterial vasodilators (Ca++ channel blockers [CCB], ACE inhibitors) DECREASE afterload and decrease the workload of the heart.

Contractility

Contractility of the cardiac myocardium independent of Starling mechanism

- Ability of heart to change force of inherent contraction strength as needed.
- Influenced by Ca++ in action potential…Therefore, how will calcium channel blockers (CCB) influence contractility? (They will DECREASE contractility and must be used with caution in those with heart failure).
- Decrease in contractility (inotropic effect) DECREASES cardiac workload and O2 demands.
- Negative inotropic meds: CCB, beta blockers
- Positive inotropic: Digoxin, Dopamine and Epinephrine gtts.

Ejection Fraction–% (EF)

- Echocardiogram: 60–70% normal.
- With each contraction 60–70% of the blood in the LV is ejected into circulation.
- As this percentage goes down, it reflects the loss of cardiac contractility and degree of heart failure.

- 30–35% EF is half normal cardiac output.
- 10–15% EF end-stage heart failure-terminal.

I. Angiotensin Converting Enzyme (ACE) Inhibitors

- Captopril (Capoten)
- Enalapril (Vasotec)
- Lisinopril (Prinivil)

Mechanism of Action

A plasma protein, renin is secreted by the kidneys when BP falls. This converts inactive liver protein angiotensinogen to angiotensin I. The conversion to angiotensin II is enhanced by angiotensin-converting-enzymes (ACE) from the lungs to be one of the most potent vasoconstrictors in the body. The effects of angiotensin II are:

- Vasoconstriction of arterioles and veins (increases afterload)
- Stimulation of the sympathetic nervous system (SNS) (increases workload of heart)
- Retention of water by the kidneys due to aldosterone a hormone secreted by the adrenal glands (increases preload)

In heart failure (HF), each of these normal physiologic actions will worsen underlying HF and must be counteracted. This is why ACE-I are the first medication used in HF.

ACE inhibitors block the conversion of angiotensin I to angiotensin II. This inhibition decreases angiotensin II concentrations and causes:

- Vasodilation, which decreases SBP (decreases afterload) and decreases sodium and water retention (decreases preload)

Uses

HTN, HF, coronary artery disease (CAD)

Side Effects–Most Common

Hypotension, dry cough, dizziness

- Angioedema (life-threatening) laryngeal swelling that can cause asphyxia. Facial swelling is also a concerning precursor and a clinical RED FLAG.

Nursing Considerations

- Obtain BP before administering–hold typically if SBP <90.
- Change position slowly–especially with elderly to prevent orthostatic changes.
- Monitor for decreased WBC count, hyperkalemia as well as liver function, and creatinine (metabolized by liver-excreted by kidneys).

II. Beta Blockers

- Metoprolol (Lopressor)
- Atenolol (Tenormin)
- Propranolol (Inderal)
- Labetolol (Trandate)

Mechanism of Action

Selectively inhibits or blocks beta (sympathetic/fight or flight) receptors primarily of the heart (Beta 1). Sympathetic nervous system (SNS) stimulation normally causes:

- Increased heart rate
- Increased BP
- Increased myocardium contractility and oxygen demand
- ALL THESE EFFECTS INCREASE WORKLOAD OF THE HEART!

By blocking the SNS, it effectively causes the opposite effects and DECREASES workload of the heart…decreased heart rate, decreased BP, and decreased contractility. This is why it must be used with caution in those with history of HF. They have excessive activation of SNS which will worsen CHF over time. B-Blockers very effective to manage this complication of HF, and will commonly be used in addition to ACE-I.

Uses

HTN, HF, acute MI, CAD, ventricular dysrhythmias

Side Effects–Most Common

Bradycardia, hypotension, fatigue, weakness

Nursing Considerations

- Obtain BP and HR before administering–hold typically if SBP <90. HR <60.
- Change position slowly–especially with elderly to prevent orthostatic changes.
- Contraindicated in worsening HF, bradycardia, heart block…use with caution in diabetes, liver disease (1)

III. Calcium Channel Blockers

- Diltiazem (Cardizem)
- Verapamil (Calan)
- Nifedipine (Procardia)
- Amlodipine (Norvasc)

Mechanism of Action

Inhibits or "blocks" the influx of extracellular calcium into the membranes of the heart and vascular smooth muscle cells of heart and body. This blocking of calcium ions is responsible for causing the following:

- Dilation of coronary and systemic arteries w/resultant decrease in BP (improves cardiac oxygen supply and decreases afterload)
- Decrease of myocardium contractility (decreases workload)
- Slows AV node conduction (decreases heart rate)
- Diltiazem most commonly used to slow HR and AV node conduction in atrial fibrillation

Uses

HTN, angina, controlling rapid heart rate in SVT or atrial fibrillation.

Side Effects–Most Common

Peripheral edema, hypotension, constipation.

Nursing Considerations

- Change position slowly–especially with elderly to prevent orthostatic changes.
- Measure I&O closely and fluid status due to potential for edema.
- Monitor liver and kidney function (metabolized in liver–excreted by kidneys).
- Obtain BP and HR before administering–hold typically if SBP <90. HR <60

IV. Nitrates

- Nitroglycerine subl. (Nitrostat)–SHORT acting
- Isosorbide Mononitrate (Imdur)–LONG acting
- Isosorbide Dinitrate (Isordil)–LONG acting
- Nitrodur topical patches–LONG acting

Mechanism of Action

Able to relax and dilate both coronary arterial vessels and systemic venous smooth muscle.

- Dilation of veins reduces amount of blood that returns to heart (decreases preload). With less blood to pump, cardiac output is reduced and workload of the heart is decreased, lowering myocardial oxygen demand.
- Dilation of coronary arteries can help improve blood flow to heart as well as well as relieve angina caused by coronary artery vasospasm.

Uses

Angina

Side Effects–Most Common

Hypotension, tachycardia, dizziness, headache (dilates cerebral vessels causing mini migraine)

Nursing Considerations

- Tolerance common and serious problem with long-acting nitrates. Nitrates lose their effectiveness if transdermal patches remain on continually. Patches must be taken off at night and reapplied in the morning.
- Contraindicated if client taking any erectile dysfunction meds as these are a similar nitrate that improves blood circulation to the penis–synergistic effect can cause dramatic hypotension

V. Diuretics

- Furosemide (Lasix) -most potent
- Bumetanide (Bumex) -most potent
- Hydrochlorathiazide (HCTZ)-mod. potency
- Spirinolactone (Aldactone)-mild potency-K+ sparing

Mechanism of Action

- **Loop diuretics**–Most potent diuretics that prevent sodium reabsorption in the loop of henle, causing rapid/large diuresis with resultant loss of K+, and smaller amounts of Mg+, and Na+. Because of their potency, they are not typically used for maintenance but when large diuresis is desired, such as in acute HF exacerbation (decreases preload).
- **Thiazide diuretics**–Increases excretion of sodium and water by inhibiting sodium reabsorption in distal tubule. Most common maintenance diuretic. K+ loss needs to be monitored.
- **Potassium sparing diuretics**–Weakest of all diuretics. Does not block reabsorption of sodium. Used when patient is at risk for developing hypokalemia. Must also assess for development of hyperkalemia.

Uses

HTN, HF, renal insufficiency/acute renal failure

Side Effects–Most Common

Dehydration, orthostatic hypotension, hypokalemia, hyponatremia, hypomagnesemia with loop and thiazide diuretics, potential for hyperkalemia w/spironolactone (Aldactone).

Nursing Considerations

- Change position slowly–especially with elderly to prevent orthostatic changes.
- Obtain BP before administering–hold typically if SBP <90.
- Monitor sodium and K+ levels closely as well as GFR and creatinine.
- Aldactone and ACE inhibitors can cause resultant hyperkalemia.

- If on Aldactone–make sure does not use potassium-based salt substitutes or foods rich in K+ (Vallerand, Sanoski & Deglin, 2013).

CHAPTER 5 HIGHLIGHTS

- The nurse must understand the mechanism of action of the most commonly used medications to strengthen critical thinking.
- There are five foundational questions that the nurse must be able to answer when passing medications that are most commonly used in the clinical setting. This includes identifying the pharmacologic class, why the patient is receiving it, the expected patient response based on the mechanism of action, the assessments you need to know before you administer, and if this is a safe dose.
- Make a list of the most commonly used medications in your clinical or practice setting. Make it a priority to understand and memorize the mechanism of action and answer the other pharmacologic questions.
- In order to understand the most commonly used cardiac medications, the pathophysiology principles of cardiac output, stroke volume, preload, afterload, and contractility must be understood in order to critically think and provide safe patient care.

Additional Resources

- Book: *Nursing Pharmacology Made Incredibly Easy* (3rd ed.)
- Book: *140 Must Know Meds* by Jon Haws
- Book: *Memory Notebook of Nursing: Pharmacology & Diagnostics*
- Flashcards: *Mosby's Pharmacology Memory Note Cards: Visual, Mnemonic, and Memory Aids for Nurses*
- Book: *Memory Notebook of Nursing Vol. 1*
- Book: *Memory Notebook of Nursing: A Collection of Visual Images and Mnemonics to Increase Memory and Learning, Vol. 2*
- Flashcards: *Mosby's Pathophysiology Memory NoteCards: Visual, Mnemonic, and Memory Aids for Nurses, 2nd ed.*

Chapter Reflections

1. Is understanding pharmacology and the mechanism of action a struggle for you?

   If so, what will you do to make this your strength?

2. Can you name the most common or most important medications in your current clinical setting?

   If known, write them down below and use your drug guide to answer and then memorize the foundational five questions for each of these medications.

   1.
   2.
   3.
   4.
   5.
   6.
   7.
   8.
   9.
   10.

> *Don't mess with me. I am a nurse and get paid to stab people with sharp objects!*

Chapter 6
Fluid and Electrolyte Content You NEED to Know

Fluids and Electrolytes (F&E) is a challenging subject because it requires application of chemistry, acid/base knowledge, and physiology. It is also relevant and foundational to practice and must be DEEPLY understood by every student so that this knowledge can be used/applied at the bedside.

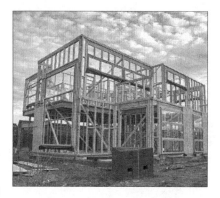

Laboratory values provide an EARLY window to physiologic status changes that may not be initially evident in vital signs or assessment data collected by the nurse. Examples of this in clinical practice are TRENDS of an elevated serum lactate in any shock state, elevated neutrophils, bands, or WBC's that are typically seen in sepsis, or elevated serum creatinine in acute renal failure or severe dehydration.

For example, in acute renal failure (ARF), would you be able to identify the relationship between ARF and an elevation in creatinine, BUN, potassium, and decrease in CO_2 (serum bicarbonate)? Would you be able to anticipate the expected electrolyte derangements most often seen with dehydration caused by severe vomiting and diarrhea and know WHY they are present?

You must be able to APPLY knowledge to practice by identifying the most important labs for your patients and why. You must also be able to use this knowledge to recognize basic clinical relationships, such as the electrolytes most likely to be depleted with diuresis when furosemide is given. When you have this level of understanding, you will be a PROACTIVE nurse in practice because you will be able to use your knowledge, anticipate what to expect, and understand WHY.

In comparison, students who are unable or who have not been taught to contextualize content at this level will be REACTIVE nurses in practice. They will likely respond only AFTER a problem has developed, and recognize it later rather than sooner. Their patients will be more likely to experience adverse outcomes because of the nurse's delayed reaction or complete failure to rescue.

Danger...TMI in Clinical!

Once students are in the clinical setting, content overload is a given! They will encounter an overwhelming amount of clinical data in the medical record. Patricia Benner's novice-to-expert research identified that because new nurses have a lack of knowledge and clinical experience, they struggle with identifying the most important data in the clinical setting and tend to see EVERYTHING as equally relevant (Benner, 1982)! This includes the numerous lab values found in the most commonly ordered lab panels.

Routine laboratory panels are difficult for students to sort through because of the sheer amount of data. Students will have difficulty identifying the most important labs and values relevant to the primary problem.

For example, a basic metabolic panel (BMP) is the most commonly ordered lab panel and has the following 10 lab values:

- Sodium
- Potassium
- Chloride
- Carbon dioxide (CO2-bicarb)
- Glucose
- Blood urea nitrogen (BUN)
- Creatinine
- Glomerular filtration rate (GFR)
- BUN/creatinine ratio
- Anion gap

Do every one of these lab values have equal relevance and importance to nursing practice? I would emphatically state NO. From my perspective, I could easily filter half of these lab values in a BMP as NEED to know and emphasize them as relevant to nursing practice. The other half of these values are NICE to know and will have at times situational relevance, but do not need to be considered for most patients.

As I reflected upon the filtering of clinical data that I use in practice, I have noted that there are lab values that I consider ALWAYS relevant because of their physiologic importance and relevance to homeostasis and well-being. As a clinical educator, I helped my students determine relevance by compiling a SHORT list of lab values that have universal relevance. If they are present in the medical record, they MUST be seen as clinically significant and noted even if they are normal.

Students tend to think that it is only the ABNORMAL labs that are significant and must be noted. But if a lab value is ALWAYS relevant, even if it is normal, it has clinical significance because of its importance and what it represents. For example, a normal WBC and neutrophil count after surgery represents the absence of a systemic infectious or inflammatory response.

I have compiled my list of always-relevant lab values that provide a foundation for novice nurses to build upon. If present in the chart, my students were expected to note these lab values and more importantly to TREND the direction they were going over the last day or two. In my list below I have also included my rationale as to why they have relevance, even if they are normal.

Always Relevant Laboratory Values

Though a BMP and CBC are the most common lab panels ordered, I have compiled a short list of additional labs that if present in the chart are always relevant and must be noted by the nurse because of their clinical significance.

Basic Metabolic Panel (BMP)/Chemistries

Potassium (3.5-5.0 mEq/L)

- Essential to normal cardiac electrical conduction. If too high or low, can predispose to rhythm changes that can be life threatening! Potassium tends to deplete more quickly with loop diuretic usage than magnesium.

Sodium (135-145 mEq/L)

- I consider sodium the fluid balance "Crystal-Light®" electrolyte. Though this is simplistic, it does help to understand in principle how basic sodium is to fluid balance. When you add one small packet of Crystal Light to a 16-ounce bottle of water, the concentration is just right. This is where a normal sodium will be (135–145).

- Where free water goes, sodium will follow to a degree. Therefore, if there is a fluid volume deficit due to dehydration, sodium will typically be elevated because it's concentrated (less water in the bottle!). If there is fluid volume excess, sodium will be diluted and will likely be low (too much water in the bottle!). It is the "foundational" fluid balance electrolyte!

Glucose (Fasting: 70-110 mg/dL)

- Required fuel for metabolism for every cell in the human body, especially the brain.

- Relevant with history of diabetes or stress hyperglycemia due to illness. Elevated levels post-op can increase risk of infection/sepsis.

Creatinine (0.6-1.2 mg/dL)/Glomerular Filtration Rate (GFR) (>60 mL/minute)

- GOLD STANDARD for kidney function and adequacy of renal perfusion. The functioning of the renal system impacts every body system; therefore, it is ALWAYS relevant!

- When creatinine is elevated, this can be due to damage done to the fragile capillary membrane screen of the glomerulus which is like a screen door with larger holes that are letting things through that they shouldn't, such as protein and glucose.

Complete Blood Count (CBC)

White Blood Cells (WBC) (4500-11,000/mm 3)

- ALWAYS RELEVANT based on its correlation to the presence of inflammation or infection. Will usually be increased if infection present, though it may be decreased in the elderly or peds <3 months.

Neutrophils (50-70%)

- ALWAYS RELEVANT for same reason as WBCs. They are the most common leukocyte and their role as a FIRST RESPONDER to any bacterial infection within several hours is always relevant.

- The more aggressive or systemic the infection, the higher the percentage of neutrophils and WBCs. Immature neutrophils (bands) greater than 8 are also clinically significant and must be clustered with WBC and neutrophils to determine if sepsis is a clinical concern.

Hemoglobin (Male: 13.5-17.5 g/dL & Female: 12.0-16.0)

- GOLD STANDARD to determine anemia or acute/chronic blood loss.

Platelet count (150–450 x 103/µl)

- Relevant whenever there is a concern for anemia or blood loss or a patient on heparin. If platelets are low, it will obviously be significant and must be noted. Any patient on heparin products must also have this noted because of the clinical possibility of heparin-induced thrombocytopenia (HIT), which develops when the immune system forms antibodies against heparin that causes small clots and lowers platelet levels.

Cardiac

Troponin (<0.4 ng/mL)

- When ordered to rule out myocardial infarction, it is ALWAYS RELEVANT. It is the most sensitive cardiac marker and will be elevated if there is cardiac muscle damage. Can take up to six hours after chest pain to elevate so labs are always ordered every 6–8 hours x 3 and each is carefully trended to the prior to see if trend is increasing and positive.
- Very sensitive cardiac marker that can be slightly elevated and positive in heart failure and unstable angina.
- Those with renal disease, usually CKD III-IV, will be unable to clear troponin by the kidneys and may have a baseline that is a low level positive. This is why it is so important to TREND the current level to the most recent in the chart and determine if there is a clinical elevation in this context.

CPK-MB (<5%)

- Specific iso-enzyme for cardiac muscle. If this is elevated, confirms presence of MI. Because troponin can be sensitive, many physicians order both troponin and CPK-MB to correlate. If troponins are slightly positive but CPK-MB negative, most physicians would not diagnose an MI.

BNP (B-natriuretic Peptide) (<100 ng/L)

- What troponins are to MI, BNP is to heart failure. It is a neurohormone secreted by myocytes in the ventricles. When ventricles are stressed and overloaded, BNP is a compensatory hormone that is a vasodilator and also diuretic to help the body naturally decrease the workload of the heart. It will be elevated in heart failure exacerbation.

Coagulation

PT/INR (0.9–1.1 nmol/L)

- Measures time required for a firm fibrin clot to form and measures the clotting cascade. Is dependent on vitamin K synthesis from the liver. Therefore, will be elevated in liver disease without being on warfarin. Standard anti-coagulant ordered for those on warfarin (Coumadin) to maintain therapeutic goal of INR 2–3.
- Relevant and must be noted for any patient on warfarin but especially when a bleeding complication secondary to warfarin presents. Warfarin can be reversed quickly if patient is actively bleeding by administering vitamin K IV and/or fresh frozen plasma.

Miscellaneous Chemistries

Magnesium (1.6-2.0 mEq/L)

- Essential to normal cardiac electrical conduction. If too high or low, can predispose to rhythm changes that can be life threatening!

Lactate (0.5–2.2 mmol/L)

- Not routinely done, but when present in chart, it is there for a reason! Remember Krebs cycle and lactic acidosis in A&P due to anaerobic metabolism? GOLD STANDARD lab to trend with any shock state, especially sepsis! Elevated levels correlate with higher likelihood of dying. For example, in septic shock, a level >4 reflects a 28 percent mortality. Lactate builds up within the serum and can be seen as a marker of strained cellular metabolism (Van Leeuwen & Poelhuis–Leth, 2009).

Lab Planning

Another way that nurses in clinical practice establish care priorities is based on the knowledge of RELEVANT, abnormal labs on their patient. I call this "lab planning." It is not enough to identify that a lab value is abnormal. Is it RELEVANT to the patient and the primary problem? If the answer is yes, the nurse must be able to identify what to DO about it by asking what assessments and interventions must be implemented as a result of this relevant, abnormal lab. This is an excellent example of how the nurse must be able to USE knowledge and APPLY it in the clinical setting, not just memorize content in order to pass a test.

An abnormal lab value in and of itself does not mean it is significant or a relevant finding. The ability to recognize the relevance of abnormal clinical data requires time and experience to develop in the clinical setting. By putting this content into context in practice, students will be able to identify and recognize the relationship between the primary problem and the most relevant clinical data.

For example, a student is caring for a patient who has been admitted for heart failure exacerbation and collects the following clinical data from the chart:

- Creatinine increased from a baseline of 1.4 and is now 2.5
- B-Natriuretic Peptide (BNP) increased from a baseline of 180 and is now 1255

The nurse can use these relevant, abnormal findings to create a "lab plan of care" that will dovetail with traditional nursing care priorities based on the primary problem. Because creatinine is a key indicator of renal function and kidney perfusion and the BNP represents the degree of ventricular stretch and overload, the nurse must recognize the clinical significance and relationship of these labs to the primary problem. If this is done, the nurse will be able to use this knowledge to develop a "lab plan of care" with needed nursing assessments and interventions.

For example:

Lab Plan of Care: Creatinine 2.5

Relevant Lab:	Nursing Interventions:
Creatinine: 2.5 (0.6-1.2 mg/dL)	1. Assess urine output and I&O. Determine if minimum of 30 mL/hour of urine output is present 2. Fluid restriction if ordered 3. Assess for signs of fluid retention/edema 4. Assess daily weight and trend daily

Lab Plan of Care: BNP 1255

Relevant Lab:	Nursing Interventions:
BNP: 1255 (<100)	1. Assess respiratory status for tachypnea and breath sounds for basilar or scattered crackles (may be fine or course crackles depending on severity) 2. Assess HR and SBP carefully to promote decreased cardiac workload (goal is heart rate <80 and SBP <140) 3. Assess tolerance to activity 4. Assess I&O and urine output 5. Assess lower extremities for any pitting edema present

As a clinical educator, I quickly realized that most students struggled with this nurse thinking strategy because it is NOT taught in most nursing textbooks, though it is used intuitively in clinical practice by experienced nurses. Therefore, I created a handout that my students could use to situate the most common abnormal lab values that are relevant to practice and essential nursing assessments and interventions to create their own "lab plan" for their patient. This handout, "Clinical Lab Values and Nursing Responsibilities," is found in appendix E.

To develop a deep understanding of the most important labs in your clinical setting, I have created a simple worksheet, "Lab Planning: Laboratory Tests That Must Be Mastered" worksheet" that is also available in appendix E. It is a blank worksheet that allows you to use a nursing lab manual and fill in the normal range, critical RED FLAG values, relevance to practice, and most importantly, the "lab planning" or nursing assessments/interventions required based on this lab derangement.

Lab Panel Summaries

In addition to always-relevant labs discussed earlier, there are labs that have situational relevance depending on the primary problem of the patient. In the most common lab panels that are ordered, the remaining labs listed below must also be DEEPLY understood by students because of their physiologic significance. The normal ranges are listed for each lab, but note that these ranges can vary slightly between institutions, so validate what is normal for your practice setting.

The following lab panels are covered in this section:
- Basic Metabolic Panel (BMP)
- Miscellaneous Chemistries
- Complete Blood Count (CBC)
- Liver Panel (LFT)
- Urinalysis (UA)
- Cardiac Markers
- Coagulation

In addition to identifying labs that have situational relevance, I have included a brief rationale to present the "essence" of this NEED to know content. I have found that as a nurse educator, LESS can be MORE. Though a lab manual goes into needed additional depth, if you can grasp and understand the essence of the short descriptions of each lab panel described below, you will be able to use and apply this knowledge readily to the bedside.

Basic Metabolic Panel (BMP)

Chloride (95–105 mEq/L)
- Relevant if NG suction or frequent vomiting is present due to loss of hydrochloric acid. Chloride is the Cl- of hydrochloric acid.

CO2 (22–28 mEq/L)
- Relevant when there are acid-base concerns. Though it is CO2 on a BMP and students may assume it is carbon dioxide, it is actually reflecting the amount of HCO3-!

Anion Gap (AG) (7–16 mEq/l)
- This is the difference between primary measured cations (Na+ and K+) and the primary measured anions (chloride Cl- and bicarbonate HCO3-) in serum. Useful with acid/base concerns typically seen in renal failure.

Calcium (8.4–10.2 mg/dL)
- Relevant with renal failure and ETOH abuse. Low albumin can cause hypocalcemia, while elevated levels can be seen with cancer (with and without bone metastases).

BUN (7–25 mg/dl)
- I use creatinine/GFR as most relevant/important lab to determine renal function. I do not consistently use BUN in practice as it can be elevated for other reasons rather than renal, though it is relevant with renal failure to trend with creatinine and will also be elevated with dehydration.

Miscellaneous Chemistries

Phosphorus (2.5–4.5 mg/dl)
- 85 percent stored in bones. Primary intracellular anion and responsible for cellular metabolism and formation of bones and teeth. Relevant in renal failure and will be increased due to decreased renal excretion.

Ionized Calcium (1.05–1.46 mmol/L)
- Represents Ca++ that is metabolically available compared to serum Ca++ that is more generalized. This value is more accurate determinate of calcium. If low, serum calcium is usually also decreased.

Amylase (25–125 U/l)
- Digestive enzyme to break down complex carbohydrates. Primarily formed in pancreas and will "leak" into circulation with pancreatic inflammation.
- Relevant with pancreatitis/cholecystitis and obstruction of common bile duct that leads to pancreatic inflammation.

Lipase (3–73 units/L)
- Glycoprotein produced primarily in pancreas to break down fats. Will "leak" into circulation with pancreatic inflammation. Relevant with pancreatitis/cholecystitis and obstruction of common bile duct that leads to pancreatic inflammation.

Ammonia (20–100 mcg/dL)

- Blood ammonia comes from two sources: deamination of amino acids during protein metabolism and degradation of proteins by colon bacteria. The liver converts ammonia in the portal blood to urea, which is excreted by the kidneys. When liver function is impaired, ammonia levels rise. Ammonia is potentially toxic to the central nervous system and causes acute confusion and altered mental status. Is a contributing factor to hepatic encephalopathy in end-stage liver disease.

Complete Blood Count (CBC)

Hematocrit (male: 39–49% female: 35–45%)

- In comparison to hemoglobin, hematocrit is not as relevant, though elevation can confirm fluid volume deficit–will be concentrated and elevated in this context.

RBCs (male: 4.3–5.7 (x108/µl) female: 3.8–5.1 (x108/ µl)

- Identifies the number of RBCs in a cubic millimeter. In anemia or when there has been a significant blood loss, hemoglobin is the GOLD STANDARD that must be noted. I rarely find this value relevant as most practitioners emphasize the hemoglobin in practice.

WBC Differential

Band forms (3–5%)

- Immature neutrophils that are elevated in sepsis as the body attempts to fight infection and releases these prematurely. If elevated, it's a clinical RED FLAG in the context of sepsis. If elevated to >8, it is considered a "shift to the left," which indicates impending sepsis.

Lymphocytes (23–33%)

- Relevant when there is a known or suspected VIRAL infection.

Monocytes (3–7%)

- Phagocytes similar to neutrophils, but not as dominant, nor are they as clinically significant and relevant to practice as neutrophils.

Eosinophils (1–3%)

- Elevated with parasitic infections or allergic responses.

Basophils (0–1%)

- Phagocytes, but not as dominant, nor are they as clinically significant and relevant to practice as neutrophils.

Liver Panel (LFT)

Relevance in this panel will depend on the primary problem and chief complaint, but if patient has Gastro Intestinal (GI) or liver problem, they are ALL relevant!

Albumin (3.5–5.5 g/dL)

- Is a large colloid plasma protein made by the liver. Because it is comprised of protein, it will be decreased in malnutrition. Therefore, it can be a contributing factor to ascites or edema.

Total Bilirubin (0.1–1.0 mg/dL // 0.0–0.3 mg/dL)

- Total of both direct/indirect bilirubin. Bilirubin is metabolized by the liver and broken down by-product of heme protein in RBCs. Relevant in any liver disease.

Alkaline Phosphatase (male: 38–126 U/l female: 70–230 U/l)

- Nonspecific hepatic iso-enzyme that has a large concentration in liver, but found in other parts of the body. If there is a primary liver disease, focus on ALT and AST as these are much more specific to liver function.

ALT (8–20 U/L)

- Relevant with any primary liver disease. Enzyme found in liver. Is released into circulation when liver cells are damaged. Has a higher specificity to liver than AST.

AST (8–20 U/L)

- Relevant with any primary liver disease. Enzyme found in liver. Is released into circulation when liver cells are damaged.

Urinalysis

Color (yellow)

- Clear to pale yellow is usually seen with aggressive diuresis. Orange color typically due to bilirubin in urine with liver disease. Dark amber is commonly seen with dehydration or fluid volume deficit.

Clarity (clear)

- Though the context here is a UA, students must recognize the importance of always evaluating the clarity in the tubing of any patient with a Foley catheter. If urine is cloudy or has sediment, patient may have possible urinary tract infection (UTI) and UA should be obtained, especially if new finding.

Specific Gravity (1.015–1.030)

- Measures the kidney's ability to concentrate or dilute urine in relation to plasma. Increased with dehydration and decreased with diuresis.

Protein (neg)

- Relevant when positive in any patient with renal disease. If kidneys have been damaged or there is a new finding of renal failure, proteins, being a large colloid, should be filtered by glomerulus. If there is damage to the glomeruli, the inability to adequately filter urine will be present and therefore will be positive. However, in active young adolescent females there is a phenomenon that produces a higher protein in the urine. A first voiding of the day should be measured with these individuals.

Glucose (neg)

- Relevant if diabetic. Degree of presence in urine reflects poorly controlled diabetes. Also same rationale as protein above. Glucose is also a large particle that should be filtered by glomerulus.

Ketones (neg)

- Ketones are formed from metabolism of fatty acids. Relevant and most commonly seen in DKA and dehydration.

Bilirubin (neg)

- Must be noted and relevant with liver disease. Should be negative, but with liver disease may be positive.

Blood (neg)

- Will typically be positive if patient has UTI or renal calculi.

Nitrite (neg)

- To rule out UTI or determine its presence, nitrites, LET, and WBC micro must be assessed together. Nitrites are relevant because, if positive, they reflect the presence of gram-negative bacteria in the urinary tract, the most common being E. coli. By itself, it is not a predictable indicator of urinary infection.

LET (Leukocyte Esterase) (neg)

- To rule out UTI or determine if present, nitrites, LET, and WBC micro must be assessed together. LET is relevant–it is an enzyme that is present if WBCs are in the urine. By itself is not a predictable indicator of urinary infection.

UA Micro

RBC (<5)

- Must be noted if UTI or renal calculi–this gives amount of RBCs present which can correlate with severity.

WBC (<5)

- ALWAYS RELEVANT and GOLD STANDARD that by itself indicates the presence of UTI if patient has symptoms. Most clinicians will diagnose UTI if >5 WBCs present in urine and symptomatic. Amount of WBCs present indicates severity. To rule out UTI or determine if present, nitrites, LET, and WBC micro must be clustered and assessed together.

Bacteria (neg)

- Does not consistently correlate to presence of infection, though it can be clustered with WBC, LET, and nitrites.

Epithelial (neg)

- Skin cells are present but not relevant in itself.

Cardiac

CPK total (Male: 38–174 U/l Female: 26–140 U/I)

- Enzyme that is found in muscle fibers of the body. Is not generalized to cardiac muscle. CPK is used as a ratio to MB to identify if the ratio of CPK to CPK-MB is clinically significant and positive for a MI (Van Leeuwen & Poelhuis–Leth, 2009).

CHAPTER 6 HIGHLIGHTS

- Though there are numerous lab values and chemistries in the most common lab panels, there are only a handful that are consistently relevant.
- In a basic metabolic panel (BMP), the most important labs that are consistently relevant to the nurse include sodium, potassium, glucose, and creatinine.
- In a complete blood count (CBC), the most important labs that are consistently relevant to the nurse include the total white blood cell count, neutrophils, hemoglobin, and platelets.
- It is not enough to simply identify an abnormal lab. The nurse must know what to do with this information.
- Lab planning is an essential nurse thinking skill that is used when the nurse identifies relevant abnormal labs, and interventions and assessments to use in response to an abnormal finding.

Additional Resources

- Book: *Lab Values: 63 Must Know Labs for Nurses* (2015) by Jon Haws
- Book: *Fluids and Electrolytes: The Easy Guide to Understand Fluids and Electrolytes* (2015) by Dr. Russell
- Flashcards: *Mosby's Fluids & Electrolytes Memory NoteCards: Visual, Mnemonic, and Memory Aids for Nurses, 2nd ed.*
- Web PDF: Lab Values: Interpreting Chemistry and Hematology for Adult Patients.

Chapter Reflections

1. Is understanding laboratory values and the application of fluid and electrolyte content a current struggle for you?

   If so, what will you do to make this your strength?

2. Do you know what the most common or most important laboratory values are in your current clinical setting?

   If known, write them down below and use your lab manual to answer and then memorize the essence of "lab planning" to identify nursing interventions for these labs that are abnormal.

   1.
   2.
   3.
   4.
   5.
   6.
   7.
   8.
   9.
   10.

Web MD...
Something that makes a mild cold into a deadly disease that will kill you in the next 24 hours.

Chapter 7
Concepts You NEED to Know

There are currently two primary approaches that nursing programs use to teach the vast body of nursing knowledge:

1. **CONTENT, or traditional textbook knowledge for each topic taught.** This can lead to content overload as students are expected to know broad amounts of content for each specialty (fundamentals, med/surg, pediatrics, OB, mental health). This approach typically results in superficial depth of knowledge of a broad body of content knowledge, but not the DEEP learning of what is truly most important to each topic.

2. **CONCEPT-based curriculum that emphasizes conceptual learning.** A concept is simply a framework or classification of information that looks at the "bigger picture" of theoretical content. Once concepts are understood, the student can make links and readily translate this knowledge to other areas and specialties of nursing practice (Giddens, 2013).

More than 50 nursing concepts have been identified. Examples of concepts include nutrition, elimination, safety, gas exchange, and perfusion. Concepts often have relationship to one another and must not be seen as individual "silos." An excellent example of how concepts are often interrelated is found with sepsis. The interrelated concepts of infection, inflammation, and immunity are all impacted by an underlying systemic infection.

One of the strengths of conceptual learning is that the student is able to deeply understand the essential components of nursing practice and see the bigger picture of nursing theory without becoming overwhelmed in the details of each clinical specialty. For example, under the concept of perfusion, when hypovolemic shock and the principles behind it are deeply understood, this knowledge can translate to identifying universal signs and symptoms of shock regardless of the cause. This includes a child who is severely dehydrated from gastroenteritis, a woman who has a severe postpartum bleed and is in hemorrhagic shock, or a postoperative patient who is sliding into septic shock. Each of these presentations will have the same underlying pathophysiology and compensatory response.

Throughout this book I have also discussed nursing concepts that must be understood and incorporated into your practice. These concepts include fluid and electrolyte balance, professionalism, clinical judgment, leadership, and patient education. But for the sake of this chapter I want to emphasize additional key concepts that are foundational to everything that the nurse does in practice and must be DEEPLY understood.

Foundational Concepts to Nursing Practice
• Safety
• Gas Exchange
• Perfusion
• Infection/Inflammation/Immunity

Safety

Safety is the unifying thread of nursing practice that ties everything together. Once you have received report at change of shift, if you are the primary nurse, you are responsible for any inherited errors that may be present in the patient's room. In order to provide safe care, I have derived the following safety topics from my own practice that can help you to develop your own safety "checklist" of essential safety assessments to review as you enter the patient's room for the first time. Modify this list as needed, depending on your clinical practice setting.

General Safety Principles

Tab alarms

- Make sure that any device that is related to preventing a patient fall works properly. Tab alarms must be properly secured to the patient in order for them to release and alarm.

Level of bed/side rails

- Be sure to note if the bed is down at the lowest position. Note also if the side rails are up or down, depending on the need and concern for safety.

Miscellaneous

- Are assistive devices available to the patient and at the bedside?
- How many staff are needed to transfer the patient safely?
- Any adaptive equipment needed and in place for bathroom safety?

Room order

- Do a "once over" of the room. Though your patient may not currently need oxygen or suction, is there an oxygen flowmeter or suction canister in the room? What about an ambu bag or other supplies that are standard but may not have been replaced?
- Though you may have inherited a messy room, it is not okay to leave it that way! A room that is clean and in order is a room that promotes a healing environment. This emphasis goes all the way back to Nightingale! Therefore, this should always be a priority for the nurse. Do what is needed to bring order and cleanliness to every patient's room.
- Make sure that the patient has fresh water and all old trays and food that may no longer be safe are removed.
- Remember that the floor of any care setting is obviously dirty and contaminated. One of my pet peeves is the frequency I find sequential compression device (SCDs) sleeves that go around the lower legs of the patient on the floor when they are not in use! Do not be that nurse. Keep them off the floor and as clean as possible!

Safety Assessments

Assessment of IV Site

Make it a priority to determine if the IV site is patent or not.

- From my clinical experience I have seen an IV patent and in a few minutes it can be leaking and obviously infiltrated. The most common signs that you will see clinically with IV infiltration is leakage of fluid at the insertion site, pain, and obvious swelling distal to the insertion site.

- Flush all saline locks to ensure patency at the beginning of your shift. Since a saline lock has nothing running through it, it can be dislodged and appear just fine. By identifying a problem before you need to administer a medication intravenously, you are beginning the habit of being a proactive and not reactive nurse!

Is IV well secured?
- It is not uncommon for a peripheral IV to be poorly secured or to find the tape peeling off when you assess it for the first time. Carry tape and secure all IVs securely.

Is IV dressing intact?
- The clear Tegaderm® dressing can peel on the edges to such a degree that the insertion site is compromised. This is especially important to determine site integrity with any type of central line or peripherally inserted central catheter (PICC) because of the risk of sepsis. If the dressing is peeling on the edges but the site is intact, reinforce with tape. If site is compromised or bloody, change dressing per hospital protocol ASAP!

Assessment of IV Fluids

Determine that the IV solution is exactly what is ordered on the Medication Administration Record (MAR).
- A common error that I have observed is related to the similarities of many IV fluids such as D5 0.9% NS vs. D5 0.45% NS.

Assessment of IV Rate

Confirm that the IV rate is exactly what is ordered on the MAR.
- These rates can change frequently and might have been missed by the prior nurse. Double-check the MAR with the correct rate is an essential safety check at the beginning of your shift.

Oxygen Assessments
- This is especially important if the patient has a history of COPD and is on a specific flow rate at home. This flow rate must be the same to ensure adequate oxygenation if their oxygenation needs have not increased as a result of being hospitalized.
- If there is no specific rate that the physician has ordered but instead has an order to keep oxygenation greater than 92 percent, once a complete assessment of your patient has been made, do not hesitate to wean and decrease the flow rate if the oxygenation is greater than the minimum percentage ordered to advance the plan of care. For example, I have cared for many patients who are on oxygen per nasal cannula with O2 sat of 100 percent who had been documented for two to three shifts at 100 percent and were able to be promptly weaned to room air with no significant drop in O2 sat.

Naso-gastric (NG) Tube Assessments
NG to Correct Suction
You must confirm from the chart and physician order the correct amount of suction.

- The most common settings are low continuous suction, or low intermittent suction. Determine from the suction unit on the wall if the correct suction is currently applied.

Correct Placement

Determine the correct centimeter markings from the prior assessment and recheck to make sure nothing has changed.

- Follow your hospital or institution's policy for verifying placement once the tube has been established. After I have confirmed placement, I have found it beneficial to place a pen mark just below the tape that is attached to the tube so I have a visual identifier. Every time I enter the room, I can quickly determine that the tube is still properly placed.

Properly secured

- This same principle is also essential for a peripheral IV. It is not uncommon for the tape or securement device to become moist and the tube barely holds on to the nose. It is also important to make sure that the tape attached to the tube below the nostril holds the tube firmly and does not allow it to slide. The nurse needs to physically grasp the tube to see if it has any movement back and forth. I have seen tubes appear to be in place but, because this aspect of the tube is not secure, the tube slowly slides out.

Enteral formula correct

- Same principle under IV fluids.

Tube feeding at correct rate

- Same principle under IV rate.

Flush nasogastric tube

- Flush naso-gastric tubes every four hours to ensure patency. Though fluids may be running through the tube, remember the thickness and consistency of what is going through the tube. Regardless of your institution policy, there is no harm done gently flushing the tube every four hours with 20–30 mL of water unless contraindicated.

Chest Tube Assessments

Chest tubes banded

- To simplify my assessment of a patient with a chest tube, I start with the patient and work my way down to the water seal chamber. My first priority is to make sure the chest tube has the white thin plastic "zip tie" bands where it is secured to the tubing that is coming from the water seal unit. It must be secured on each side of the connector. If this band is missing, the chest tube could become disconnected and a pneumothorax could result.

Chest tube secured

- Chest tubes are painful if they move excessively. Make it a priority to securely tape it to the chest, ideally with foam tape if it is loose.

Crepitus

- Gently palpate the chest at the insertion site for the presence of crepitus. The presence of crepitus means that air is leaking into the subcutaneous tissue. The extent of crepitus must be identified. It is not typically a critical event, but the physician should be notified if newly present, and documented in the chart. Crepitus has the potential to compromise the patient's airway. Patients have developed an "Incredible Hulk" look caused by the crepitus under the skin! Crepitus can create a medical emergency by occluding the airway through soft tissue swelling that can radiate from the chest tube insertion site. Don't minimize this problem if it presents!

Correct suction

- With a wet suction water seal chamber, the correct amount of suction is determined by the amount of water that is present in the suction chamber. It is not uncommon for this to be less than the typical -20 cm of suction. If it is low, add enough sterile water to bring it up to -20 cm.
- Newer models of the Atrium water seal units are dry suction and no longer require water level to determine suction. They are also completely quiet and make no aquarium-like "bubbling" noises. Instead, an orange bellows fully inflates and sticks out horizontally when proper suction is applied. Determine there is proper suction going to the unit by ensuring that the orange bellows is sticking out.

Presence of air leak

- Determine the presence of an air leak by looking for small bubbles in the water seal chamber. The water level commonly fluctuates with inspiration and expiration but no bubbles should be seen. If an air leak is present and this is new, as long as there is no respiratory distress from the patient, this is not a critical event. However, the physician should be notified and the leak documented in the chart.
- It is more concerning to have a continuous air leak than an air leak that is present intermittently or only with a deep cough. Note the characteristics of the air leak and document this and report to the primary care provider as needed.

The following concepts must be understood because they are the essence of the ABC's of nursing prioritization. This is the importance of airway, breathing, and circulation priority setting of a patient problem or change of status. Priority setting using the ABC's is foundational to practice as well as for the NCLEX licensure examination.

A/B: Gas Exchange

Gas exchange can be defined as the process when oxygen is transported to cells and carbon dioxide is transported from cells. Gas exchange is foundational to almost all illnesses and diseases because all cells in the human body depend on gas exchange and the ability of the body to remove waste gas such as CO_2 (Giddens, 2013).

It is important to remember the interrelationship of body systems to deeply understand this concept. Though it is obvious that the respiratory system is critical to gas exchange, the importance of the circulatory system to pump oxygen-carrying hemoglobin to every body cell must also be considered under this concept.

In order to further understand gas exchange, there are three subcategories that you must understand. This includes ventilation which is the process of inhaling oxygen into the lungs and exhaling the waste gas of carbon dioxide. Transport refers to the availability and ability of hemoglobin to carry oxygen from the lungs and then to remove the waste gas of carbon dioxide for elimination. Perfusion which will be discussed in more detail, refers to the ability of the body to deliver oxygen containing hemoglobin to the cells and return the waste gas of carbon dioxide back to the right side of the heart to be re-oxygenated once again (Giddens, 2013).

Most Common Problems of Ventilation:

Chronic obstructive pulmonary disease (COPD)

Pneumonia

Asthma

Respiratory syncytial virus (RSV-peds)

Most Common Problems of Perfusion:

Heart failure

Shock

Most Common Problems of Transportation:

Anemia

Sickle cell disease

Here is an application exercise to put this foundational content into context!

Patient Scenario
Joann Walker is an 84-year-old female who has had a productive cough of green phlegm 4 days ago that continues to persist. Though she has had intermittent chills, she first noticed a fever last night of 102.0. She has had more difficulty breathing during the night and has been using her albuterol inhaler every 1–2 hours with no improvement.

Complete Blood Count (CBC:)	Current:	Most Recent:
WBC (4.5–11.0 mm 3)	14.5	12.9
Hgb (12–16 g/dL)	9.7	11.1
Platelets (150–450 x10$_3$/μl)	185	188
Neutrophil % (42–72)	92	89

Arterial Blood Gas:	Current:	Baseline:
pH (7.35–7.45)	7.25	7.38
pCO2 (35–45)	85	60
pO2 (80–100)	75	78
HCO3 (18–26)	42	38
O2 sat (>92%)	90	95

Based on your knowledge of the concept of gas exchange, and the interpretation of these laboratory values, is the primary problem one of ventilation, perfusion, or transportation? Or is there a combination of more than one problem related to gas exchange?

If you answered more than one you are correct. The primary problem is gas exchange with arterial blood gases that reflect a clear problem of ventilation. This patient is also anemic with a hemoglobin of 9.7. Though this is a secondary problem, it has relevance as a component of gas exchange. In order to identify and recognize the significance of Joann's current respiratory distress, the interrelated concept of acid base balance must also be understood to correctly interpret these arterial blood gas results that demonstrate a problem of gas exchange.

What is your interpretation of the baseline ABG result?

What is your interpretation of the current ABG result?

Let's look at each ABG step-by-step to correctly interpret:

Baseline ABG

Arterial Blood Gas:	Baseline:
pH (7.35–7.45)	7.38
pCO2 (35–45)	60
pO2 (80–100)	78
HCO3 (18–26)	38
O2 sat (>92%)	95

1. **What is the pH?** It is normal, but why?
2. **What is the pCO2?** It is significantly elevated. Knowing that this patient has COPD, this is expected because of the damage to the alveoli that impact diffusion of both O2 and CO2. Because the CO2 is elevated, the nurse must note the HCO3 to see if it is elevated and compensating.
3. **What is the HCO3?** It is elevated, but why? CO2 is an acid, and HCO3 is a metabolic base that is secreted by the kidneys, but it takes 24 hours to compensate when there is an acidotic state present. This elevation is expected with COPD and represents compensated respiratory acidosis.
4. **What is the pO2?** It is low, but not by much and with COPD, this finding is expected.

ABG Interpretation: Compensated Respiratory Acidosis

Respiratory Distress: Current ABG

Arterial Blood Gas:	Current:	Baseline:
pH (7.35–7.45)	7.25	7.38
pCO2 (35–45)	85	60
pO2 (80–100)	75	78
HCO3 (18–26)	42	38
O2 sat (>92%)	90	95

In order to recognize the significance of the present problem of gas exchange with the current ABG, each component of the ABG must be trended and compared to the baseline ABG to identify the aspects of ventilation that have changed, and what have remained the same.

1. **What is the pH?** It has now become acidotic, but why?
2. **What is the pCO2?** It is significantly elevated and much higher than her baseline. Because the CO2 is elevated, the nurse must note the HCO3 to see if it is elevated and able to compensate.
3. **What is the HCO3?** It is elevated slightly from the baseline but not by much. HCO3 is clearly not compensating with this new elevation of pCO2.
4. **What is the pO2?** It is low, but compared to her baseline, not by that much. Her problem of gas exchange and ventilation is not primarily a problem of oxygenation, but one of CO2 retention and an inability to remove this waste gas from the body. As the CO2 elevates, in addition to respiratory distress, the patient will exhibit decreased level of consciousness and lethargy. If Bi-pap is unable to improve CO2 ventilation, this patient will need to be emergently intubated.

ABG Interpretation: Uncompensated Respiratory Acidosis

C: Perfusion

In addition to oxygen, every cell in the human body requires a constant blood supply to deliver oxygen to cells. If there is a lack of perfusion to any portion or organ of the body, ischemia and cellular death will soon follow. Tissue perfusion can be defined as the flow of blood through arteries and capillaries that deliver oxygen and nutrients to cells and the consequent removal of cellular waste products (Giddens, 2013). The ability of the heart and cardiovascular system to maintain adequate cardiac output are foundational to adequate perfusion.

It is important to remember that problems of perfusion encompass a spectrum from ischemia (blood supply is present but decreased) to infarction (no blood supply that causes cellular death). Ischemia can cause cellular death over time if the underlying problem is not corrected. Angina, chronic renal insufficiency and transient ischemic attacks (TIA) are common examples of ischemia. Myocardial infarction (MI), cerebral vascular accidents (CVA), and pulmonary embolus (PE) are the most common illnesses that represent infarction.

There are two determinants of perfusion: central perfusion and tissue perfusion. Central perfusion is related to the ability of the heart to generate adequate cardiac output and can also be influenced by the vascular system that may cause a decrease in central perfusion due to vasodilation that is seen in septic shock. Tissue perfusion is the volume of blood that is needed to flow through target organs and is supplied by arteries to capillaries. Because the kidneys and brain require higher amounts of blood flow to remain adequately perfused, these systems are especially vulnerable to any problem of perfusion.

Most Common Problems of Central Perfusion

- Cardiac arrhythmias
- Heart failure
- Shock states

Most Common Problems of Tissue/Organ Perfusion

- Atherosclerosis/hyperlipidemia
- Hypertension
- Myocardial infarction
- Stroke
- Chronic renal insufficiency

Here is another application exercise to put this foundational content into context!

Patient Scenario
Carlos Boccerini is a 68-year-old male who has a 5-year history of systolic heart failure secondary to ischemic cardiomyopathy with a current ejection fraction (EF) of 15%. He presents to the emergency department (ED) for shortness of breath (SOB) the past 3 days. His shortness of breath has progressed from SOB with activity to becoming SOB at rest. The last 2 nights he had to sleep in his recliner chair to rest comfortably with his head partially elevated. He is able to speak only a partial sentence and then has to take a breath when talking to the nurse. He has noted increased swelling in his lower legs and has gained 6 pounds in the last 3 days.

Does this scenario represent a problem of central perfusion or tissue/organ perfusion?

If you answered central perfusion, you are correct. A 15 percent ejection fraction is a finding consistent with end-stage heart failure, and Carlos is clearly in crisis as he is in heart failure exacerbation. Why is Carlos experiencing shortness of breath and orthopnea? Is this a problem of organ/tissue perfusion? To answer this question correctly, the nurse must have a deep understanding of the pathophysiology of heart failure.

The shortness of breath is present because of an impairment in gas exchange, the first concept that was discussed. In acute heart failure, the failure of the left ventricle causes increased hydrostatic pressure in the left atrium that transfers to the pulmonary veins. This increase in pressure pushes fluid into the alveoli, which impairs gas exchange.

Heart failure is an excellent clinical example of how the primary problem of central perfusion affects other organ systems and other concepts relevant to nursing such as gas exchange. But heart failure does not just impact gas exchange and the lungs, it can also impact tissue/organ perfusion of other body systems. This is why a deep knowledge of fluids and electrolytes and its application to the nurse's ability to correctly interpret lab values is also central to practice. In this same scenario, the primary care provider orders a basic metabolic panel.

Basic Metabolic Panel (BMP)	Current
Sodium (135–145 mEq/L)	133
Potassium (3.5–5.0 mEq/L)	5.5
Glucose (70–110 mg/dL)	105
Creatinine (0.6–1.2 mg/dL)	2.7

What lab(s) have identified a current problem of tissue/organ perfusion as a result of the impairment of central perfusion due to heart failure and what body system does it represent?

The creatinine and potassium are relevant abnormal labs and represent an impairment of organ/tissue perfusion to the kidneys. These physiologic impairments are classic and commonly seen in clinical practice. It is not enough for the nurse to identify the concepts and abnormal lab values that are relevant to any disease, but understand WHY these derangements are present. For example, why is the potassium elevated in acute or acute on chronic renal failure? When the function of the renal tubules and how potassium is excreted by the kidneys is understood, this answer becomes evident.

C: Infection/Inflammation/Immunity

Sepsis is the most common complication after any invasive procedure and is responsible for more deaths than heart disease in the United States. Sepsis begins as a localized infection that goes throughout the body causing a systemic inflammatory response syndrome (SIRS). In order for an infection to establish a foothold in the body, the individual's immune system is impaired in some way causing the patient to be a susceptible host.

Though infection, inflammation, and immunity are separate concepts, they are interrelated and each must be understood to acquire the deep knowledge that is required to think critically and recognize sepsis EARLY, before it progresses to the life-threatening complication of septic shock.

The following definitions will help to distinguish what is similar and unique about each of these concepts:

Infection

Infection is invasion of microorganisms in the body (bacterial, viral, fungal, protozoal) that dramatically multiply. The evidence of this infection may be without obvious clinical symptoms, which can result in a local or systemic infection.

Inflammation

Inflammation is an expected and protective physiologic response to any type of cellular injury that allows the body to heal and repair after any type of injury. The inflammatory response neutralizes or removes the pathogen, which results in restoration of homeostasis. It is important to remember that although inflammation is always present with an infection or injury, it can also be provoked in the absence of infection.

Inflammation can be either acute or chronic. Common examples of acute inflammation include acute infection that remains localized such as cellulitis, appendicitis, tonsillitis, or an acute infection that progresses to sepsis. Ulcerative colitis, atherosclerosis, COPD, and cirrhosis are examples of chronic inflammation most commonly seen in clinical practice.

Immunity

The immune response is an incredibly complex response to defend the body against any foreign microorganism invaders. I liken this response to one of my favorite movies, *Braveheart*, starring Mel Gibson. If you are familiar with the plot of this historically based movie from the 1400s, Scotland is invaded by the English. William Wallace is a Scots leader who attempts to resist the invasion of the English, but he and his followers are ultimately overcome by a superior military. Wallace and many others die trying.

This is the essence of how the immune system was designed to respond, as well as white blood cells and neutrophils, which are the quickest to respond in high numbers to ultimately sacrifice themselves to contain the invading pathogens.

Numerous factors influence the normal immune response and increase the susceptibility of a person. The reasons for an altered immune response include the following:

- Infants less than 2 months
- Adults older than 60 years
- Malnutrition
- Chronic illnesses
    - ✓ COPD
    - ✓ Diabetes mellitis
    - ✓ Cancer
    - ✓ Human immunodeficiency virus (HIV)
- Medications/Treatments
    - ✓ Radiation therapy
    - ✓ Chemotherapy
    - ✓ Prednisone

Patient Scenario
Jimmy Jones is a 38-year-old African-American male with a relevant history of C-4 quadriplegia 2 years ago secondary to a car accident. He was seen today in outpatient clinic for a wound check for a baseball-sized stage 4 decubiti on his coccyx that he developed 6 months ago. He developed chills and a fever yesterday. His current VS: T: 100.5 (o) P: 94 R:20 BP: 90/52 O2 sat: 99% RA. He has a large amount of yellow/green drainage on the dressing and the drainage has a strong odor.

Use your knowledge of these concepts to identify relevant clinical data is, but then differentiate the clinical data that represents the concept of infection, inflammation, and immunity from the following clinical scenario:

What data from this scenario is important and RELEVANT and has clinical significance to the nurse?

RELEVANT Data from Present Problem:	Clinical Significance:	Concept:

Clinical Data Collected:

Current VS:
T: 101.2 (oral)
P: 110 (regular)
R: 22 (regular)
BP: 92/50
O2 sat: 95% RA

Complete Blood Count (CBC:)	Current:
WBC (4.5–11.0 mm 3)	12.9
Hgb (12–16 g/dL)	11.8
Platelets (150–450 x10³/μl)	188
Neutrophil % (42–72)	89
Band forms (3–5%)	1

Basic Metabolic Panel (BMP:)	Current:
Sodium (135–145 mEq/L)	135
Potassium (3.5–5.0 mEq/L)	4.2
Glucose (70–110 mg/dL)	95
Creatinine (0.6–1.2 mg/dL)	0.4

RELEVANT Clinical Data:	Clinical Significance:	Concept:

Based on your knowledge of infection, inflammation, and immunity, how did you do? Here is the data you should have identified as relevant, and WHY:

RELEVANT Clinical Data from Present Problem:	Clinical Significance:	Concept:
C-4 quadriplegia two years ago secondary to car accident.	*Immobility increases susceptibility to decubiti that become breaks in skin integrity and potential source of infection.*	*Immunity (susceptible host)*
He was seen today in outpatient clinic for a wound check for a baseball-sized stage 4 decubiti on his coccyx that he developed six months ago.	*This problem has unfortunately developed. Stage 4 is full thickness and through muscle.*	*Immunity (susceptible host)*
He developed chills and a	*Chills and fever represent an expected*	*Inflammation*

fever yesterday.	*response when the inflammatory response is activated. Infection is the most likely reason in this scenario.*	
His current VS: T: 100.5 (o) P: 94 R:20 BP: 90/52 O2 sat: 99% RA.	*This finding clearly confirms the current source. The color of drainage and foul-smelling odor is consistent with pus.*	*Inflammation Perfusion*
He has a large amount of yellow/green drainage on the dressing and the drainage has a strong odor.	*Drainages that is yellow, green, or a combination of the two is pus that is composed primarily of dead neutrophils that have sacrificed themselves to neutralize an infection. The odor is also consistent with what is expected with an infection of any kind.*	*Infection*

RELEVANT Clinical Data:	Clinical Significance:	Concept:
T: 101.2 (oral)	*When the inflammatory response is activated, fever is expected to help mobilize additional WBCs to fight the invaders as well as make it less hospitable for microorganisms to thrive.*	*Inflammation*
P: 110 (regular)	*Though an elevated HR is expected with fever, this elevation could be compensatory response to decreased cardiac output.*	*Perfusion*
R: 22 (regular)	*RR will be elevated with increased metabolism due to elevated temp. Watch closely for increased tachypnea secondary to progression of sepsis.*	*Perfusion*
BP: 92/50	*This BP is low, but knowing that this patient is a quadriplegic, this may be his norm. Assess closely for further decrease that could be related to sepsis.*	*Inflammation*
WBC: 12.9	*Systemic inflammatory response to a localized infection. Expected but continue to trend over time.*	*Inflammation*
Neutrophil %: 89	*Systemic inflammatory response to a localized infection.*	*Inflammation*

	Neutrophils are dominant first responders of inflammatory response. Expected but continue to trend over time.	
Creatinine: 0.4	Knowing that kidneys are sensitive to low levels of perfusion, this normal finding suggests that his current BP is likely WNL. Continue to trend closely for any elevation.	Perfusion

Closing Thoughts

When the most important concepts related to nursing are deeply understood, this provides another way of thinking that the nurse can use to strengthen the critical thinking that is required for practice. My goal with this chapter was to highlight the concepts that represent A, B, C priorities and make them practical with common scenarios seen in clinical practice. For more information on concepts in nursing, I highly recommend *Concepts for Nursing Practice* by Jean Giddens.

CHAPTER 7 HIGHLIGHTS

- Concepts are frameworks or classification of content that looks at the bigger picture of nursing theory.
- Though there are over 50 identified concepts relevant to nursing. The most important concepts related to clinical practice include safety, gas exchange, perfusion, and infection/inflammation/immunity.
- These concepts are foundational because they are directly related to safe patient care, but also incorporate the ABC's of nursing priority setting, which is airway, breathing, and circulation.

Additional Resources

- Book: *Concepts for Nursing Practice* (2012) by Jean Giddens
- eBooklet: *6 Easy Steps to ABG Analysis* by David Woodruff

Chapter Reflections

1. Do you consistently utilize the safety principles and assessments that were listed at the beginning of the chapter in your practice?

2. Which safety assessments/principles do you find difficult to incorporate into your practice?

3. How well do you understand the ABC's of clinical concepts and their pathophysiology?

   What will you do to address areas you don't understand to make them your strength?

4. Identify the most common illnesses/diseases/problems in your current clinical or practice setting. Use your nursing resources or an online data base such as http://emedicine.medscape.com/.
   1.
   2.
   3.
   4.
   5.
   6.
   7.
   8.
   9.
   10.

5. With each problem, make it a priority to truly understand the pathophysiology and write a brief paragraph in your own words.

I'm sorry honey. Mommy is a nurse so we only go to the doctor when we're dying.

Part III

GET SET...

Essentials of
Clinical Practice

Though knowing and understanding the right content and concepts are important, the nurse must be able to use and apply this knowledge to the bedside of every patient. It is not about memorizing content in order to pass a test! The primary responsibility of the professional nurse is the ability to think like a nurse and make correct clinical judgments by using the knowledge in the earlier chapters as well as in your program.

Thinking like a nurse is complex and is much more than the five steps of nursing process. In chapter 8, I break down three primary components of nurse thinking that includes nursing process, critical thinking, and understanding and identifying the clinical relationships of data that you will collect. Once these relationships are identified, like pieces of the puzzle, your patient and current priorities will begin to become more readily apparent.

Clinical reasoning is the essence of nurse thinking and is the topic of chapter 9. Clinical reasoning is the ability of the nurse to think in action and reason as a situation changes. What will you do when the status of your patient suddenly changes with an elevation in temperature or decrease in blood pressure? Being able to anticipate and respond by thinking in action – using clinical reasoning – is an essential nurse thinking skill that must be deeply understood.

Once you are in the clinical setting, chapter 10 addresses the essentials of real-world clinical practice that includes practical "pearls" on completing your head-to-toe nursing assessment. I share principles that I have learned over my 30 years in clinical practice that will help you strengthen this foundational skill. The importance of priority setting and time management, embracing the responsibility of being an educator to your patient and family, delegating appropriately, and how to lead as a nurse in practice are also addressed.

Chapter 11 ties everything together that we have covered to this point with my unique clinical reasoning case studies that require you to use and apply knowledge. I use the priority setting approach of the ABC's and provide three case studies that address each of these priorities separately. There are no multiple-choice questions. You must be able to use and apply what you have learned in your nursing program and in this text to identify relevant clinical data and clinically reason in order to make a correct clinical judgment. These three case studies are found in the attachments in the eBook and can be easily downloaded to print and then work through.

Chapter 8
How You Need to THINK

The "roof" of thinking like a nurse is extremely important and crucial to the strength of the "living" house that each student represents. In a building, the roof trusses tie the four walls and the rest of the structure together. The same is true for the "roof" of nurse thinking. It ties the walls of the applied sciences and the foundation of the "art" of nursing together. If the roof is not strong and well developed, the entire structure of the "living" house is impacted adversely and weakened.

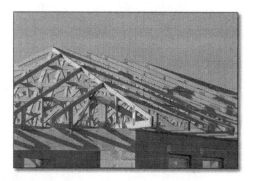

It is easy to get caught up with the new technical skills that you are learning, such as Foley catheterization and naso-gastric tube insertion. These skills are important, but do not define the primary responsibility of the professional nurse. The distinguishing characteristic of the professional nurse is the ability to THINK like a nurse by using knowledge to improve patient outcomes and advance the plan of care.

Thinking like a nurse is a skill that requires clinical experience and practice to develop. The developed skill of nurse thinking is the essence of what is required to be safe in practice. Though the "art" of nursing is foundational to my "living house" metaphor of nursing education, it is the roof of NURSE THINKING or lack of it that can make the difference between life and death. This can happen when a student fails to use and apply content knowledge, think like a nurse, and rescue a patient with a change in status.

Novice Nurse Thinking

Patricia Benner identified five distinct stages of knowledge and expertise acquisition that represent the growth and development over time, beginning as a student. An inexperienced novice nursing student can progress over time to become an expert nurse. To progress through each of these five stages requires time and clinical experience.

The five stages of nurse proficiency are (Benner, 1982):

1. Novice
2. Advanced beginner
3. Competent
4. Proficient
5. Expert

As a nursing student, you are in the first or novice stage because of your lack of experience. Knowledge alone will not propel a nurse through each of these sequential stages. As a student or new nurse, you must have realistic expectations of your current professional development. I will discuss this essential theory in additional depth later in the book.

How a Novice Nurse Thinks

There are predictable patterns that represent how a new student nurse thinks and processes clinical data while providing patient care. See if you can identify with any of these characteristics of a novice nurse:

- Experiences anxiety and lack of self-confidence in the clinical setting
- Relies heavily on textbooks and other resources
- Tends to be a concrete learner whose knowledge is organized as facts and follows policies and standards by rote
- Is comforted by clear-cut rules of what to do and does not appreciate clinical ambiguity
- Focuses on the tasks that need to be done and struggles to see the holistic needs of the patient. As a result, tends to forget to assess thoroughly before doing an intervention.
- Relies on step-by-step procedures (task oriented) and may neglect the patient response to the procedure (Alfaro-LeFevre, 2013)

Did you identify with the aspects of novice nurse thinking that define your current approach to thinking and priority setting in the clinical setting? I am confident that you saw yourself in most if not all of these traits. It takes about two years of clinical experience as a student to develop to the next stage of advanced beginner. Then another two years to progress to the next stage of competence. As you enter into your first year of practice, don't be hard on yourself that you are not progressing as fast as you would like! The content in the next two chapters is written in a manner that recognizes your comfort level with step-by-step ways of thinking and uses this knowledge to guide and strengthen your ability to think like a nurse.

Four Roof Trusses of Nurse Thinking

Thinking like a nurse is extremely complex and something that experienced nurses tend to take for granted. But the "roof" of "nurse thinking" must be built from scratch because the born nurse does not exist! It is a work in progress for novice students who will continue to develop this aspect of practice years after they graduate.

As I reflect upon my own clinical experience and practice, thinking like a nurse requires at least four separate "roof trusses" of nurse thinking. Each truss of nurse thinking must be DEEPLY understood and then applied to practice.

Four Components (roof trusses) of Nurse Thinking
1. Nursing Process
2. Critical Thinking
3. Identify Relationship of Clinical Data
4. Clinical Reasoning

In nursing education, the two "roof trusses" that have been consistently emphasized are nursing process and critical thinking. Identifying the relationship of clinical data and clinical reasoning are also essential to thinking like a nurse and must also be emphasized to thoroughly prepare you for professional practice.

Roof Truss #1: Nursing Process

Nursing process is the foundation of thinking like a nurse. It is typically introduced and taught at the beginning or fundamental level and is the nurse thinking skill that most students are familiar and comfortable with. In this brief review, I will share some additional insights on each step of the nursing process.

Assessment

Comprehensive, systematic assessment is the first step in delivering nursing care that includes collecting and recognizing RELEVANT clinical data. This includes not only physical assessment data, but also psychological, sociocultural, spiritual, economic, and lifestyle assessment data as well.

Nursing Priority/Diagnosis

This is the priority that is identified once clinical data from the chart as well as data personally collected is assimilated by the nurse. This judgment forms the basis for the plan of care. Critical thinking and clinical reasoning must also be incorporated and are essential skills that are needed to recognize the correct nursing priority.

I took the liberty to more accurately relate step 2 of the nursing process to clinical practice by emphasizing and establishing a nursing PRIORITY, which is a key component of clinical reasoning and de-emphasizes nursing diagnosis. You cannot have a nursing diagnosis without NANDA-I. Though NANDA-I is a taxonomy that remains relevant to nursing practice and priority setting, there are other ways that a nurse in practice establishes care priorities besides NANDA-I.

Outcomes/Planning

Based on the assessment and establishment of nursing priorities, a plan of nursing care is established. The nurse also sets measurable and achievable short- and long-range outcomes.

Implementation

Nursing care is implemented according to the care plan, which is specific to the patient and focuses on achievable outcomes.

Evaluation

The patient's status and the response to nursing care must be continuously evaluated, and the care plan modified as needed to determine if outcomes have been met ("The Nursing Process," n.d.). Clinical reasoning, which will be discussed in the next chapter, emphasizes thinking in action, must also be incorporated and applied to this final step.

Why NANDA-I Can Be a NO-NO

I believe that NANDA-I has relevance to clinical practice, but clinical reasoning needs to be emphasized and integrated within the nursing process, especially step 2 (nursing diagnosis/priority) to develop students' ability to think like a nurse in practice. If NANDA-I is primarily emphasized as the ONLY or primary way that students are allowed to establish a care priority throughout the nursing program, this can be a barrier that will limit their ability to think like a nurse.

One of the limitations of NANDA-I is that many of the nursing diagnostic statements are best suited for stable patients with expected outcomes. But when the status of the patient changes and is in need of rescue, there are often no salient NANDA-I nursing diagnostic statements that consistently capture the essence of the problem. Practical nurse thinking does not lend itself to a three-part NANDA-I nursing diagnostic statement with "related to" and "as evidenced by" that lay the foundation of traditional care planning in nursing school.

NANDA-I and "Failure to Rescue"

Though NANDA-I nursing diagnostic statements has been an established taxonomy to identify nursing priorities for over 40 years, del Bueno (2005) identified a relationship between the use of NANDA-I nursing diagnostic statements and the nurse's inability to readily recognize a change of status.

Del Bueno (2005) found that 65% of new nurses were unable to exercise correct clinical judgment at a basic level to "rescue" (identify the problem and then intervene) their patient in a simulated scenario due in part to the inappropriate use of NANDA-I nursing diagnostic statements to make them "fit" when there was a change in status (del Bueno, 2005).

For example, when a patient had a condition change consistent with a stroke, the nurse used the NANDA-I statement "alteration in sensory perception" or "alteration in nutrition." In another patient having symptoms consistent with a myocardial infarction, the nurse used "activity intolerance related to pain." Del Bueno (2005) summarizes her research findings with the following statement, *"Many inexperienced RN's also attempt to use a nursing diagnosis for the problem focus. Whatever the original intent for its use the results are at best cumbersome and at worst risible"* (p. 280).

Roof Truss #2: Critical Thinking

The essence of critical thinking as it relates to nursing practice is the ability of the nurse to APPLY nursing theory to the bedside and USE this knowledge to advance the plan of care. Potter & Perry (2009) define critical thinking as *"a commitment to think clearly, precisely, and accurately and to act on what you know about a situation"* (p. 216). This definition recognizes the importance of accuracy and making a correct clinical judgment as well as the importance of APPLICATION of knowledge to the bedside where it matters most.

Communication and Critical Thinking

In addition to being able to apply knowledge, the nurse must also be able to communicate effectively with the patient, family, primary care providers, and members of the health care team. Critical thinking depends on the mutual exchange of both verbal and nonverbal messages and having them accurately understood and interpreted. In order for the nurse to communicate effectively, he/she must actively listen.

This is done when the nurse is open, authentic, and free from any bias. The nurse must also listen empathetically, by intending to understand the patient's perspective and experience (Alfaro-LeFevre, 2013). The stakes are highest at change of shift report and when communicating directly with primary care providers. Lack of communication or miscommunication in these contexts can adversely impact patient outcomes because important information may not be accurately communicated.

Linda Caputi (2011) identified that it is essential that the nurse integrates the following practical critical thinking skills into their practice:

- Assess the patient systematically and comprehensively.
- Cluster related information. This essential nurse thinking skill identifies clinical relationships and will be discussed in greater detail later in this chapter.
- Collaborate with co-workers.
- Determine the importance of information by distinguishing relevant from irrelevant information.
- Gather complete and accurate data, then act on that data.

Another simple approach to effectively communicate the essence of critical thinking is to emphasize the HABITS of critical thinkers. According to Bittner and Tobin (1998), these habits include the following characteristics that you want to develop as you progress through your program. Be patient with yourself because these habits are developed with clinical experience, NOT textbook or classroom learning:

- **Confidence.** There is no substitute other than clinical experience to develop this!
- **Flexibility.** Are you able and willing to "roll with the changes"?
- **Inquisitiveness.** Clinical curiosity regarding new illnesses/medications or anything else you do not know. Are you able to state the WHY?
- **Open-mindedness.** Consider all clinical possibilities vs. narrow/closed minded.
- **Reflection.** Reflect continually to learn from what you did well, and what you can learn when things did not go so well!

Roof Truss #3: Identify Relationships of Clinical Data

The nurse must be able to step back and see the "big picture" of patient care and the essence of the current clinical picture. The nurse must be able to recognize relationships, patterns, and how pieces of clinical data "fit" together to establish nursing priorities, make correct clinical judgments, and think like a nurse.

Clustering related clinical data so that patterns can be identified is essential to recognize and identify clinical relationships. When collected clinical data begins to "fit," the clinical puzzle begins to come together. In order for the puzzle to be CORRECTLY assembled, the clinical data must be first sorted and filtered by the nurse to determine if it is relevant or most important. The ability to critically think by applying nursing theory to recognize relevant clinical data is needed to make correct clinical judgments that will form the foundation for clinical reasoning in practice.

There is a series of questions that the nurse can ask to determine if a clinical relationship is present. Though these questions are derived from my extensive clinical experience, they are not unique to me. They are also used intuitively by experienced nurses to help guide the thinking that is required to put any clinical puzzle together that each patient represents.

The first five relationships address the primary medical problem. The last two relationship questions address the nursing priority in the context of the medical problem and how they are related and intersect and the relationship of the primary nursing priority to other identified nursing priorities.

SEVEN CLINICAL RELATIONSHIPS OF NURSE THINKING

Medical Problem:

1. Identify the RELATIONSHIP of what current medications are treating past medical problems.
2. Is there a RELATIONSHIP between the past medical history and/or psychosocial needs that may have contributed to the development of the current primary problem?
3. What is the RELATIONSHIP between the primary problem and the current chief complaint?
4. What is the RELATIONSHIP between relevant clinical data and the primary problem?
5. What is the RELATIONSHIP between any new orders and the primary problem?

Nursing Priorities:

6. What is the RELATIONSHIP between the primary medical problem and nursing priority(s)?
7. What is the RELATIONSHIP between the primary nursing priority and secondary nursing priorities?

These seven clinical relationships will help develop "big picture" nurse thinking that are further defined and explained below.

1. *Identify the RELATIONSHIP of what current medications are treating past medical problems.*

This is the most basic clinical relationship that beginning students can be guided to recognize. In order to identify the clinical relationship of what current medications are treating past medical problems, the nurse must know not only what the medication is for, but based on the patient's history, why is he receiving it. For example, if a patient is receiving atenolol, he most likely has a history of hypertension. But if the patient has no history of hypertension but does have atrial fibrillation, would you be able to identify the clinical relationship between atenolol and atrial fibrillation?

If you DEEPLY understand the mechanism of action of a beta blocker, you will be able to connect this knowledge to atrial fibrillation. Atrial fibrillation can cause a rapid ventricular response or HR>100. Atenolol is indicated to keep the heart rate within normal limits. Once this clinical relationship is recognized, you will be able to see the "fit" and put these two clinical "puzzle" pieces together. This will build your confidence to help you recognize the significance of the next clinical relationship.

2. *Is there a RELATIONSHIP between the past medical history and/or psychosocial needs that may have contributed to the development of the current primary problem?*

In order to recognize this clinical relationship, students must have a strong "wall" built of applied pathophysiology. Pathophysiology must be DEEPLY understood so students can identify the contributing risk factors of the most common disease processes. Another way to view this relationship is the "domino effect." When one domino (problem) begins to fall (develop), it affects the next domino and causes another problem to develop as a consequence.

For example, if you have a patient who is admitted with heart failure exacerbation and has a history of:

- Hypertension
- Hyperlipidemia
- MI
- Ischemic cardiomyopathy with ejection fraction of 20%

Would you be able to recognize the clinical relationship between any or all of these problems? These problems did NOT develop in isolation, but every one of these illnesses has a relationship to the other. To take this clinical relationship identification one step further, could you list these illnesses that have relationship to one another in the chronological order they most likely occurred from first to last?

In this example, this is the relationship order that is most likely:

1. Hyperlipidemia as well as hypertension caused underlying damage to the arterial vessels that accelerated the development of atherosclerosis.
2. This caused the next domino to fall, which is an acute MI.
3. Because of chronic ischemia secondary to progressive atherosclerosis and MI, the ischemic cardiomyopathy domino has now fallen.
4. Finally, as the cardiomyopathy progresses, the ejection fraction domino falls and is reflected by a deterioration of function from a normal range of 60–65% to now only 20%.

Psychosocial Needs

In addition to the more obvious physiological problems that may have been influenced by the past medical problem, the patient must be viewed holistically. The relationship of psychosocial needs, including relevant mental health problems, must be identified and addressed by the nurse. If a patient has a history of depression, anxiety, or schizophrenia, these mental health problems can also directly or indirectly influence physiologic health.

If a patient is a native of another country, the influence of culture, and the ability to understand English may influence her or his ability to value or understand the plan of care to maintain health. Educational needs, emotional support, current stress level, and recent losses including the death of a loved one must be on the nurse's radar so they are recognized, identified, and remedied before discharge. These psychosocial needs are not often as obvious as the pressing physiologic needs, but when they are intentionally assessed and identified, they will guide the nurse to consistently deliver holistic care.

3. *What is the RELATIONSHIP between the primary problem and the current chief complaint?*

In order to recognize this clinical relationship, pathophysiology needs to be applied to the bedside. For example, what if the same patient who was situated in relationship #2 presented to the ED with an exacerbation of heart failure, and the following presenting symptoms:

- SOB
- Orthopnea
- Decreased tolerance to activity
- 2+ pitting edema in lower legs

- Weight gain of five pounds in the last two days

When the pathophysiology of left-to right-sided heart failure exacerbation is deeply understood, the relationship of these symptoms becomes evident. Shortness of breath and orthopnea are classic signs of left-sided failure, while pitting edema and weight gain reflect right-sided heart failure. When this relationship is recognized, two more pieces of the clinical puzzle for this patient are connected!

DEEP understanding of pathophysiology and the ability to critically think in practice will lay the foundation to recognize this relationship in clinical practice. For example, if you have a patient whose primary medical problem you have not seen before, make sure you go to access a database to understand the pathophysiology as well as the rationale for the primary care provider's plan of care. My favorite web-based database to DEEPLY understand pathophysiology that is oriented to physicians and other health care professionals is http://emedicine.medscape.com/

4. What is the RELATIONSHIP between relevant clinical data and the primary problem?

In order to recognize this clinical relationship, students must be able to identify the most important clinical data and tie it to the primary medical problem. Relevant clinical data would include physical assessment findings, vital signs, and laboratory values.

Using the same example of a patient with heart failure exacerbation, you have now collected the following relevant clinical data:
- 2+ pitting edema in lower legs
- Coarse crackles half–way up bilaterally
- Respiratory rate 24/minute with O2 sat 88% on room air
- BP: 178/88
- Creatinine: 1.9/last creatinine was 1.1
- BNP: 1125/last BNP was 210

Based on this relevant clinical data and a DEEP understanding of pathophysiology, would you be able to identify the clinical data that supports right-sided heart failure, and the data that reflects left-sided heart failure (2+ pitting edema is right-sided failure, while the crackles reflect left)?

Is there a relationship between left-sided failure, crackles, RR 24, and O2 sat of 88%? Is the blood pressure too high? What is the significance of increased afterload for this patient? Finally, the laboratory values must be understood and situated with the primary medical problem.

Why would the creatinine be elevated? If you can recognize the relationship between decreased cardiac output from heart failure exacerbation and kidney perfusion, you are on your way to thinking like a nurse! The BNP is also elevated. WHY? The relationship of left ventricular stress and overload and this neurohormone must be recognized.

In addition to recognizing that the BNP is elevated in heart failure exacerbation, could you state the physiologic effects that BNP has on the body during heart failure? This, too, must be understood. (The body was designed with a number of compensatory mechanisms, and BNP acts as a vasodilator and has diuretic effects that lower preload as well as afterload and the workload of the heart when it is failing.)

5. *What is the RELATIONSHIP between any new orders and the primary problem?*

Though the nurse is not a primary care provider, she or he must be able to understand the rationale for all procedures and medications ordered and how they relate to the patient's primary medical problem. This is an excellent example of critical thinking and the ability to use knowledge at the bedside. By questioning an order that does not make sense based on the primary problem and recognizing the importance of this relationship, the nurse can prevent an error that could have devastating consequences when the WHY or rationale of all orders are clearly understood. This is an example of why a nurse must be able to understand the essence of physician practice in order to be a better nurse.

Let's continue with the same patient who has heart failure exacerbation. The primary care provider writes the following new orders:

- Furosemide (Lasix) 40 mg IV push
- Nitroglycerin IV gtt-titrate to keep SBP <140

In order to recognize the clinical relationship of these orders to the medical problem, you must also have a strong "wall" built of applied pharmacology and pathophysiology and understand the mechanism of action for every medication administered. Ask yourself, "Why would the primary care provider order these medications in someone with heart failure?" When you are able to apply your knowledge of the mechanism of action for each of these medications, and how they will help resolve the primary problem, this relationship becomes evident.

For example, furosemide (Lasix) is a loop diuretic that will promote potent diuresis and decrease preload. But WHAT IF the patient has 1000 mL of urine output two hours following administration, and the most recent potassium was 3.5? Identifying the relationship of the loss of electrolytes, including potassium, with increased urine output is essential to safe practice and thinking like a nurse.

The nurse must also recognize that even though the potassium was normal, it was in the low normal range before diuresis. Therefore, the nurse must make a correct clinical judgment and use an SBAR to contact the primary care provider to recommend a recheck of the serum potassium if increased premature ventricular contractions (PVC) are noted. In addition, the nurse must be able to situate F&E and recall the most common signs and symptoms of hypokalemia, especially if muscle weakness and increased ventricular ectopy have just started to develop!

Why would the primary care provider want the systolic blood pressure (SBP) <140 and how will nitroglycerin IV drip accomplish this stated objective? Does an elevated SBP and increased afterload increase the workload of the heart? Is this going to help or hurt this patient with heart failure? Nitroglycerin dilates coronary arteries for those with angina, and also dilates systemic venous circulation, which will benefit the patient by decreasing preload as well as afterload. This will also decrease the workload of the heart, the primary objective with exacerbation of heart failure.

Another benefit that a DEEP understanding of pharmacology and pathophysiology offers is that it will deepen students' critical thinking. This is done by recognizing any possible implications or contraindications of medications that are ordered. For example, many heart failure patients develop atrial fibrillation. The mechanism of action of medications used to control this rhythm such as diltiazem (Cardizem) or metoprolol (Lopressor) must be situated to practice.

Do both of these medications affect cardiac contractility? (Yes.) Could this be a potential problem with a patient in heart failure? (Absolutely!) In addition to lowering heart rate and blood pressure, beta blockers and calcium channel blockers also decrease cardiac contractility. Therefore, the effect of these medications could worsen heart failure and commonly seen symptoms such as shortness of breath.

6. *What is the RELATIONSHIP between the primary medical problem and nursing priority(ies)?*

I have addressed five clinical relationships that emphasize a medical problem-based approach to the patient requiring care. This aspect of patient care is important so critical thinking can take place. But once these first five relationships are deeply understood by the nurse, the nurse must transition and recognize the relationship of the primary problem to the nursing priority.

For example, in this scenario of heart failure, using the ABC's of nursing priority setting, the NANDA-I nursing diagnostic statement of impaired gas exchange represents the essence of the physiologic changes that are present. The nurse needs to understand the pathophysiology and recognize the relationship between impaired gas exchange (fluid in the alveoli secondary to fluid volume overload) and biventricular heart failure. Once this relationship is recognized, the nurse will be able to anticipate an expected improvement in the plan of care as excess volume is diuresed and pulmonary edema resolves and oxygenation improves as a result.

7. *What is the RELATIONSHIP between the primary nursing priority and secondary nursing priorities?*

Though it is essential to identify the primary nursing priority, every patient in need of care has several nursing care priorities that often have relationship to one another. When this relationship is recognized and understood, another piece of the clinical puzzle fits. This aids the nurse's ability to visualize the bigger picture of the current clinical scenario. When the current nursing priority is resolved and progression in the plan of care is realized, the additional nursing problems or diagnostic priorities that are secondary will also likely improve or resolve as well.

For example, in the same scenario of heart failure, as the patient is successfully diuresed and the secondary nursing priority of fluid volume excess is resolved, the number one nursing priority of improving gas exchange will occur and additional secondary nursing diagnoses/problems will also be resolved. As oxygenation improves, fatigue, activity intolerance, and ineffective tissue perfusion will improve. These secondary nursing priorities do not exist in isolation but have relationship to each other.

A novice nurse tends to focus on the tasks that involve the most pressing physiologic needs. However, once these physiologic priorities have been addressed, the nurse must be able to step back and recognize the possible impact of the medical problem to the holistic care needs of the patient and address emotional and even spiritual needs. Relevant NANDA-I nursing diagnostic statements that need to be considered for each patient include fear, anxiety, ineffective coping, hopelessness, and spiritual distress.

- Thinking like a nurse is extremely complex and includes four distinct thought processes that include nursing process, critical thinking, identifying relationships of clinical data, and clinical reasoning.
- Nursing process and written care plans that utilize a NANDA-I nursing diagnostic statement are common in nursing education, but if NANDA-I nursing diagnostic statements are the primary method to identify care priorities, this can be a potential barrier to develop nurse thinking.
- In order to think critically, the nurse must be able to apply knowledge to the bedside and use this knowledge to advance the plan of care. This is why the most important content of nursing theory must be deeply understood.
- Patient care can be likened to putting a clinical puzzle together. The majority of clinical data has relationship to one another and literally fits together.
- There are seven clinical relationships that, when understood, will help guide the nurse to put the clinical puzzle together.

Additional Resources

- Book: *Thinking as a Nurse* (2009) by Bruce Austin Scott

Chapter Reflections

1. What habits of critical thinkers are your strengths?

2. What habits do you need to address to make them your strengths?

You know you're a nurse when...
You start to worry if your patient hasn't urinated in a few hours, but you went the entire shift without making it to the bathroom.

Chapter 9
Clinical Reasoning Is Nurse Thinking

"Constant attention by a good nurse may be just as important as a major operation by a surgeon."
–Dag Hammarskjöld

Though the nurse must use all four "trusses" of thinking that include nursing process, critical thinking, recognizing clinical relationships, and clinical reasoning in order to think like a nurse, clinical reasoning is not consistently emphasized in nursing education. Yet it most closely mirrors how a nurse thinks in practice. Clinical reasoning complements these other aspects of nurse thinking and captures the essence of the thinking in action that is needed to make a correct clinical judgment.

Roof Truss #4: Clinical Reasoning

Patients do not stay static. Their condition can gradually improve or it can slowly or suddenly worsen. How well will you be able to think on your feet and recognize the nursing priority when the status of your patient changes? You must be able to THINK IN ACTION and be able to readily transfer classroom learning to the bedside.

The most important role of the professional nurse is NOT performing tasks. Nurses are knowledge workers who use the information they have been taught as well as what they have learned from clinical experience and translate this knowledge into action to deliver safe patient care (Porter-O'Grady, 2010). In order to think like a nurse, students must understand and incorporate clinical reasoning into their practice.

But in order to deeply understand and then apply clinical reasoning it must first be properly defined. The most descriptive and practical working definition of clinical reasoning is found in the work of pre-eminent nurse educator and scholar Patricia Benner (Benner, Sutphen, Leonard, & Day, 2010) and (Benner, Hooper-Kyriakidis, & Stannard, 2011).

CLINICAL REASONING DEFINED
Ability of the nurse to think in action and reason as a situation changes over time by:
• Filtering clinical data to recognize what is most and least important
• Capturing and understanding the significance of clinical trends
• Grasping the essence of the current clinical situation
• Identifying if an actual problem is present

Though recognizing and identifying a problem is an important aspect of clinical reasoning, the nurse must also be able to think globally and accurately INTERPRET the situation to identify possible reasons WHY the problem is present.

For example, if a nurse is caring for a patient who recently had an open hysterectomy who is beginning to complain of increasing lower abdominal pain, though pain is expected after surgery, what if the pain continues and even gets worse despite opiate narcotics that had controlled the pain earlier?

Is the problem increased pain that needs a higher dose of narcotics or does the nurse need to investigate and collect additional clinical data? Internal bleeding or ileus are common complications that could be present. If the nurse practices with tunnel vision and does not widen the funnel and use clinical reasoning, increasing the pain medication dosage if these problems are present will ultimately cause more harm than good.

Attitudes Required to Clinically Reason

In addition to being able to apply and use knowledge at the bedside, the nurse must bring the right ATTITUDE to the clinical setting in order to THINK like a nurse. Take a moment to pause and reflect to determine if these attitudes are a weakness or strength by answering the question that follows. Pesut & Herman (1999) identified six attitudes that are needed in order for the nurse to clinically reason:

1. **Intent.** Excellent and correct nurse thinking is not random and does not just happen by accident, but is intentional. When you are intentional in clinical practice, you understand the rationale of how nursing interventions will advance the plan of care. The nurse has a deliberate plan of thinking and reasons with the end in mind by having a clearly defined purpose or outcome guiding the plan of care.
   - *How well do you understand the rationale and reason for nursing care priorities with each patient in your care?*
   - *Do you have a clearly-defined outcome that you are working toward with each patient?*

2. **Reflection.** This is an essential skill that is foundational to clinical reasoning as well as making a correct clinical judgment. Everything that the nurse does in practice, must also be reflected upon by the nurse to determine if the actions and interventions are effective and working toward the outcome outlined by the plan of care. Clinical reasoning is strengthened and developed when you are able to reflect on past and current clinical experiences and situations and know WHY you are engaging and choosing specific nursing interventions. Stated another way, reflection is thinking about your thinking and determining what can be learned, affirmed, or done differently to grow and develop as a nurse.
   - *How well are you able to integrate reflection and learn while you care for patients?*

3. **Curiosity.** The nurse must be eager to ask questions and acquire needed information and knowledge. The origin of curiosity is "cura," which means to care. Reflection and curiosity are a perfect fit and need to be used together. Nursing is curiosity or care with a purpose. When the nurse is inquisitive about everything that takes place in the clinical setting including the ways that the patient acts, thinks, and presents, the less judgmental the nurse will be. The greater the level of curiosity, the more compassion the nurse will possess.
   - *Do you have a strong desire to deeply understand aspects of your patient that you do not understand?*

4. **Tolerance for ambiguity.** This is the ability of the nurse to feel comfortable even when the current situation is unclear and the best outcome is undefined or unknown. Since students are concrete, textbook learners (Benner, 1982), this aspect of practice can be difficult for them to adjust to. The textbook tends to be concrete and clinical situations are rife with ambiguity, moral and ethical conflict, as well as family dynamics that are interrelated and contribute at times to ambiguity and volatility in practice.

   - *What is your comfort level in the clinical setting when ambiguity is present?*

5. **Self-confidence.** The nurse must possess a certain amount of "mojo" that is balanced and healthy. Believe in yourself, feel good about your abilities as a nurse though you may be inexperienced. Be confident that you have what it takes to be a nurse! An important aspect of self-confidence is to know your strengths as well as weaknesses, and be willing to do what is needed to turn those weaknesses into a strength.

   - *Are you your own worst enemy or do you have a healthy sense of your abilities as a nurse?*

6. **Professional motivation.** The nurse must be committed to the vision, values, and mission of the nursing profession embodied in the code of ethics. These values must be known, assimilated, and lived out by the nurse. You must choose to act differently and hold yourself to the highest level of moral and ethical practice. This means that you become self-monitoring and will self-report if a medication error is made or other deficiency in practice occurs. By using the attitude and skill of reflection, you will learn from any error made and be the better as a result.

   - *Do you consistently hold yourself to the highest standards of ethical conduct and have a strong desire to be the best nurse possible?*

Key Components of Clinical Reasoning

The essence of clinical reasoning and how it must be used in bedside practice consists of four components. Just as a roof truss consists of multiple pieces of lumber that provide bracing for strength, the following four components are the pieces of lumber that represent and comprise the essence of clinical reasoning (Benner, Sutphen, Leonard, & Day, 2010):

- Priority setting
- Rationale for everything
- Identify and trend relevant clinical data
- Grasp the essence of the situation

Priority Setting

Setting priorities with your patient is determined by differentiating between problems that need immediate attention and problems that can wait. Once a problem has been identified, does it need to be documented in the medical record or does the physician need to be notified? Developing this aspect of practical priority setting in your practice is crucial. If you give equal attention to both major and minor problems, you will not have the time to manage what is most important (Alfaro-LeFevre, 2013).

As a novice nursing student, one of the challenges you will experience when establishing nursing care priorities is that all tasks and priorities seem to be of equal significance. Knowing which interventions are a priority is not always readily apparent. A novice nurse has difficulty seeing the big picture and identifying what is clinically significant. Novice nurses are also TASK-oriented and focus on the tasks that need to be done, not necessarily what is most important (Benner, 1982).

Setting priorities is also a key component of Management of Care, the client need category of the NCLEX that comprises the largest percentage of the exam (17–23%). In order to be prepared for professional practice as well as the NCLEX, this aspect of clinical reasoning must be deeply understood. Practical priority setting is discussed in additional depth in chapter 10.

Rationale for Everything

You must be able to understand and answer the rationale or WHY of everything that is done in the clinical setting. As a clinical instructor, I have felt at times like a two-year-old asking the following "whys" of my students:

- WHY are you giving these medications?
- WHY will these nursing interventions advance the plan of care?
- WHY did the primary care provider order these labs, treatments, or medications?

Am I just antagonizing my students, or do I have a rationale for asking these WHY questions? Understanding the WHY is the foundation for SAFE patient care. It is only when a student has a DEEP UNDERSTANDING of the rationale for everything that is done in practice, that the student is SAFE.

If a new order or medication does not make sense based on the student's understanding or rationale, it must be questioned and not followed blindly. The ability to use and apply classroom theory to the bedside is also the essence of critical thinking. Make the most of any down time in clinical to expand and develop your knowledge base so you can build your ability to DEEPLY understand the rationale for everything that is done in clinical practice.

Identify and Trend Relevant Clinical Data

Identifying the MOST important clinical data and trending it by comparing it to the most recent data is an essential component of clinical reasoning and thinking like a nurse in practice. Because students tend to see ALL clinical data as relevant, they will have difficulty sorting out the least from the most important (Benner, 1984). In order to "rescue" a patient with a change in status, the nurse must be able to recognize SUBTLE changes in a patient's condition over time.

It is the EARLY changes in a patient status that are subtle and, therefore, must be recognized before a problem progresses and an adverse outcome results. In addition to trending VS and nursing assessment data, nursing interventions and laboratory values must also be consistently compared and trended.

Nurse Collected Data that Must Be TRENDED

What clinical data needs to be trended? The short answer is just about everything! The following is a summary of the clinical data that must always be compared and trended with the most recent data in the chart:

Vital Signs

- Temperature
- Heart rate
- Respiratory rate

- Blood pressure
- O2 saturation
- Pain

Nursing Assessment

Respiratory
- Breath sounds
- Rhythm/character
- O2 amount/delivery (if applicable)

Cardiac
- Heart sounds
- Strength/regularity of peripheral pulses
- Cap refill
- Color/temperature extremities
- Telemetry rhythm (if applicable)
- Edema—location/amount/pitting vs. non-pitting
- Breath sounds
- Rhythm/character

Neuro
- Alert/oriented x 4 (person-place-time-situation)
- Level of consciousness (LOC)
- Movement/sensation in extremities

GI
- Appearance of abdomen
- Tenderness w/palpation
- Bowel sounds/flatus/LBM (last bowel movement)

GU
- Urine amount/color/clarity
- Foley—secured/urethral drainage?

Skin
- Color/temperature
- Skin integrity—redness/blanchable over pressure points if present

I&O
- Shift and 24-hour trends if relevant
- Daily weights. Remember, every 1 kg. of weight loss or gain represents 1000 mL of volume.

Psychosocial
- Cultural needs
- Emotional support/needs
- Spiritual care/needs
- Educational priorities

Determining Acceptable Ambiguity

To determine the relevance of each patient's clinical data and then trend this data over time, the nurse needs to develop the important understanding of the degree of acceptable ambiguity. To a new nurse in practice, it will soon become apparent that not all patients have textbook norms of clinical data. Depending on the patient's past medical history or current illness, she may have elevated heart rate, respiratory rate or high blood pressure.

For example, a patient with chronic COPD will have a lower than normal oxygen saturation and may be slightly tachypneic. The nurse must identify the normal baseline of all clinical data that is collected and determine the significance of any changes based not on textbook norms, but on the norm for this patient.

To determine acceptable ambiguity for each patient you care for, go back 24 to 48 hours in the medical record and compare and contrast textbook norms for vital signs and assessment parameters with your patient. Then ask yourself the following questions:

- What degree of ambiguity is present between textbook norms and your patient?

- What degree of ambiguity is expected and would be acceptable?

- When would you become concerned (Koharchik, Caputi, Robb, & Culleiton, 2015)?

If ambiguity is present, it is important to determine the clinical significance for the variations that are present and what is responsible for the ambiguity. The following are the most common reasons for abnormal clinical data:

- Past medical history
- Current problem
- Medications
- Abnormal diagnostics

The most difficult aspect of accurately interpreting the significance of clinical data when ambiguity is present is that since a deviation from what is normal is already present, when would the nurse become concerned and decide to intervene? For example, if your patient with COPD has a baseline respiratory rate of 22 and oxygen saturation of 88–90%, when the respiratory rate increases to 28 and his oxygen saturation drops to 84% with activity, is this expected, or a cause for clinical concern? It depends.

By completing a thorough physical assessment, if the patient is in distress and appears anxious with increased wheezing, the nurse must intervene. But if the patient is in no distress and there is no change in breath sounds, this may be his normal response to activity due to lowered pulmonary reserves.

Grasp the Essence of the Situation

Once the priority is identified, rationale for the plan of care understood, and relevant clinical data is trended the nurse should be able to grasp the essence of the current clinical situation. Essence is the ability of the nurse to identify the most significant aspect of the current clinical situation. But it is really much more. It is the ability to break down the patient and current needs to the lowest common denominator of what is needed and what must be done to advance the plan of care. Essence is closely related to priority setting.

As I look back at my own professional development, being able to grasp the "essence" of a clinical situation is the skill that took the most time for me to develop. Unfortunately, it is not going to be strongly developed in a typical five- to ten-week clinical rotation of any clinical unit in nursing school! This takes months and typically more than a year of clinical experience in the same practice setting. The ability to see the whole of patient care and grasp the essence is a characteristic of proficiency, the fourth stage of clinical competence (Benner, 1984). Essence is developed by repeatedly seeing patients with similar problems and the patterns that are seen with the typical chief complaint, nursing assessments, VS, lab values, and expected medical treatment.

Clinical Reasoning & Nursing Process

Though clinical reasoning has not been emphasized in nursing education as long as nursing process, these two important aspects of nurse thinking complement one another in clinical practice. Reviewing the five steps of nursing process will make this relationship apparent.

Assessment: Recognize RELEVANCE

As novice nurses, students tend to see EVERYTHING that is collected in the clinical setting as relevant and important (Benner, 1984). They do not have the experience to guide them to FILTER clinical data by what is most important or relevant. Make it a priority throughout each level of your program to APPLY classroom and clinical knowledge. When content is placed into context and applied to the bedside, this assessment will guide you to recognize what is most and least important so you can identify if an actual problem is present (Benner, Sutphen, Leonard, & Day, 2010).

Remember that clinical data does NOT need to be abnormal to be RELEVANT. Vital signs are ALWAYS vital, and even when normal, are always relevant. For example, consider a patient who just arrived to the floor from the OR who has a temperature of 98.6, HR of 80, RR of 20, BP of 120/80, and O2 sat of 95%. Though all normal parameters, each vital sign parameter is relevant because they support a nursing judgment of clinical stability.

Assess Systematically and Comprehensively

In order to systematically and comprehensively collect assessment data, the nurse must have a thorough and consistent approach in the clinical setting. In order to make a correct clinical judgment, the nurse must have thoroughly collected all patient assessment data. Missing or inaccurate assessment data will lead to an error in clinical judgment and decision making (Alfaro-LeFevre, 2013).

For example, if the nurse does not listen thoroughly to all auscultation sites in a respiratory assessment and fails to recognize new crackles in the bases of her patient with heart failure, this will result in progression of left-sided heart failure that will become insidiously worse over the course of the day until the patient becomes short of breath. This is the reason why a nursing assessment is often called a "head-to-toe assessment." It is meant to be done systematically from the top down! When this is done in practice, it will lead to a thorough and rich collection of data that will recognize clinical problems and advance the plan of care.

Nursing Priority: What Is My PRIORITY?

It is only when students are able to translate classroom theory to the bedside and identify relevant clinical data and prioritize its importance that they will be able to identify the presence of a problem and establish proper nursing priorities. Failure to rescue a patient with a worsening change of status is really a failure to apply clinical reasoning to the assessment and nursing priority steps.

To make priority setting practical, it is imperative that the nurse step back after preparing to assume patient care and ask:

What is the one thing (priority) that I can/must do today to advance the plan of care?

Outcomes/Planning: Think in ACTION

Unless the nursing priority is recognized through assessment of relevant clinical data and a correct judgment made, identified outcomes and planning will be inaccurate. Assessment is like the first of several dominos set upright. Get it right and the series of dominos will fall correctly and in the right direction.

But if the nurse misses relevant data and a problem goes unrecognized, the dominos will also fall, but in the wrong direction! This will ultimately lead to failure to rescue in a patient with a change of status by making an incorrect judgment, leading to the wrong nursing priority, which will lead to an incorrect plan and implementation.

Implementation: Failure to Rescue

Implementation is only as good as the assessment, correct nursing priority, and resultant plan of care. If clinical reasoning has not been correctly situated, patient outcomes will be impacted by NOT implementing needed interventions. This will ultimately lead to failure to rescue. This chain of events can be readily seen during simulation when students are allowed to continue even when essential data is missed and the Sim-Man reflects a status change that can ultimately progress to a full arrest! Unfortunately, this can also happen in practice and can lead to the same outcome!

Evaluation: Think in ACTION

The ability to think in action is also the essence of evaluation. Clinical data is continually collected and response to the plan of care is evaluated by the nurse. But unless the nurse recognizes the relevance and significance of evaluative data that is collected, a change of status, if present, will remain unrecognized. This is why EARLY assessment findings of common complications must be identified so that students will recognize the significance of subtle but significant changes earlier vs. later, when it may be too late.

An excellent example of this principle in practice is when a patient develops sepsis. If early signs of sepsis that include tachycardia but a normal blood pressure are not recognized, when the nurse evaluates the next set of vital signs and finds that the blood pressure has dropped to 78/30, evaluation will identify that a problem is present. Unfortunately, it may be too late to prevent an adverse outcome.

"Five Rights" of Clinical Reasoning

As a nursing student you have memorized the five to ten "rights" of safe medication administration in order to safely administer medications. But are you aware that there are "five rights" of clinical reasoning (Levett-Jones et al., 2010)? These five rights are as important as the rights of safe medication administration to promote patient safety.

Familiarize yourself with these five rights. Incorporate and recite them just as fluently as the medication rights that your program emphasizes! Knowledge of these five rights will deepen your understanding of applied clinical reasoning to practice. These five rights are another way to deeply understand the essence of clinical reasoning and are an easy acronym to guide nurse thinking in the clinical setting.

1. RIGHT Cues

This is the clinical data that is collected and clustered by the nurse. Recognizing the RELEVANCE and RELATIONSHIP of this data and contextualizing it to your specific patient is the essence of this "right." EARLY cues that are missed or not identified and allow a complication to progress is a classic example of "failure to rescue" by the nurse when this "right" is not used in practice.

2. RIGHT Patient

This "right" is not about checking the name and date of birth of your patient, but the ability of the nurse to identify a patient who is high risk for developing a potential complication. The nurse must be able to recognize that an 18-year-old with an appendectomy is not as likely to develop a complication as a patient with the same problem who is 88! Patients who are susceptible hosts due to chemotherapy, radiation, or medications such as prednisone also fall under this "right" as patients at risk.

3. RIGHT Time

This refers to the timeliness of identifying a change of status. Recognizing EARLY signs of a complication and then initiating nursing interventions at the RIGHT time and in the RIGHT sequence is imperative to prevent a bad outcome. Remember that "failure to rescue" occurs not only by missing a complication that develops, but also when nursing/medical interventions are implemented too late.

4. RIGHT Action

Once a clinical judgment is made, the right action or intervention must be initiated. Clinical data that suggest a potential complication must be acted upon. The consequences of an incorrect clinical judgment can make the difference between life and death. In one study, one-half of patients who had cardiac arrests on the hospital floor had clinical signs of deterioration 24 hours before the arrest. These signs were NOT recognized and acted upon by the nurse (Thompson et al., 2008).

5. RIGHT Reason

The right reason is not just making the correct reasoning that leads to a correct nursing judgment, but understanding the RATIONALE or WHY of everything that is done in practice. In order to do this consistently, the nurse must be able to apply key aspects of clinical reasoning, which include grasping the essence of the current situation to put the clinical puzzle together.

Clinical Example

In order to see the relevance of these five rights to clinical practice, I will use the clinical scenario I used in the introduction. Ken was an elderly male patient who had a perforated appendix and was post-operative day #2. Ken was a RIGHT PATIENT who was at high risk for a possible change of status because he was elderly, had an invasive procedure, and his ruptured appendix spilled bacteria into a sterile peritoneum.

Ken developed the RIGHT CUES. He became restless for no apparent reason, his initial BP was normal but his HR was in the 100's. Tachycardia with a normal BP is a classic presentation of EARLY shock as the body compensates for a low output state by increasing heart rate.

If the nurse had correctly interpreted these clinical cues, she would have recognized the possibility of sepsis in the RIGHT TIME and contacted the primary care provider as a RIGHT ACTION to address this concern.

Instead, Ken was given pain medication for restlessness, albuterol neb for tachypnea, and the RIGHT ACTION for the RIGHT REASON did not take place. Had these five rights been correctly acted upon in this scenario, Ken would likely still be alive today.

Why the Patient's Story Matters

Each patient is unique and has a story that the nurse must know. It is not enough to know the primary medical problem and the pathophysiology of this problem. The expert nurse comes to know his or her patients through the stories they share about their health care experiences (Benner, Tanner, & Chesla, 1996). These stories are important because they are unique and represent the journey that gives context to the current clinical scenario. This is an important component of the art of nursing that involves making meaningful connections through listening to and learning from the patient's story (Pesut & Herman, 1999).

When the patient's story is known and understood by the nurse, the next step is to frame the patient's story. Framing creates meaning out of the patient's story and helps distinguish the central or core problem from those that are peripheral. Framing the current clinical situation is like having a lens through which the nurse views the patient's story and is best done through the use of reflection (Pesut & Herman, 1999).

If the nurse does not frame or view the patient's story correctly, the clinical reasoning and judgments that follow will be incorrect as a result. For example, a surgical patient who is in need of pain control may also have a past history of misusing narcotics. If the current story is not properly framed and identified, the nurse has the choice to view this scenario in two different ways.

The nurse could identify frequent requests for pain medications as possible drug-seeking behavior. Or the nurse could see the situation as an appropriate use of pain medications as a result of opioid tolerance and will do what is needed to control the pain.

Make it a priority to engage with and know the story of your patient. This will help you frame each patient appropriately and correctly enhance your ability to be thorough in your thinking and make the correct clinical judgment. This is an excellent example of how the art of nursing must be incorporated into every aspect of the nurse's practice and why it is relevant to everything that the nurse does in practice.

How to Obtain the Story

As an inexperienced or novice nurse, it is all too common to focus on the tasks of patient care and not be tuned in to the patient in your care. In order to frame your patient's current clinical scenario correctly, you must make an effort to engage person to person and allow this patient and his/her story to matter to you as a nurse. This was discussed at length in chapter 3.

The saying that people don't care how much you know until they know how much you care has relevance here. The patient's story can only be known and framed when caring and trust have been established and the patient feels safe sharing with the nurse.

In order to do this, you must avoid all assumptions or judgments that may have been made and come to this person with a clean slate. To obtain the story, while you are providing care or if you are able to sit at the patient's bedside, put down your stethoscope, make eye contact, and ask the following questions. Let the patient lead and share his/her story so you can frame the current situation.

- Tell me about your family (spouse, children, grandchildren, etc.)
- Tell me about your work and what you do (or did) for a living?
- Were there any contributing factors that may have influenced your need for care?
    o Financial
    o Personal stress
    o Chemical dependency (ETOH, etc.)

After collecting this information and framing the patient's story, you are now able to incorporate a framework of clinical reasoning that will guide the step-by-step thinking required to rightly interpret the clinical data that is collected.

Clinical Reasoning Step-by-Step

I have presented an overview of clinical reasoning applied to practice. Though understanding the "big" picture is needed, I have found that this theoretical knowledge does not readily translate to DEEP student understanding and practical application of clinical reasoning to the bedside. Let's make clinical reasoning practical and bring it to the bedside of the next patient you care for in the clinical setting.

I reflected on how I have prepared to care for any patient over my 30 years of clinical practice while collecting data from the chart and in report. What were my priorities when I saw a patient for the first time? From my lens of clinical practice and drawing from the literature, I created a handout (found in appendix E), "Clinical Reasoning Questions to Develop Nurse Thinking" that breaks down clinical reasoning step-by-step. It identifies how a nurse systematically sets and establishes care priorities when preparing for patient care as well as throughout the shift.

These twelve clinical reasoning questions have been derived and adapted from the work of leading nurse educators such as Patricia Benner, Linda Caputi, and Lisa Day, as well as observations from my practice. Therefore, it is grounded on a best practice theoretical foundation and filtered through my lens of extensive clinical experience.

This template is divided into two sections. First, there is a series of eight questions that represent the sequential thinking that is required BEFORE a patient is seen by the nurse. As the nurse reviews the chart and obtains reports, these eight questions must be answered. This section emphasizes the following aspects of clinical reasoning:

- Relevant data collection
- Care planning priorities/interventions
- Nurse vigilance by identifying the worst possible or most likely complication and what to do if it presents

The second half of my template has four questions to guide nurse thinking AFTER the patient is seen for the first time and the nurse has collected clinical assessment data firsthand. These four questions emphasize the following aspects of clinical reasoning:

- Relevance of VS, assessment data collected
- Nursing priority…has it changed?
- Priority educational needs to address
- Rationale of primary care provider's plan of care

These clinical reasoning questions can also be used to replace the traditional care plan (recommend at advanced level) because it combines care planning, nursing process, and clinical reasoning in one form. I have received numerous anecdotal reports from faculty who have successfully incorporated this template into their clinical setting with students instead of a traditional care plan.

Clinical Reasoning Step-by-Step

Formulate and reflect on the following BEFORE providing care:

1. What is the primary problem and what is its underlying cause or pathophysiology?
2. What clinical data from the chart is RELEVANT and needs to be trended because it is clinically significant?
3. List all relevant nursing priorities. Which nursing priority captures the "essence" of your patient's current status and will guide your plan of care?
4. What nursing interventions will you initiate based on this priority and what are the desired outcomes?
5. What body system(s), key assessments, and psychosocial needs will you focus on based on your patient's primary problem or nursing care priority?
6. What is the worst possible/most likely complication(s) to anticipate based on the primary problem?
7. What nursing assessments will identify this complication EARLY if it develops?
8. What nursing interventions will you initiate if this complication develops?

Formulate and reflect on the following WHILE providing care:

9. What clinical assessment data did you just collect that is RELEVANT and needs to be TRENDED because it is clinically significant to detect a change in status?
10. Does your nursing priority or plan of care need to be modified in any way after assessing your patient?
11. After reviewing the primary care provider's note, what is the rationale for any new orders or changes made?
12. What educational priorities have you identified and how will you address them?

To deepen your understanding of this step-by-step template of clinical reasoning and thinking like a nurse in practice, let me briefly explain what is most important and relevant for each of these questions. Then you will be able to incorporate this information into your practice.

Part 1: Reflect on the Following BEFORE Providing Care:

1. *What is the primary problem and what is its underlying cause or pathophysiology?*

This is typically going to be the admission medical problem or diagnosis. The most important aspect of this question is your ability to truly UNDERSTAND the pathophysiology of the illness or the patient's problem. This understanding will lay the foundation for critical thinking by recognizing the clinical relationship and establishing correct nursing care priorities.

As a nurse in practice, you will routinely encounter diseases you barely remember covering in school or not at all. Treating the clinical experience as a puzzle that needs to be solved or viewing the nurse as a detective who needs to understand and uncover the clinical mystery will encourage "clinical curiosity" that must be a central part of every student's practice. Make it a priority to promote your learning by using any available resources or the Internet to research what you do not know or understand about your patient's primary problem. (http://emedicine.medscape.com/ is my favorite resource for this purpose.)

2. *What clinical data from the chart is RELEVANT and clinically significant that needs to be trended?*

This was addressed at length earlier. But one observation I have made as a nurse educator is that students will take as much time as you give them in the clinical setting to collect data on their patient from the medical record. As novice nurses, students do not have an experiential base to recognize relevant clinical data and, therefore, will tend to write down any and everything that is present in the medical record. The ability to filter clinical data and focus on what is RELEVANT takes time and clinical experience to develop. This question is also one of the five "rights" of clinical reasoning, the importance of the nurse to recognize the right cues of clinical data, when a complication begins to become evident (Levett-Jones et al., 2010).

3. *List all relevant nursing priorities. What nursing priority captures the "essence" of your patient's current status and will guide your plan of care?*

Make a list of all relevant nursing care priorities based on your patient's primary medical problem. With most patients, you should be able to identify at least five relevant care priorities. For example, a patient admitted to the med/surg floor with an acute COPD exacerbation would likely have the following nursing priorities:

- Fatigue
- Anxiety
- Activity intolerance
- Impaired gas exchange
- Self-care deficit
- Risk for impaired skin integrity

Once you have made a list of all relevant nursing care priorities, which one captures the essence of the current medical problem? You can use two approaches to make this determination.

Identify a nursing priority/diagnostic statement that is related to an ABC priority. When the primary medical problem is understood, and resultant relationship of the nursing diagnosis of impaired gas exchange is interpreted as a clear "B" breathing priority, this nursing priority would be the best to center the plan of care around because none of the other nursing priorities are a "B" or even "C" priority.

Another way to frame the nursing priority is to identify the relationships between these six care priorities. Which of these nursing priorities have a relationship, connection, or association with one another? The nursing diagnostic statement of impaired gas exchange has a direct relationship to the other diagnostic statements of fatigue, anxiety, activity intolerance, and self-care deficit. This approach will identify impaired gas exchange as the PRIMARY nursing priority with the most direct connections or relationships.

Though not clearly stated in this question, the nurse addresses not only the primary priority and resultant plan of care, but the other nursing care priorities remain relevant and must be included in the plan of care for that day.

I have seen my students struggle with establishing appropriate care priorities in the clinical setting when NANDA-I has been the only way taught to establish nursing priorities. There are some NANDA-I statements that do capture the essence of the nursing priority such as "acute/chronic pain" or "fluid volume excess/deficit", but NANDA-I must not be the only way to establish nursing care priorities for your patient. Nurses in practice don't think this way exclusively and neither should you! There are numerous clinical situations where NANDA-I does not "fit" or even come close to describe the care priority.

I use applied clinical reasoning. I allowed my students to use a concise statement that captures "the essence of the current clinical situation" (Benner, Hooper-Kyriakidis, & Stannard, 2011) that may or may not be a NANDA-I nursing diagnostic statement.

4. *What nursing interventions will you initiate based on this priority and what are the desired outcomes?*

It is important to recognize that questions 2–4 integrate the essence of nursing process by expecting the student to:

- Identify relevant assessment data (assessment)
- Identify correct nursing priority (nursing diagnosis/ priority)
- Initiate nursing interventions (implementation)
- Identify desired or expected outcomes

This is the essence of the nursing care plan, but it is positioned within the framework of applied clinical reasoning. Another aspect of clinical reasoning that is inferred but not clearly specified is the importance and expectation that students are able to identify the RATIONALE for every intervention that is implemented. Correctly stating the rationale ensures safe practice.

5. *What body system(s), key assessments, and psychosocial needs will you focus on based on your patient's primary problem or nursing care priority?*

Though students are taught to perform a systematic head-to-toe assessment for every patient they care for, they must also be able to identify the priority body system as well as psychosocial needs that must be more thoroughly assessed, based on the patient's primary problem or nursing care priority. This is the first step of a two-step process.

Once the priority body system(s) have been identified, the second step is to identify the specific key assessments. This is an essential skill that nurses use in practice, especially when caring for multiple patients. For example, in a patient who is anxious with heart failure exacerbation, the nurse would identify the following priority body systems and perform these key assessments:

Respiratory
- Anterior/posterior breath sounds
- Work of breathing/presence of retractions
- RR/O2 sat

Cardiovascular
- Cardiac rhythm
- BP/HR
- Color
- Cap refill/strength of peripheral pulses
- Edema

Holistic care is the hallmark of nursing practice. Psychosocial needs that include emotional as well as spiritual needs must be considered as no less significant than the physical needs that demand immediate attention. Any physiologic problem can cause anxiety, fear, and stress. How is your patient coping as a result of requiring medical and nursing care? This must be considered and assessed as well as the more pressing physical needs. In this same scenario of heart failure exacerbation, the following psychosocial assessments:

Psychosocial
- Encourage verbalization of feelings/anxiety to assess underlying influencing factors
- Determine if anxiety is related to SOB or primary problem

6. *What is the worst possible/most likely complication(s) to anticipate based on the primary problem?*

Identifying the most likely or worst possible complication BEFORE patient care is assumed is an essential critical thinking skill applied to practice. This is the importance of being PROACTIVE vs. REACTIVE and it can make a difference in improving patient outcomes. When a problem is anticipated and identified EARLY in practice, the nurse is one step ahead. But when the nurse is caught completely off guard by a sudden change of status, they are caught "flat-footed" and are one step behind. The problem will likely be more serious because it has been recognized LATER. Sepsis that progresses to septic shock is a common clinical occurrence with potential life-threatening consequences if treatment is delayed.

7. *What nursing assessments will identify this complication EARLY if it develops?*

Once the worst possible/most likely complication is identified, the specific assessments to recognize it correctly must be determined. EARLY recognition of any complication is essential to good patient outcomes. If early signs that tend to be more subtle go unrecognized, an adverse outcome and even death is possible.

For example, if sepsis/septic shock is the most likely complication, the EARLY assessments that the nurse would need to cluster to confirm its presence and then initiate "rescue" are

- Temperature: fever >100.8 or <96.8

- HR: >90
- BP: downward trend with mean arterial pressure (MAP) <65
- WBC <4,000 or > 12,000

8. What nursing interventions will you initiate if this complication develops?

If you look at these last three questions (6–8) closely, they follow the pattern of putting nursing process and nursing plan of care in the context of the most likely/worst possible complication. The potential PRIORITY complication is identified, assessments to conclusively recognize are listed so this problem does not remain hidden, and then nursing interventions to initiate "rescue" can be implemented if needed. This is another "nurse thinking" skill that is not typically taught in nursing education, yet it captures the essence of how nurses in practice prioritize and provide safe care.

Nurse as Lifeguard

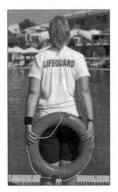
Have you ever thought of the similarities that a nurse has with a lifeguard? Just as a lifeguard continually and vigilantly scans the water for signs of a struggling swimmer, the nurse must also look vigilantly to assess for a deteriorating change of status, in order to rescue a patient who may be experiencing a complication. TRENDING all clinical data and assessing EARLY signs and symptoms must be done so that a complication is not allowed to needlessly progress. There is a short distance and time frame between the body's ability to compensate and the "swirl" of decompensation (Scott, 2009). For example, in sepsis that progresses to septic shock, the body can briefly compensate by elevating heart rate and maintaining blood pressure – but not for long before the bottom literally falls out!

A distinction between a novice and more experienced nurse is that a more experienced nurse anticipates potential problems, recognizes the significance of clinical cues, and practices PROACTIVELY to PREVENT a possible patient complication (Levett-Jones et al., 2010). Novice nursing students tend to practice REACTIVELY. They don't anticipate potential problems, and react to them after they have already developed (Levett-Jones et al., 2010).

Because of clinical inexperience, there is a lack of clinical reasoning skills by the novice nurse. This can contribute to adverse patient outcomes that can progress to a bad outcome and even patient death. The primary reason for these adverse outcomes include failure to properly identify the problem after it develops, failure to initiate appropriate nursing interventions, and inappropriate management of the complication once it is present.

When analyzing a new graduate's ability to think critically, especially in the context of a change of status, del Bueno (2005) identified the following four questions that help a nurse anticipate a change of status. You will see that there is some overlap and correlation to these questions and the essence of clinical reasoning. Following each question are additional subtopics that will practically situate this content:

1. Can the nurse recognize there is a problem?

Until the problem is recognized, no action will be taken by the nurse. To recognize a problem, the nurse must do the following:

- Recognize RELEVANT clinical data.
- INTERPRET clinical data correctly (Tanner, 2006)
- Identify medical/nursing PRIORITY
- Identify the most likely WORST POSSIBLE COMPLICATION for your patient.
- Intentional vigilance. LOOKING for this complication and trending all RELEVANT clinical data and required assessments over time.

2. Can the nurse manage the problem safely and effectively?

- Proper nursing interventions initiated based on current problem once identified.

3. Does the nurse have a relative sense of URGENCY?

- Lack of clinical experience often causes students to not recognize the need for urgency. I have seen new nurses have a patient with a status change of sepsis, yet have no sense of urgency when his BP has dropped to 70/30!

4. Does the nurse take the right action for the right reason?

- Once the problem is identified the RATIONALE for nursing/medical interventions is able to be stated.
- Nurse contacts the physician promptly to initiate needed interventions.

Del Bueno's research identified the importance of a nurse's ability to RECOGNIZE a problem before rescue can take place. It is only when a problem is recognized that the nurse will intervene and do something about it. How does one not only identify a problem but at the same time specify the desired outcome? Problems and outcomes are complementary and need to be considered concurrently. When the desired outcome is juxtaposed with the current clinical status, this will create a contrast that will guide nursing interventions and progression in the plan of care (Pesut & Herman, 1998).

To help you DEEPLY understand the importance of early identification of a complication and initiate "rescue" if needed, I will use a metaphor of "Jason," the serial killer from the "Friday the 13th" horror movie series. Remind yourself that Jason is still out there...

Looking for "Jason"...the Worst Possible Complication

Do you remember "Jason" from the original *Friday the 13th* slasher/horror movies from the 1980s? Teenagers are murdered one by one as they attempt to reopen an abandoned campground. Since I graduated from high school in 1981, and the first of many in this series started in 1980, I remember all too well the classic ending from the original when it first came out.

Only Alice survived the terrifying night at Camp Crystal Lake. As morning came, she was on a small boat in the middle of the lake. All is calm and quiet, the birds are singing and she has no reason to be concerned. Out of nowhere, Jason leaps out of the water and grabs Alice and takes her down...but it was only a dream and a movie.

No reason to fear and look for Jason any longer, right? WRONG! Jason is still out there and lurks around the corner of every clinical setting! Who is "Jason"? He is a metaphor for the worst possible/most likely complication any patient may experience. "Jason" is still very deadly, and he has new identities such as sepsis, septic shock, post-op bleed, pulmonary embolism, and cardiac arrest, to name only a few.

Clinical vigilance is required to keep "Jason" from harming your patients. If you are looking for him, you will recognize the "Jason" of the worst possible complications before it is too late! It is only when the nurse loses this sense of vigilance and forgets that "Jason" is still out there that complications go unnoticed until it is often too late.

Even if everything appears uneventful and your patient appears stable, just like Alice on the boat, things can change quickly. That is why nurse vigilance is always required in practice.

Sepsis is the most common "Jason" and hides early with subtle changes such as a low-grade temperature, slight hypotension, and tachycardia. When the nurse does not recognize the significance of these findings, tachycardia will persist as "Jason" continues to have his way and sepsis progresses to septic shock. It is only when "Jason" is RECOGNIZED that his power to destroy is broken and your patient can be RESCUED from an adverse outcome.

Most Common "Jasons"

At the large metropolitan hospital where I practice there is a "Rapid Response Team" (RRT) that rounds the hospital 24/7, circulating and responding to calls from nurses who identify a possible change in status that may indicate a need to rescue. Based on statistical data compiled where I practice as to why a RRT is paged, students can anticipate these most common changes of status in the acute care setting (see table).

In addition to discussing the implications for each of these most common changes in patient status, I will highlight the most important assessments that I use in practice to quickly identify the scope of the potential problem.

Most Common Patient Complications
1. Chest pain
2. Increased respiratory distress
3. Hypotension
4. Change in level of consciousness (LOC) or neurologic status
5. Falls

Top Five Change of Status in Order of Frequency

1. Chest Pain

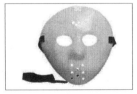

Regardless of the practice setting, the nurse needs to evaluate and assess chest pain in such diverse settings as phone triage, outpatient clinics, and community health clinics. In acute care, this is by far the most common reason an RRT is paged. The good news is that most chest pain is NOT cardiac. However, it can still be a potential problem because pneumonia and a pulmonary embolus can also cause this complaint. I encourage the use of mnemonics such as W-I-L-D-A or P-Q-R-S-T (these will be discussed later) to help you concisely and systematically assess and document any complaint of pain.

If a patient has a complaint of chest pain, it is essential to perform the following assessments to differentiate cardiac vs. noncardiac chest pain. If available in your practice setting, a 12-lead EKG is a standard tool to determine if there are new changes consistent with ischemia. What are these changes? In early ischemia, the T waves that are normally rounded and upright may be flattened or inverted. The ST segment after the QRS complex may be elevated or depressed more than 1 mm.

In addition to the EKG, remember to look at your patient! Does he look as if he is in distress? Has his color changed from pink, warm, and dry to pale, cool, and diaphoretic? Is he anxious, restless? Are other subtle but apparent changes present? If present, this validates that his current complaint is likely more serious. In addition to an EKG, the following nursing assessments must be implemented to put this clinical puzzle together and differentiate the primary problem.

Take a deep breath
- If taking a deep breath causes the pain to dramatically increase, then this chest pain is most likely noncardiac. But pleurisy, pneumonia, and a pulmonary embolus also cause pleuritic chest pain. The next assessment to help clarify the cause of this chest pain is palpation.

Palpate the area of pain for reproducible tenderness
- Gently but firmly palpate the location of where the pain is present. If the pain is reproducible with palpation, this is most likely noncardiac and is likely pleurisy, an inflammation of the pleura that is non-emergent.

Location of the pain
- There are gender differences of cardiac chest pain. For example, women tend to have a higher likelihood of nonclassic symptoms that include epigastric pain as well as referred pain with no anterior chest pain. For most patients though, cardiac chest pain will be anterior chest pain in a large, general area of the chest. If the pain is localized to a very small area that the patient can point to, this is typically NOT associated with angina.

Presence of other complaints consistent with cardiac ischemia
- In addition to the primary location of chest pain, cardiac chest pain typically consists of referred pain to the neck, back, jaw, or arms. It is important for the nurse to determine the presence of this referred pain. Shortness of breath (SOB) is also a common component of cardiac chest pain related to coronary artery disease, myocardial ischemia, or pulmonary embolus.

Length of pain
- This will help differentiate cardiac from noncardiac chest pain because angina will typically last longer than five minutes. If the patient reports that her pain lasts for just a few seconds at a time, or less than a minute, this pain is likely noncardiac.

Character of pain
- It is important to distinguish if the nature or character of this pain is similar to any prior history of heartburn or GERD. If it is, this again is likely noncardiac. Cardiac chest pain is most commonly a diffuse pressure, tightness, squeezing, or achiness.

2. *Increased Respiratory Distress/O2 sat <90%*

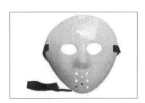 If a patient complains of shortness of breath and/or has decreased oxygenation, immediate intervention and relevant assessments are required. Use the same principle of, "How does my patient look?" If he looks like he is in distress, he most likely is! In addition to general appearance, the following are the most relevant assessments that must be closely trended over time:

Respiratory rate

- Rate > 20 is a clinical RED FLAG and likely represents distress, anxiety, or both!

Heart rate

- Rate >100 is a clinical RED FLAG and will be elevated with physiologic distress caused by sympathetic nervous system stimulation. The nurse must be able to situate knowledge and determine the most likely reason WHY!

O2 saturation

- Saturation <90% is a clinical RED FLAG that is reflecting hypoxia in a non-COPD patient. With any complaint of SOB, immediately obtain the oxygen saturation to determine the baseline with this change of status, and then administer supplemental oxygenation and titrate to oxygen saturation greater than 92%.

Breath sounds

- Posterior auscultation FIRST if possible, then anterior. There is less subcutaneous fat posterior and you'll be able to detect adventitious breath sounds more readily. Listen carefully to all lobes, especially the bases. Compare each lobe right to left.
- Rales or crackles typically represent fluid seen in the alveoli with heart failure. Rhonchi is most commonly seen with pneumonia. Wheezing or very-diminished aeration is typical with asthmatic or COPD exacerbation. However, an audible wheeze may be present in heart failure due to fluid in the alveoli causing bronchial constriction. This is referred to as cardiac asthma.

3. Hypotension

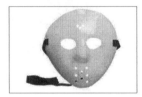

This can be caused by many things, but the most common is fluid volume loss/deficit related to bleeding, dehydration, or sepsis. If the nurse has been carefully trending the systolic blood pressure and it is running 30+ points lower than baseline, or if the systolic blood pressure is less than 100, this is a clinical RED FLAG. If the systolic blood pressure has been trending 130–140 consistently and now it is 100–110, though not less than 100, this is still a RED FLAG. The nurse must step back and ask WHY?

Remember the relevance of this formula of cardiac output to clinical practice:

$$CO=SV \times HR$$

With any shock or volume-depleted state, the earliest compensatory response by the body is to INCREASE heart rate in response to DECREASED cardiac output. The finding of low blood pressure with tachycardia demands an immediate response. When a low blood pressure trend is identified, the following priority assessments must be clustered and trended with the current blood pressure to determine the most likely complication that is beginning to manifest.

General appearance

- Does he appear in any distress or is the patient tolerating the decrease in BP? The nurse needs to make a clinical judgment if the patient is unstable. This finding will help determine the urgency you need to have in this clinical situation.

Skin

- If he is in distress with sympathetic nervous system stimulation, he will likely be pale, cool, and diaphoretic. In early shock, his extremities will be cooler when compared centrally by touching his forehead. If a patient is cool centrally and this is a new finding, this is an urgent situation and must be recognized as such.

Pulses

- The pulses must be taken while assessing the coolness or warmth of the extremities. If the pulses are already more difficult to palpate than a prior assessment, this is a critical RED FLAG. It most likely represents a shock state as the body shunts volume centrally from the periphery. Palpate pulses together at the same time to assess any significant differences.

Temperature

- A complete set of vital signs, including the temperature, is essential with a low blood pressure. The most common complication that must be ruled out is SEPSIS. An elevated temperature with a low blood pressure is a classic finding with sepsis. With the elderly, it is not uncommon to have a temperature less than 96.8 when septic. This is a clinical RED FLAG that must be recognized.

Heart rate

- The expected physiologic response to volume depletion and a low blood pressure is tachycardia, which is an early sign of physiologic compensatory mechanisms. If the patient is NOT tachycardic with a low blood pressure, it is important for the nurse to look at his daily medications. What medication will influence the finding of a normal heart rate in a shock state? Any beta blocker will prevent the heart rate from being elevated, even when the sympathetic nervous system is activated!

Respiratory rate

- It is important to note the respiratory rate because of its relationship to shock. If your patient is in any form of progressive shock state, he will likely be tachypneic.

Blood pressure

- The most important finding related to blood pressure is the current trend and the direction it is going. Remember that even if the SBP is >100 but has dropped by 30+ mm/Hg recently from prior assessments, the nurse should recognize this as a clinical RED FLAG.

4. *Change in LOC or Neurologic Status*

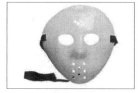 Whenever there is a change in neurologic status, it is important for the nurse to determine the most obvious reason. For example, if a patient just received a dose of IV hydromorphone (Dilaudid) and now is more lethargic and difficult to arouse, narcotic over-sedation is the most likely cause. Instead of beginning with the assumption that this is a stroke, begin with this obvious assumption and cluster clinical data from there. Since the brain is dependent on adequate blood pressure for optimal function, a change in LOC and even confusion can result from a sudden decrease in blood pressure from the patient's norm or low blood glucose.

Though narcotic over-sedation is the most common reason for a clinical change and altered level of consciousness, the nurse must also be vigilant for the possibility of a stroke with any of the following NEW assessment findings:

Facial droop

- This is always a clinical RED FLAG. If facial droop is present, a complete neuro assessment must be immediately initiated. This finding can be subtle; just the corner of the mouth may be level while the other side moves or is elevated in comparison. If the nurse is suspicious that this is present, simply have the patient smile BIG and show their teeth. It will be obvious if a droop is present.

Hemiparesis

- Weakness on either side of the body that may or may not involve both upper and lower extremities is also a clinical RED FLAG. It is not uncommon for an upper extremity to have weakness, but the lower extremity of the impaired side to have normal strength.

Slurred speech

- If the patient has slurred speech or expressive or receptive aphasia, this is a clinical RED FLAG that is consistent with a stroke. The nurse must recognize the significance and the need to make this patient NPO until this has been ruled out.

Confusion or disorientation

- This finding can be generalized to other problems besides a stroke, but if present and no medications have been given that would alter the patient's level of consciousness, this becomes more concerning and a thorough neurologic assessment must be initiated by the nurse. This is also an early sign of ETOH withdrawal.

Cincinnati Pre-Hospital Stroke Scale

A simple, focused neurologic assessment that students should be taught and can quickly determine the possibility of a stroke is called the "Cincinnati Pre-Hospital Stroke Scale" (Kothari, Pancioli, Liu, Brott, & Broderick, 1999). It consists of three assessments that may indicate a patient is having a stroke. Though designed for emergency medical staff in pre-hospital care, it can guide nurses in any clinical setting if there is cause for concern with any new neurologic changes.

Patients with one of these three findings as a new event have a 72 percent probability of an ischemic stroke. If all three findings are present, the probability of an acute stroke is more than 85 percent. Even if students may not be confident in their comprehensive neuro-assessment skills, this will simplify what is NEED TO KNOW in this context of a change in neurological status.

Three Essential Assessments

1. **Facial droop:** Have the patient smile or show his or her teeth. If one side doesn't move as well as the other or it seems to droop, this is clinically significant and a possible stroke.
   - *Normal:* Both sides of face move equally.
   - *Abnormal:* One side of face does not move as well as the other.
2. **Arm drift:** Have the patient close his or her eyes and hold his or her arms straight out in front, palms up for about 10 seconds. If one arm does not move, or one arm drifts down more than the other, this is clinically significant and a possible stroke.
   - *Normal:* Both arms stay level and do NOT drift.
   - *Abnormal:* One arm does not move, or one arm drifts down compared with the other side.
3. **Speech:** Have the patient say, "You can't teach an old dog new tricks," or some other simple, familiar saying. If the person slurs the words, gets some words wrong, or is unable to speak, this is clinically significant and a possible stroke.
   - *Normal:* Patient uses correct words with no slurring.

- *Abnormal:* Slurred or inappropriate words or mute.

F–A–S–T

FAST is an easy to remember mnemonic that will also help students to recognize a neurological change of status using the same assessment data used in the Cincinnati Pre-Hospital Stroke Scale ("Spot a Stroke," n.d.).

Face

- Facial droop present?

Arm

- Arm drift?

Speech

- Slurred or aphasic?

Time

- Time is of the essence if any of these symptoms present! Get medical assistance immediately!

5. Falls

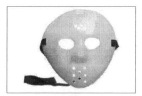
The most important nursing PRIORITY is to determine the MECHANISM OF INJURY related to the fall. If the patient fell in such a way that he has complaints of pain, or may have hit his head, he may require cervical spine immobilization by the RRT nurse. He must be kept perfectly still until this immobilization takes place and a cervical spine injury is ruled out. Additional relevant neurologic assessments that can be made by the nurse include:

- Level of consciousness (LOC)
- Movement of all extremities
- Numbness, weakness, tingling in any extremity

Part 2: Reflect on the Following WHILE Providing Care:

9. What clinical assessment data did you just collect that is RELEVANT and needs to be TRENDED because it is clinically significant to detect a change in status?

As novice nurses, students consistently struggle with recognizing what is clinically relevant or MOST important. In addition to recognizing relevant data, the student must also consistently compare or TREND the data that was collected and put it side by side with data received in report or last recorded in the chart. Has anything changed? Were any of the findings unexpected? Do they require further assessment or an SBAR to the physician? Because patients rarely stay static but can change quickly, trending all clinical data will encourage nurse vigilance, and trigger the need to "rescue" if there is a change in status.

10. Does your nursing priority or plan of care need to be modified in any way after assessing your patient (include psychosocial priorities)?

Clinical reasoning is the ability of the nurse to think in action and reason as a situation changes (Benner, Sutphen, Leonard, & Day, 2010). Nurse thinking is fluid and NOT rigid. Continually reevaluate the nursing priority and plan of care based on the data that was just collected. VS and nursing assessment must never be seen as a TASK to check off a list, but an opportunity to THINK in action and make a nursing judgment regarding the CURRENT status of your patient.

In order to advance the plan of care, the nurse must know the desired outcome(s). Once the desired outcome from the nursing priority is identified, the nurse must compare and contrast this desired outcome with clinical data that is assessed to determine clinical progression. This systematic approach will make it clearly evident if the patient is progressing as expected or not. It is then the nurse's responsibility to implement interventions to move the patient from the current problem state to the desired outcome (Kautz, Kuiper, Pesut, & Williams, 2006).

11. After reviewing the primary care provider's note, what is the rationale for any new orders or changes made?

Though the nurse is not the primary care provider, it is essential to understand the essence of the primary care provider's plan of care and the rationale for any changes in orders that have been made. The daily progress note or most recent documentation by the primary care provider is a "must read" by the nurse to clearly understand these priorities and benefit from the primary care provider's perspective on the patient. When the primary care provider note is understood and this knowledge dovetails with the data the nurse has collected, the clinical puzzle begins to come together.

12. What educational priorities have you identified and how will you address them?

The professional nurse is also an educator. Embrace the responsibility of this role. This is NOT just another task. When done in a way that promotes patient learning and understanding, it can improve patient outcomes and even prevent hospital readmissions. You cannot teach what you do not fully understand. Make this an incentive to deeply learn content so it can be taught effectively to your patients.

Every patient has a need for education to promote his/her health and care. A practical approach to assess patient knowledge when administering medications is to ask, "Do you know what this is for?" If the patient is unable to answer, you can reinforce or choose to address any knowledge deficits another time during that clinical. Additional practical information to effectively educate your patients and families will be discussed in chapter 10.

Clinical Judgment: End Result of Nurse Thinking

Making a correct clinical judgment is a complex process that is directly influenced by the clinical experience of the nurse and by what the nurse brings to the patient care scenario, including the ability of the nurse to use knowledge and grasp the essence of the current clinical scenario by using the skill of clinical reasoning. Clinical judgment is influenced by how well the nurse knows the patient based on prior clinical experience and the level of engagement that leads to recognizing subtle differences that are clinically significant (Cappelletti, Engel, & Prentice, 2014).

Though clinical reasoning has been emphasized in this chapter so it can be incorporated into your practice, it is NOT the end point of nurse thinking. It's a critical component in the equation of clinical practice to make a correct clinical judgment. What do you decide to do with the data you have collected? Will you act now, or wait? The decision the nurse makes when interpreting clinical data is the essence of making a clinical judgment.

The following summarizes the equation of nurse thinking that is required for safe clinical practice (Alfaro-Lefevre, 2013):

Critical Thinking + Clinical Reasoning = Correct Clinical Judgment

Because clinical judgment is the end result and hallmark of professional practice, it must be properly defined and understood. Tanner (2006) defines clinical judgment as an interpretation or conclusion about what a patient needs and/or the decision to take action or not. Good clinical judgment requires the nurse to be flexible, recognize what is most important, interpret the meaning of this clinical data, and respond appropriately.

Clinical decision making is when the nurse selects interventions that move the patient from their current state toward progression to the desired goal or outcome (Pesut & Herman, 1999). Another way to define nursing clinical judgment is to use clinical reflection to contrast the present clinical status and the desired state. Utilize specific criteria to identify if the desired outcome state has been achieved, and then make a conclusion or clinical judgment if the desired outcome has been attained (Kautz, Kuiper, Pesut, & Williams, 2006).

To make a correct clinical judgment, clinical reasoning selects from all alternatives, understands the rationale for each alternative, collects and recognizes the significance of clinical data, processes this information to understand the current problem, and identifies the current care priority and plan of care (Levett–Jones et al., 2010).

Clinical judgments are made on a continual and ongoing basis in practice. In one study, on a typical med/surg floor over an eight-hour shift, the nurse engaged in an average of 50 significant clinical reasoning concerns that required a clinical judgment (Thompson, Cullum, McCaughan, Sheldon, & Raynor, 2004).

Clinical Judgment Step-by-Step

Tanner (2006) has developed a model that breaks down clinical judgment in four steps. This can help students strengthen their ability to make correct judgments by identifying breakdowns and using reflection to identify areas of growth.

The four steps Tanner identified are:

1. *Noticing*

    Can the nurse identify the most relevant clinical data and why? Though this can be part of nursing assessment, it is really much more. It emphasizes the nurse's expectations of the current clinical situation. If the patient is presenting in a way that is expected or unexpected, a decision can be made based on the nurse's textbook knowledge that is used and applied as well as prior clinical experience. When the nurse contrasts and juxtaposes the desired outcome with the present status, this will help to facilitate the ability to notice what clinical data is relevant (Pesut & Herman, 1998).

2. *Interpreting*

Once the essence of the current clinical situation is grasped and relevant clinical data identified, this data must now be interpreted. What does this data mean and what is its significance? Unless a nurse has a deep understanding of the applied sciences, especially pathophysiology, the ability to correctly interpret data will be impacted.

3. *Responding*

Based on the correct interpretation, does the nurse need to ACT or rescue, or is further monitoring warranted?

4. *Reflecting*

A nurse needs to develop two aspects of reflection. Reflection-IN-action is the ability of the nurse to "read" the patient and her response to CURRENT nursing interventions and adjust what is done based on the patient's response.

Reflection-ON-action is done AFTERward. It completes the four-step cycle by determining what can be learned from what was just experienced and how that experience will contribute to ongoing clinical knowledge development. This is especially important if an error in judgment occurred. The nurse needs to learn and grow from her mistake.

In order to understand these two important aspects of nurse reflection, let's take a closer look at each of these principles to strengthen your ability to use reflection to strengthen your ability to think like a nurse.

Reflection-IN-Action

Reflection-IN-action is the nurse's ability to accurately interpret the patient's response to an intervention in the moment as the events are unfolding. You have just administered narcotic pain medication to your surgical patient and have just reassessed the response. This is the essence of reflection-in-action. It is the ability of the nurse to interpret the patient response to CURRENT nursing interventions and adjust what is done based on the evaluation of the patient's response. The medication's effectiveness of pain relief would determine your next step in making a clinical judgment.

Though this was a simple scenario, the nurse will make numerous clinical judgments throughout the shift based on every intervention that is utilized to advance the plan of care. To strengthen the ability of the nurse to accurately reflect in action and to make consistently correct clinical judgments, the nurse can use these three questions to reflect and transfer learning from each clinical experience to the next. Whenever the nurse is required to make a clinical judgment, ask:

1. What can I learn from this?
2. What would I do differently (if applicable) in this situation?
3. How can I use what has been learned from this situation to improve patient care in the future?

Reflection-ON-Action

Reflection-ON-action refers to the nurse's ability to reflect upon a situation that required a clinical judgment and identify what can be learned from it retrospectively and after the fact. This typically involves a more thorough and comprehensive reflection on a significant event in the clinical setting.

This level of reflection is needed when the nurse may have misinterpreted clinical cues that led to an adverse outcome or when an error in practice is made. Nurses will at times make mistakes in practice. This is expected, but the nurse must make it a priority to learn as much as possible from errors made in practice so it does not happen again! To guide this level of reflection that will lead to strengthening the thinking and clinical judgment of the nurse, use the following framework:

- **Description.** Describe the patient situation.

- **Feelings.** How did you feel? What were you thinking and feeling?

- **Evaluation.** How did you or others react? What problems did you experience? What challenged you?

- **Analysis.** Explore details by determining the real problem. Why was the problem encountered? What did you base judgments on? Were these assumptions accurate?

- **Conclusion.** Make a decision to determine what really happened. What was done well? What could have been done differently? Could you have responded differently?

- **Action plan.** Where do you go from here? Make a plan to do what is needed to maximize learning. Is additional knowledge or training needed? (Koharchik, Caputi, Robb, & Culleiton, 2015)

Strategies to Develop Clinical Judgment

Just as it takes time and clinical experience to develop and progress from a novice to the next stage of professional development as a nurse, the same is true with your ability to develop clinical judgment (Alfero-LeFevre, 2013). Be fully engaged in the clinical setting to maximize your learning and the clinical experience for all its worth. The following are some practical strategies to grow in your ability to make correct clinical judgments:

- **Become familiar with what is "normal" so the abnormal becomes readily apparent.** This principle is not only true for nurses but also for bank tellers! One effective strategy bank tellers are taught to identify counterfeit bills is to handle the original bills that represent what is authentic and normal. Once they become familiar with the feel and appearance of a normal bill, the abnormal counterfeit is easily recognized.

  In the same way in the clinical setting, make it a priority to establish and compare normal lab values, vital sign parameters, and assessment findings so that abnormal data collected in practice is immediately recognized. For example, once you know and understand the normal heart tones of S1S2, you compare this to every set of heart tones you listen to with your patients. Abnormal heart sounds such as murmurs and S3,S4 gallops are readily recognized when compared to what is normal.

- **Know your pathophysiology.** Once the pathophysiology of a problem is deeply understood, clinical data is correctly interpreted and signs and symptoms of a worsening progression or improvement become readily apparent. Once the pathophysiology of sepsis is understood, the significance of an elevated temperature, tachycardia, and elevated WBC and neutrophils are recognized as clinical concerns. Conversely, when the temperature, WBC, and tachycardia return to normal ranges, this clinical data can be correctly interpreted for the clinical improvement that is clearly evident.

- **Reflect on all clinical data that you collect and record.** As a novice nurse, resist the temptation to see vital signs and nursing assessments as just another task to complete and document in the chart. REFLECT on what you have collected and compare it to the most recent data to establish trends. Is the data collected expected or unexpected based on your report and the primary problem? By taking the time to REFLECT, you will be much more likely to accurately INTERPRET the data, which will make it much more likely that it will lead to a correct clinical judgment.

- **Authentically care.** When the nurse is engaged and empathetically cares, this personal/professional engagement results in heightened vigilance or attentiveness that will lead to better patient outcomes.

CHAPTER 9 HIGHLIGHTS

- The definition of clinical reasoning is the nurse's ability to think in action and reason as a situation changes over time by capturing and understanding the significance of clinical trajectories and grasping the essence of the current clinical situation.

- Clinical reasoning can be broken down into four components that include identifying the priority, rationale for plan of care, and trending relevant clinical data, which allows the nurse to grasp the essence of the current clinical situation.

- Though nursing process and clinical reasoning are separate components of nurse thinking, they complement one another in the clinical setting.

- By utilizing clinical reasoning, the nurse functions as a lifeguard in the clinical setting by recognizing a potential complication early before it is allowed to needlessly progress.

- There are 12 sequential questions that the nurse can use to clinically reason, regardless of the clinical setting.

- The most common complications in the acute care setting include chest pain, increased respiratory distress, hypotension, change in level of consciousness, and falls.

- In order to make a correct clinical judgment, the nurse must be able to utilize both critical thinking and clinical reasoning.

- The four steps that the nurse must use to make a correct clinical judgment include noticing a potential problem, interpreting clinical data, responding appropriately, and reflecting in action taken as well as reflecting on action.

- Reflection-in-action is simply the nurse's ability to interpret accurately the patient's response to intervention.

- Reflection-on-action refers to the nurse's ability to reflect upon a situation that required a clinical judgment and identify what can be learned from it.

Additional Resources

- Book: *Clinical Wisdom and Interventions in Acute and Critical Care, Second Edition: A Thinking-in-Action Approach* (2011) by Patricia Benner, Patricia Hooper Kyriakidis, & Daphne Stannard
- Book: *Critical Thinking, Clinical Reasoning and Clinical Judgment 5th ed.* (2011) by Rosalinda Alfaro-LeFevre

Chapter Reflections

1. To capture the essence of clinical reasoning, define clinical reasoning in your own words.

2. What does a nurse have in common with a lifeguard?

3. What are the most common "Jasons" in your clinical setting?

4. For those complications most commonly seen in your clinical setting, what nursing interventions will you initiate if this complication develops?

5. What nursing assessments will identify this complication EARLY if it develops?

Since I have become a nurse I triage my laundry and have decided that none of it requires immediate attention.

Chapter 10
Essentials of Clinical Practice

People will forget what you said, they will forget what you did,
but they will never forget how you made them feel!
–Maya Angelou

Nursing is a practice-based profession. It is not enough to KNOW what to do, you must be able to translate all that you have been taught in the classroom, clinical, and skills lab to the bedside of direct patient care where it matters most. In this chapter I will highlight key aspects of nursing that will strengthen your practice and confidence when you care for patients in the clinical setting. The following topics related to clinical practice will be discussed in this chapter:

- Practical pearls of physical/nursing assessment
- The nurse is an educator
- Principles of priority setting and time management
- Principles of proper delegation
- The nurse is a leader

Practical Pearls of Physical/Nursing Assessment

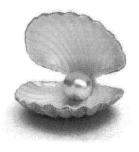 Nurses must be able to identify EARLY changes that are subtle yet clinically significant. This requires thoroughness and attention to detail as well as clinical experience. As you acquire clinical experience, pay attention to your sense of intuition, the thought or feeling that something may not be quite right. Intuition leads to further investigation, which may then lead to intervention (Scott, 2009). I have cared for patients who had just a slight change in skin color from pink to pale-pink and slightly moist skin that aroused concern and led to further investigation and identified a change in status.

Below are some "clinical pearls" that I have derived from my clinical experience and have taught to my students. These pearls on nursing assessment will help you build on what you have been taught and can use this knowledge to perform nursing assessments thoroughly and with attention to detail.

Vital Signs

- Do NOT use the heart rate found on the blood pressure machine or oximeter when you collect VS. These can be inaccurate and are influenced by a number of variables. Spend the extra 15 to 30 seconds and palpate a radial or auscultate an apical pulse to ensure accuracy.

- Validate the accuracy of every oximeter reading obtained with a radial or apical pulse. In order for an oximeter reading to be validated, the heart rate on the oximeter must be within four to eight beats of what was palpated. If the heart rates do not correlate, the oximeter reading may not be accurate. Another reason may be an irregular pulse if the patient is in atrial fibrillation. This is an especially important assessment validation to do whenever the oximeter reading is <90%!
- Be sure to use the right size BP cuff. Though this is going back to fundamentals, I routinely find cuffs in practice that are clearly too large or too small for my patients from the prior nurse. If the cuff is too large, the numbers will skew lower than actual, and if too small, the numbers will skew higher than actual.
- Remember that if your stethoscope has a bell, this should be used because it auscultates the low tones more readily than a diaphragm.
- If your patient has a PICC (peripherally inserted central catheter) in the upper arm or is obese with thick upper arms, use the lower forearm with a smaller cuff instead. As long as the cuff is the correct size and the pulse arrow is on top of the radial pulse, I have found this to be accurate with minimal difference compared to the traditional upper arm location. Be sure to document that this location was used to ensure consistency and trend of this measurement.

Pain Assessment

A thorough assessment of pain must be more than the patient's report of pain and collecting data using these mnemonics in practice. Vital signs are still vital as well as relevant neurological assessment that includes LOC as well as size of pupils with any assessment of pain. Since pain is such a common assessment, I use two mnemonics that help to concisely and systematically assess any complaint of pain:

W-I-L-D-A
W–*Words*…that describe the pain
I–*Intensity*…scale of 1 to 10
L–*Location*…specific location of pain
D–*Duration*…how long has the pain lasted/intermittent or continuous
A–*Aggravating/Alleviating factors*…what makes the pain worse or what makes the pain better

P-Q-R-S-T
P–*Provoke/Palliative*…what makes the pain worse or what makes the pain better
Q–*Quality*…words that describe the pain
R–*Radiation*…does the pain radiate to other parts of the body
S–*Severity*…scale of 1 to 10
T–*Timing*…how long has the pain lasted/intermittent or continuous

In addition to using these mnemonics to perform any pain assessment, be sure to step back and ask the following question for any patient complaint of pain:

Is this pain EXPECTED or UNEXPECTED for my patient based on the reason they are in the clinical setting? For example, incisional pain that is localized to the abdomen that is severe on day of surgery or day #1 after surgery is obviously expected. Abdominal pain three to four days later that is generalized, severe, and combined with assessment findings of firm, distended abdomen, nausea and vomiting is NOT expected and could be an ileus or bowel obstruction that must be recognized by the nurse as being clinically significant.

Head-to-Toe Nursing Assessment

Respiratory

Breath sounds

- Posterior auscultation is always preferred because there is less body tissue and adventitious breath sounds can readily be identified if present. Remember, the right lower lobe is easier to auscultate from the back. The right middle lobe is found under the axilla at the mid-line. This will be the first place that early pneumonia from aspiration is generally heard and is often missed by nurses. Because the trachea deviates slightly to the right, patients who are at risk for aspiration will usually have a right middle lobe pneumonia if they aspirate.
- If the patient has any kind of abnormal lung sounds from mucus or infection, you should always have the patient cough to clear the secretions in order to get a true picture of the lung sounds. If they have upper airway secretions, the upper airway rhonchi can radiate into the lung fields when auscultated.
- ALWAYS start at the top and compare one lobe laterally to the opposite side, listening carefully for not only the presence of abnormal sounds but also the quality of the aeration. If pneumonia or pleural effusion is present, the only assessment finding could be diminished aeration and this is the easiest way to determine if this finding is present.
- Auscultate four levels of the lung fields (anterior or posterior): upper, mid, lower, and lower lateral.
- ALWAYS listen very carefully at the mid/lower lobes because this is where most adventitious sounds start, especially crackles, because of gravity.
- If wheezing is present, be sure to note if the wheezing occurs on inspiration or expiration. Expiratory wheezes are most common, but if inspiratory wheezing is present, it can reflect a greater degree of bronchoconstriction and is a clinical RED FLAG.
- If crackles are present, the degree of coarseness correlates with the amount of fluid in the alveoli. For example, fine crackles represent small amount of fluid or even atelectasis, while coarse crackles reflect more fluid in the alveoli. This is a clinical RED FLAG.

Rhythm/character

- If respiratory distress is present for any reason, in addition to noting the rate, be sure to also determine if any retractions are present. Intercostal retractions are the earliest compensatory assessment findings seen in infants, children, and adults.
- With infants, any retractions, if present, are a clinical RED FLAG! Intercostal retractions typically represent mild to moderate distress. However, if supraclavicular and substernal retractions are present, this represents severe distress.
- If a pediatric patient presents with acute respiratory distress and wheezing, often times as they progress and worsen, the wheezing ceases because the bronchi have narrowed and the lack of aeration causes the wheezing to no longer be auscultated. This indicates a worsening in status and is a definite RED FLAG that must be recognized by the nurse.

Cardiac

General

- Diaphoresis is ALWAYS clinically significant and reflects sympathetic nervous system stimulation. The nurse must step back and ask: WHY is this present? What is most likely causing this assessment finding based on the patient's story and most likely/worst possible complication? "Jason" is likely not far away!
- Orthostatic BPs: Positive orthos…remember the number **20**. INCREASE of HR >20 or DECREASE in systolic blood pressure (SBP) > 20 from lying to standing represent a positive orthostatic BP. From what I have observed in clinical practice, with mild to moderate volume depletion, you will typically see HR increase with no change in SBP. If both the HR INCREASES and SBP DECREASES, then the fluid volume deficit is much more pronounced in severity and is a clinical RED FLAG!
- Potassium is the electrolyte that is most rapidly depleted during diuresis with any loop diuretic such as furosemide (Lasix). Therefore, if there has been a vigorous diuresis (>1000 mL/shift) and potassium was low normal, it is most likely now below normal and will need to be rechecked. Assess telemetry closely for increased frequency of premature ventricular contractions (PVCs) or other signs and symptoms of hypokalemia.

Heart Sounds

- You MUST know the location and physiologic landmarks of the four valves that are auscultated on the chest: aortic, pulmonic, tricuspid, and mitral. This is important because some patients have valvular disease or have had valve surgery and you must know the location of that valve and listen carefully for any murmurs or adventitious sounds.
- Use the mnemonic **"All Patients Take Meds" (APTM)** to help you remember the correct sequence of a cardiac valvular assessment.
  The **A**ortic valve is second intercostal to the RIGHT of the sternum. The manubrium is the "bump" on the top end of the sternum that is the landmark for the second intercostal space.

  - ✓ The **P**ulmonic valve is also second intercostal across the sternum on the LEFT side.
  - ✓ The **T**ricuspid valve is fourth to fifth intercostal on the LEFT side of the sternum. This level is also consistent with the nipple line of men, and is the lower third of the sternum to visualize for women.
  - ✓ The **M**itral valve is the same intercostal level. Just slide the stethoscope over to the LEFT mid-clavicular. On a male, this is typically right at the left nipple. This is also the location for an apical pulse.

- To be considerate of women, when auscultating the tricuspid and mitral valves, which are over the left breast, auscultate ABOVE the breast so it is not as intrusive by auscultating BELOW the breast. You can also have the patient lift her breast so you can auscultate below.
- When auscultating heart sounds, S1S2 represents a distinct "lub-dub." Most murmurs are systolic and will be heard at the first heart sound or "lub" and sound like this: "whoooosh-dub."
  - ✓ In addition to identifying S1S2, the nurse must also assess for the presence of an additional heart sound or gallop.
  - ✓ S3 is a splitting gallop of the second heart sound. Upon auscultation, this additional gallop will sound just like the state: "Ken-tuck-y."

✓ S4 is a splitting gallop of the first heart sound. Upon auscultation, this additional gallop will sound just like the state: "Ten-ness-ee."

Strength/regularity of peripheral pulses

- ALWAYS assess right and left extremity pulses at the same time to determine true equality and any subtle changes that may be clinically significant.
- Students tend to struggle in locating the pedal and post tibial pulses. Remember the pedal pulse is found in the groove between the great and second toe. Place your fingers in this groove and slide your fingers up one to three inches until you feel the pulse. The post tibial is located on the inner aspect of the malleolus at the 3 o'clock position.
- Closely assess the regularity, strength, and quality of pulses, not just the rate. If irregular, most common arrhythmia is atrial fibrillation and must be considered, especially if rate >100.

Cap refill

- Though textbook norm is <3 seconds, most patients with vascular disease are brisk and <1 second. Increase vigilance if cap refill is equal or >2 seconds.
- If your patient has fungal toenails and you are unable to visualize the color of the toenail, blanch the tip of the toe instead.

Color/temperature extremities

- ALWAYS assess warmth/coolness of both right and left extremities at the same time to determine true equality and any subtle changes that may be clinically significant.

Telemetry rhythm (if applicable)

- Regularly check monitor throughout shift. Rhythm changes occur quickly and will not always alarm. Atrial fibrillation is the most common arrhythmia seen clinically.
- Increased frequency of premature atrial contractions (PACs) represents increased atrial irritability and can be an early warning that atrial fibrillation is just around the corner if the patient is currently in sinus rhythm.
- Increased PVCs and multifocal PVCs represent ventricular irritability. Runs of ventricular tachycardia or even ventricular fibrillation may be next!
- Remember the relationship of potassium and magnesium to cardiac electrical conduction. If these electrolytes are low, increased cardiac electrical irritability may be present. Increasing PVCs, runs of ventricular tachycardia and atrial fibrillation may be present if these electrolytes are low or even low normal range.

Edema…location/degree

- Differentiate pitting vs. non-pitting edema in the lower extremities by gently but firmly placing your fingertips for two to three seconds in the tissue and then assess the depth of the "pit."
- Systematically assess for not only the depth of pitting edema but also how far up the legs it is present. Start at the feet and work your way up until there is clearly no "pit" present. During severe heart failure, you can see pitting edema into the thighs.
- Though some nursing textbooks quantify the depth of edema in 2mm increments (1+ is 2mm), the definition at your facility may be different. The most common scale I have seen is graded by ¼-inch increments instead. So 1+ pitting edema would be documented if the "pit" was approximately ¼ inch.

Neuro

a/o x4 (person-place-time-situation)

- If a patient is on narcotics, establish the baseline orientation EARLY, so if there are any subtle changes later in the shift, the nurse will know they are new and may be clinically significant.

Level of consciousness (LOC)

- If a patient is on narcotics, establish the baseline LOC early, so if there are any subtle changes later in the shift, the nurse will know they are new and may be clinically significant.
- Remember that with narcotic over-sedation, changes in LOC or orientation are the EARLY signs of CNS depression. Decreased respiratory rate (<10) is a LATE finding.

GI

Tenderness with palpation

- Always auscultate and inspect BEFORE you palpate the abdomen.
- Palpate lightly, no more than one to two inches deep systematically in each quadrant to determine if tenderness is present. I find that most students fear they will harm their patient and tend to not go deep enough and go less than an inch.
- Closely assess for softness/firmness of abdomen when palpated. A firm abdomen can reflect ileus or constipation and must be noted.

Bowel sounds/flatus/last bowel movement (LBM)

- Pay close attention to the LBM, especially if the patient is post-op. This can easily be missed and must be noted. This is clinically significant if there has been no BM in the last two to three days. Check the flow sheet to validate and always ask the patient if they can recall LBM if they are reliable.

GU

Urine amount/color/clarity

- ALWAYS assess the color/clarity as well as the continued flow and patency of urine in the clear tubing of the catheter and continue to assess it during the shift with each assessment. It is not uncommon to have the urine be initially clear and then change to cloudy or have sediment present. This could reflect a new UTI and is clinically significant.

Foley

- ALWAYS make sure that the catheter has some type of securement device; this is the best practice to prevent needless trauma and decrease incidence of urinary tract infection (UTI).
- Be sure to perform perineal care at least every shift and prn to prevent UTI.
- Evaluate the need for a catheter and remove as quickly as possible with the physician's order to prevent UTI.

Skin

Color/temperature

- Central coolness when touching the forehead can be clinically significant and must be noted. When sepsis is early, the extremities will likely be cool, but as it progresses, the core as well as the extremities will be cool/cold.

Skin integrity
- Most common pressure point to carefully assess is the coccyx and heels. Remember the significance of redness and, if present, determine if blanchable or not. If redness is slow to return (>2 seconds), this is a clinical RED FLAG that indicates tissue is close to breaking down.

Mucous membranes
- To quickly and easily identify dehydration with adults or pediatrics, assess the lips. Unusual dryness is common with mild dehydration.
- Have patient open their mouth and assess the mouth and tongue for saliva. It should appear moist and shiny. If it is dry or tacky, this is a progression of dehydration and is likely mild to moderate in severity depending on the story. I find this much easier and practical than assessing for "tenting" of skin, though they can both be done and clustered together.

Nursing Procedures
Intravenous (IV) Access

- Use the smallest IV catheter based on the IV's purpose. The larger the IV catheter, the more likely that it will cause irritation and phlebitis. For most adults, a #22 catheter is just right for IV fluids, IV antibiotics, and other medications.
- The first place I look to establish an IV is the inner aspect of the mid forearm. This is preferred because it does not bend like an IV placed in the hand or inner antecubital (elbow). The veins in this location can be readily visualized, tend to be secured by surrounding tissue, and less likely to "roll" when you attempt to cannulate the vein.
- The most common reason that an IV insertion causes the vein to "blow" and cause a hematoma is that the vein was not properly secured while attempting to thread the catheter into the vein. To prevent this from occurring, apply traction by using your nondominant hand to spread the skin laterally just above the access site. At the same time, use the fourth or fifth digits of your dominant hand that is holding the IV catheter to pull downward as you insert the catheter in the vein. This will stabilize the vein by applying traction in two directions and keep it from moving.
- Once you have applied traction both above and below the vein insertion site, place the IV catheter bevel up at a low 10 degree angle right on top of the vein and continue to insert until you see a blood flash.
- Stop and bring the IV catheter all the way down to 0 degrees and insert the catheter only 1/8 of an inch. This will ensure that the plastic catheter is completely in the vein before you attempt to advance it. Then you can slowly, gently, yet firmly advance the entire catheter in the vein.
- Flush the IV with 3–5 mL of normal saline to ensure that the IV catheter is in the vein. There should be no pain, swelling, or leakage with a gentle flush. Many patients will comment that they can taste the saltiness of the saline shortly after flushing. This is a more indirect method of assuring that the IV is properly in the vein.

NG Placement
Be sure to consult your textbook or policy and procedure manual before NG placement. The following "pearls" are principles that you can use in addition to what is in the textbook.

- Be sure to inspect the inside of the nose for any obstructions or polyps or to determine which side is larger.
- If placing a Salem® sump tube for gastric decompression, run warm water over the entire tube for at least 30 seconds to soften the relatively stiff plastic tubing, which will facilitate correct placement.
- Though most nursing textbooks state to measure the NG tube from the tip of the nose, to earlobe, to the xiphoid process, this may put the tube in the distal esophagus or very tip of the stomach. Add 2–3 cm to your final length and you will be assured that the tube will be completely in the stomach.
- The most painful and difficult aspect of NG placement is getting the tube into the posterior pharynx. When inserting the tube into the naris, point the tube, once in the naris, to the inner canthus of the opposite eye. This follows the typical anatomic structure of the nose and septum. You can also gently curve the tube prior to insertion by gently winding it around your finger. Always have a second person available to assist with placement for two reasons. First, you will need them to assist with sips of water as you guide the tube from the posterior pharynx to the esophagus. Second, I have had unexpected levels of anxiety and agitation from non-confused patients who begin to actively fight you as you attempt to place the tube. Having the second person hold the patient's hands and provide additional reassurance will make placement easier.

Nursing Informatics

Nursing informatics supports nurses to achieve desired outcomes. This support is accomplished through the use of information structures, information processes, and information technology, with electronic medical records (EMR) the most commonly used information structure to manage patient care. I discussed some of these informatics structures in chapter 5 with mobile technology, pharmaceutical databases such as Micromedex, and internet databases such as emedicine/Medscape for pathophysiology information.

Being proficient with computers and technology is a skill that every nurse must be competent with. As electronic medical records (EMR) are utilized in acute care as well as community care settings, mastering this technology will facilitate all that is done in the patient care setting. Though there is a learning curve for baseline knowledge and proficiency as a student, make this a priority and the provision of nursing care will remain primary not secondary as you struggle to correctly chart medications, vital signs, and your nursing assessment as a student.

The challenge you will experience as a student is that there is no standardized platform for EMR's in this country. Currently Cerner and EPIC are the competing platforms in acute care settings that is akin to the old Windows vs. Apple operating systems for home computing and now Android vs. Apple in cell phones. As a result, you may need to learn more than one type of platform while a student. The good news is that once you are in practice, you will have only one platform and will be able to become quickly proficient.

I want to encourage you to make the provision of patient care your priority in the clinical setting, not the documentation. Just as a novice student nurse tends to be task oriented, the task of documentation will want to compete with the provision of patient care. In order to facilitate patient centered care regardless of your clinical setting when using the EMR, I want to share a few practical pearls that will guide your practice as a student and as a nurse in practice:

- Identify the easiest ways to access the most important clinical documentation with the EMR that your institution uses and make your own "cheat sheet" to facilitate quick data collection in the clinical setting. My short list of NEED to know clinical data that must be identified to assume patient care includes the following:
  - ✓ Laboratory values
  - ✓ Radiology reports
  - ✓ Primary care provider notes/history & physical
  - ✓ Nursing notes
  - ✓ Vital signs
  - ✓ Nursing assessment
  - ✓ Medication administration record (MAR)
- Once the access of clinical data is determined, ensure that you are able to document correctly in the MAR, nursing notes, vital sign flowsheet, and nursing assessment flowsheet.
- Once collected, document as quickly as possible all clinical data collected including vital signs and nursing assessment, preferably while still in the patient's room.
- Never turn your back on your patient when documenting if there is a computer in the patient room. I have been amazed that in some settings the location of the computer in the room is not conducive for face-to-face contact with the patient. If this is the case, do your documentation outside the room and make respectful, personal care your priority!

The Nurse Is an Educator

As a student or new nurse, you may be reluctant to see yourself as an educator. I want to encourage you to embrace the role and responsibility! Patient education is a skill that requires practice to become proficient. Just as it took regular practice to become proficient with the skill of sterile technique, use each clinical to provide some form of patient education, and over time, your proficiency as an educator will increase.

If you teach well, you will make a real difference by improving patient outcomes. You will empower your patients and their families by helping them to understand their illness and take responsibility to do their part to promote and maintain their health.

Make education a natural part of your practice. Clearly communicate everything that you are doing to the patient and family and why you are doing it throughout the shift. This includes the plan of care simply stated for the day and the rationale, the data from vital signs, nursing assessment, and the administration of any medications or treatments.

If there is a change in status, matter-of-factly communicate what you are observing and why you are calling the physician. I have observed in my own practice that I can quickly establish trust and develop a therapeutic relationship with my patient and family when they clearly understand what is taking place. Consider good nursing education as an ongoing conversation with your patient and family!

When patient education is done well, it can also prevent readmission for the same problem and save limited health care dollars. Medicare alone currently spends over $15 billion a year on readmissions from chronic illnesses. Heart failure is one of the most common reasons that patients are readmitted within 30 days after their discharge. When patients as well as families are educated well, this can reduce the number of readmissions for chronic health problems and promote patient health and outcomes.

Education Made Practical

Make it a priority to make all education INDIVIDUALIZED to the patient and family needs at the moment you teach. Remember how stress and anxiety impacts you as a student learner. Determine the best time to teach based on the current reality of the patient and family. Consider the impact of emotional distress, pain, and medications ("Tips to Improve Patient Education," 2015). Though empathy was emphasized earlier, this principle is also relevant to be an effective educator. Get inside the lived experience of your patient and family by determining:

- Education level
- Age
- Mastery of English language, particularly if patients are immigrants

Once this relevant information is known, the nurse must then be able to communicate effectively in order to teach effectively. Keep all education as simple as possible to ensure that it will be understood. Remember that it is not only what you say, but how you say it!

Use principles of therapeutic communication and ensure that in all you do as an educator, communicate caring and engagement, not just getting through the task to check off the box that education was completed. Nightingale recognized the importance of effective communication when she wrote regarding patient education, "We must not talk to them or at them but with them" (Attewell, 2012, p. 53).

Explain everything that you are doing and why. As you administer medications, tell your patient what you are administering and then ask them if they know what this medication is for. If they do not know, you can briefly explain why they are receiving it and what they need to know. Or save this education later in the shift as you have time. Avoid medical terminology and abbreviations.

If teaching was not done or was not performed well, your patient may experience a decline in health and be needlessly readmitted. Knowledge is power, and as a "knowledge worker" (Porter-O'Grady, 2010) you must use this power to your patient's advantage. Your patient and his family should be considered a partner in care and work together as able in the clinical setting. Patients are now expected to learn about their own health to be able to participate in health care decisions as partners. The goal of patient education is to assist a patient and his family to learn about his health care to improve his own health. The principles of simplicity and reinforcement will guide and empower you to embrace this important responsibility.

Simplicity

1. Teach the simple concepts about a topic first, and then move to the more complex concepts.
2. Use language that your patient will find easy to understand and avoid medical terminology whenever possible. Consider the age, level of education, and current profession to determine the level at which to teach (Freda, 2004).

Reinforcement

1. Teach the one concept you want your patient to learn FIRST.
2. Ask your patient to restate in their OWN words what you have taught, so you can be sure he understood. Engage in dialogue to determine effectiveness of education, not just yes or no answers. If any knowledge gaps are identified, address them immediately.
3. Use visual aids for teaching; identify the preferred learning style of those you are teaching and adapt your teaching to accommodate.
4. Always use written educational materials for the client to take home, if available (Freda, 2004).

Here are additional principles that I have found helpful and meaningful in promoting patient engagement.

- Identify the desired outcome with what you will be teaching. Is it knowledge to be learned or a skill that needs to be demonstrated?
- Include the FAMILY as much as possible in education. The spouse or significant other is likely going to be needed to reinforce what you are teaching once the patient is home.
- Define the priority educational needs and desired outcome of education.
- Minimize any/all distractions and teach at a time that is best for the patient.
- If there are relevant risk factors present that must be managed to promote health and disease progression, be sure that they are taught and understood.
- Assess what the patient/family already knows and what must be REINFORCED.
- Assess for any barriers to learning such as language, level of education, hard of hearing (HOH), and motivation.
- Summarize main points and keep it as simple as possible!
- When administering medications, assess knowledge by asking the question, "Do you know what this is for?" If the patient is unable to answer, you can reinforce or choose to address any knowledge deficits another time.

Practical Principles of Priority Setting

Setting priorities with your patient is determined by differentiating between problems that need immediate attention and problems that can wait (Alfaro-LeFevre, 2013). If the nurse is unable to recognize the current priority, it can delay needed intervention that can result in an adverse outcome for the patient. That is why it is imperative to set correct priorities and accomplish the most important interventions first.

As a student you likely had no more than one or two patients at a time and had plenty of time to accomplish what needed to be done with your patients. Once you graduate, you will be responsible for much higher patient loads, depending on the clinical setting. Think of your patient assignments as a deck of cards that is continually being shuffled. The top card represents the highest priority. Once this priority task is done, it goes to the bottom of the deck and the next important priority now needs to be completed.

To keep your sanity with multiple patients and ever-pressing needs, remember one word that is also the essence of emergency care – TRIAGE. Triage is the process of sorting through the medical needs of patients to determine which patient has priority based on the severity of their condition. Triage was originally performed on the battlefield with mass casualties. Doctors and nurses determined which wounded warriors could be saved and would be seen first, who was likely to die and would receive no treatment, and who had minor wounds and could wait for treatment with no adverse outcome.

As an emergency nurse, the ability to triage patient needs is especially important. In comparison to other care units in a hospital that have unchanging patient assignments, ED patients are continually coming and going, walking in or transported by paramedics. The deck of cards is shuffled at a much higher pace. Recognizing which patient is most concerning and what is the most important task to be done provides a sense of calm in the midst of the storm, knowing that the rest can wait because of the lack of an emergent clinical concern.

Practical priority setting using the principle of triage depends on the nurse's ability to recognize which patient concern/task needs immediate attention, what interventions need to be done FIRST, and what can wait. Proper priority setting is also a component of clinical reasoning. Review the earlier chapter on this foundational concept to develop not only nurse thinking but priority setting in practice.

To triage and set priorities correctly in the clinical setting, requires time and clinical experience. As a student or new graduate, you do not currently have this needed experience. You must be patient and know that this skill is something you will develop as you acquire additional clinical experience. Give yourself grace as a new nurse to develop this salience, and do all you can to make this weakness a strength over time!

In order to recognize which patient is your highest priority, you must be able to use one key aspect of clinical reasoning: RECOGNIZE the RELEVANCE or significance of clinical data that is in the chart or collected by the nurse that may represent a clinical problem. If relevant clinical data is not recognized or acted upon, the priority patient is not recognized. This can contribute to a delay of care for a patient who may have a critical concern.

Listen to your Gut!

Another important principle of priority setting that must not be minimized is the importance of listening when your gut instinct tells you something is not quite right with your patient. Though you may not be able to put your finger on the specific problem, you must pay close attention to this feeling and investigate and assess further to delineate your concern. Even if you are not able to identify a concrete assessment finding that confirms your feeling, there is a reason you are feeling what you are experiencing and it likely represents a potential problem.

Therefore, this patient must be a priority and you must continue to make assessments and watch them closely to TREND relevant assessment data. Subtle assessment findings that may represent a change in status such as skin that was dry but is now slightly moist or a slight increase in heart rate are subtle signs that may represent a much larger problem. When the nurse is able to recognize the significance and the rationale for assessment findings that are slightly abnormal, this provides context to recognize the significance of your observations.

For example, sympathetic nervous system stimulation is not expected in a patient who is recovering from surgery. Tachycardia, subtle change in skin color, moist or diaphoretic skin with normal blood pressure due to the compensatory response of an elevated heart rate are all EARLY signs of any shock state. But if you recognize and understand the significance of these findings, you will be able to accurately INTERPRET this clinical data which is an essential component of clinical judgment making.

To help develop your ability to recognize and establish priorities, the following principles of priority setting will prepare you for professional practice as well as for the NCLEX!

Priority Patient

If you have more than one patient in the clinical setting, who will be seen first and why? The following principles will guide the development of this essential nurse thinking skill.

- **How old is the patient?** The older the patient, the higher risk they are to develop complications. Therefore, if all considerations are equal, see the oldest patient FIRST.
- **When were they admitted?** The more recent the day of admission, the more likely the patient is higher acuity and at risk for a change of status. Therefore, if all considerations are equal, see the most recently admitted patient FIRST.

- **When did they have surgery?** The more recent the day of surgery, the higher the acuity and risk for a change of status. Therefore, if all considerations are equal, see the most recent surgical patient FIRST.
- **How many body systems are involved?** Chronic renal failure patients are an excellent example of patients who typically have multiple body system derangements because of systemic metabolic changes influenced by renal disease. If medical complexity is present and all other considerations are equal, this patient should be seen FIRST.

Priority Assessments

Though a head-to-toe assessment is done on every patient, do you know when to modify this assessment based on the patient's primary problem? For example, a patient admitted with COPD exacerbation will require a much more thorough and detailed respiratory assessment and less attention can be paid to the GI system.

Nursing Priority

The ABC's of priority setting are always relevant and must remain in this order. If a patient has airway, breathing, or circulatory priorities, set priorities in the sequence of alphabetical order! Encourage nurse vigilance with an awareness of the most likely or worst possible complication for your patient as a means to establish a care priority. This was discussed earlier in the prior chapter.

Priority Interventions

Priority interventions are implemented once the nursing process has been utilized to correctly identify the priority patient, correct priority assessments, nursing priority, and the interventions needed. If the nursing priority is NOT correctly identified, the interventions that follow will not benefit the patient and advance the plan of care.

Priority Setting Scenario

To tie this important content together, the following is a scenario of patients you have been assigned to care for on a cardiac telemetry floor. Based on the principles discussed in this chapter, which of these three patients do you see first, and why?

Patient #1

Mark Sullivan is a 78-year-old man who had coronary artery bypass graft x3 vessels. He transferred out of ICU earlier today and is postoperative day (POD) #2. He has no history of dementia or ETOH use/abuse. He has been forgetful and does not consistently remember why he is in the hospital. He requires frequent orientation. You can hear Mark yelling, "I got to get out of here! I need to get back home right now. My wife needs me!"

Patient #2

Mary Johnstone is a 65-year-old woman who was admitted from the ED earlier today. She has a history of hyperlipidemia, hypertension, myocardial infarction, and coronary artery bypass graft surgery x3 vessels six months ago. The past week she has had mid-sternal chest pressure that radiates into the left arm with exertion, but relieves when she rests. She came into the ED when she experienced the same pressure while at rest this morning.

She put on her call light and states that she is still having chest pain. She is on a nitroglycerine intravenous (IV) gtt at 20 mcg/hour, as well as a heparin IV gtt at 1200 units/hour.

Patient #3

Joe Sandberg is a 52-year-old male who has no prior cardiac history who was admitted yesterday to cardiac telemetry for mid-sternal chest pressure that radiated to his neck the past two weeks with moderate levels of exertion. Coronary angiogram identified a 90% proximal right coronary artery lesion. He had a PTCA and placement of a drug eluding (DES) coronary artery stent to the RCA with a residual stenosis of 5%.

The angiogram revealed the following hemodynamics:

- 55% ejection fraction
- Cardiac output: 5.9
- Cardiac index: 3.1
- Pulmonary artery pressures: 35/15

He has just arrived to your telemetry unit from the cath lab. He has no report of pain. His right arterial and venous sheaths were removed in the cath lab. Groin site is soft, and distal pulses are 2+ and palpable.

Who Do You See First?

1. Based on the recognition of relevant clinical data, which patient would you see first?

2. What clinical data did you identify as relevant to support your clinical judgment?

3. Who would you see second?

4. What clinical data did you identify as relevant to support your clinical judgment?

5. Who would you see last?

6. What clinical data did you identify as relevant to support your clinical judgment?

Answer Key

1. Based on the recognition of relevant clinical data, which patient would you see first?
    Patient #2, Mary Johnstone

2. What clinical data did you identify as relevant to support your clinical judgment?
    *   *Recent transfer from the ED*
    *   *Relevant cardiac history with chest pain that is likely cardiac in origin.*
    *   *Recognize an ACTUAL problem vs. potential problem to guide priority setting. This is an NCLEX principle. Must accurately interpret clinical data.*
    *   *Remember ABC's! This patient has a clear "C" priority of cardiac chest pain that needs to be further assessed by the nurse.*

3. Who would you then see second?
    Patient #1, Mark Sullivan

4. What clinical data did you identify as relevant to support your clinical judgment?
    *   *Due to recent change in mental status that is consistent with delirium, his increased agitation must be recognized as a safety concern and is a fall risk.*
    *   *This too could lead to an actual problem, but when the nurse has two competing priority problems or patients, the use of the ABC's must be utilized. Since Mary has a "C" priority this must be attended to.*
    *   *Nurse must delegate appropriately and could have an aide or other nurse assist immediately in order that you can assess your patient with chest pain.*

5. Who would you then see last?
    Patient #3, Joe Sandburg

6. What clinical data did you identify as relevant to support your clinical judgment?
    *   *Though he just arrived from the cath lab post procedure, an initial assessment has been completed and there are no clinical concerns. This patient is stable.*

Practical Principles of Time Management

The following are practical principles to help you see the big picture of managing your time in the clinical setting:

*   What must be done right now vs. what can wait (example: pain meds).
*   What must be done in a specific time frame to ensure patient safety (example: blood glucose before meals).
*   Identify tasks that can be appropriately delegated and do so respectfully!

Increase Your Efficiency!

*   Get in the habit of documenting VS and nursing assessment in the chart as soon as possible, preferably before going to your next patient.

- Group patient care tasks together as much as possible.
- If doing a procedure or providing care, visualize what you need and bring all that is needed into the room the first time.
- Complete one task before starting another.

How to Prepare to Assume Care

In nursing school you may have had an hour or more to prepare for a patient care assignment. In clinical practice you will not have this luxury and will need to quickly, concisely, and systematically collect relevant clinical data on each patient in your care. How you prepare to assume a patient care assignment will depend on the clinical setting. My frame of reference as a nurse is acute care, but the following principles can be adapted regardless of your clinical setting.

The nurse must first know the "big picture" or the essence of the primary problem and what brought the patient to the clinical setting. Once the bigger picture is clearly understood, then the nurse can focus on specific clinical data that will help put the current picture in context.

Become proficient in accessing the most important clinical data in the medical record. Electronic medical records (EMRs) are becoming the standard for reviewing and documenting in acute care. Your goal is to collect all needed data on your patient preparation sheet in five minutes or less for each patient. Just as you want to have a systematic approach to giving report, you want to have a similar consistent approach to collecting clinical data.

To make sense and bring order to your data collection, you need to have something to write this information on. That is why you must create your own patient preparation worksheet. In order to quickly and efficiently identify relevant clinical data from the medical record and time map your clinical day, a well-designed patient preparation worksheet can help facilitate the collection of clinical data with multiple patients. I have a simple one-page worksheet that allows me to quickly note last set of vital signs, patient assessment, relevant lab values to facilitate trending, as well as essential kardex data. I have included my worksheet in appendix E. Feel free to modify or use it as-is to meet your needs!

Big Picture Clinical Data

In order to quickly identify the big picture of your patient story, this essential data collection has already been done for you by the primary care provider in the admitting history and physical (H&P) and/or the primary care provider's most recent progress note. This is the FIRST place the nurse must go to in the medical record and note what is most relevant to visualize the big picture. The nurse can quickly gather the following data and note it on the patient preparation worksheet.

Primary Care Provider's Progress Note

- Patient name, age, primary medical problem, day of admission
- RELEVANT past medical history that is related to primary medical problem. The patient may have ten medical problems, but I want to know about the one or two that are influencing the current problem.
- Concise summary of this admission and any problems as well as progress towards the current plan of care from the physician's perspective.

Specific Clinical Data

Once the big picture or essence of the current clinical situation is identified, RELEVANT specific clinical data will begin to make sense and you can begin to put the clinical puzzle together. Use the following sections of the chart or EMR to access and note the following essential clinical data.

- **Lab Values.** Remember the principles of clinical reasoning discussed earlier. Identify the specific lab values that are most important, based on your knowledge of the primary problem. TREND these most important lab values, even if they are normal, because they have clinical significance and note the direction of the trended labs. Determine if they are improving or reflect a possible problem. It is especially important to do this with the most recent lab values and those that were collected on your shift.
- **Medication Administration Record (MAR).** What prn medications were given in the past shift? Clarify with the nurse in report what prn medications are working and what needs to be done differently based on evaluation (pain meds/pain control, etc.)
- **Kardex.** Focus on kardex data that includes code status, contact precautions, primary physician/group, location of IVs and any infusions, new orders, activity, labs to be drawn on next shift.
- **Vital Sign Flowsheet.** Note and write down the last set of vital signs and any clinical trends that may be significant over the last shift. Identify patient ambiguity for vital signs that may be outside textbook norms.
- **Intake and Output (I&O).** Note I&O if relevant by documenting the output over the last 8/24 hours and trend of daily weights.
- **Nursing Assessment.** Highlight head-to-toe nursing assessment with data that includes an emphasis on the most relevant body system based on primary problem as well as abnormal assessment findings. Identify patient ambiguity for vital signs that may be outside textbook norms.
- **Your Evaluation.** Once this clinical data is assimilated, you will begin to get a sense of the nursing priorities for your patient. Begin to formulate these priorities and when you obtain a nurse-to-nurse report, you will be able to clarify your thoughts as needed with the prior nurse. Once the essence of the current nursing priority is identified, the plan of care follows with resultant interventions and outcomes that will advance the plan of care on your shift.

Principles of Collaborative Communication

Think of any interaction with another member of the health care team as akin to a baton handoff in a track and field race. Each runner in the relay is part of the team. In order to successfully complete the race, there must be a smooth and seamless handoff of the baton from one runner to another. If the baton is inadvertently dropped during the handoff, it is disastrous and results in failure. In the same way, if the primary nurse is unable to concisely and effectively communicate with any member of the health care team, disastrous consequences can follow that ultimately impact the patient.

Respectful and effective communication between all members of the health care team is foundational to not only advance the plan of care but also to ensure and guard patient safety. If you are an international student, encourage the feedback of other students or faculty to reflect and assess your ability to be consistently understood if there is any question that your accent impacts communication. If your language and communication skills need to be strengthened, make this a priority and use the resources that are available at your college to ensure that you are consistently understood by not only the health care team but your patients as well.

Since nurses most often communicate with other nurses and primary care providers such as physicians, I will discuss ways that I have found most effective to communicate with these two groups within the health care team. These principles are also universal and translate to any member of the team with whom the nurse needs to communicate.

How to Communicate Effectively with Nurses When GIVING Report

I have observed over my 30-plus years of clinical practice that how nurses give report can be as diverse and unique as nurses themselves. Nurse-to-nurse report at the end of the shift captures the essence of the metaphor of a good baton handoff! In order to ensure a clean handoff, use the following principles:

- **Always maintain an attitude of mutual respect.** Respect for colleagues regardless of any personality or personal differences must be a given.
- **Keep your report concise with NEED to know information relevant to the patient and advancing the plan of care.** I find that some nurses feel the need to elaborate on details related to the patient or the unique family dynamics that are extraneous and may have no benefit to the next nurse assuming care. Include this if it is relevant information, but otherwise stay on task in all aspects related to report.
- **Have a consistent and systematic approach to your report.** Just as a consistent and systematic approach to priority setting and nurse thinking with each patient will soon become ingrained, so should your bedside report. The same clinical data you must incorporate into your nurse-to-nurse report is also essentially the same clinical data that must be noted when you assume care.

In my acute care practice setting, I use the following approach to cover what I share in my nurse-to-nurse report. Adapt this as needed and place in an order that works for you!

✓ Patient name, age, primary medical problem, day of admission
✓ RELEVANT past medical history that is related to primary medical problem. The patient may have ten medical problems, but I want to know about the one or two that are influencing the current problem.
✓ Concise summary of this admission and any problems as well as progress toward the current plan of care.
✓ State nursing priority and plan of care with goals/outcomes for the shift, and how it was advanced and what yet needs to be done.
✓ What prn medications were given and, based on your evaluation, what is working and what needs to be done differently (pain meds/pain control, etc.).
✓ RELEVANT normal/abnormal lab values. Use the content from chapter 6 to identify relevant labs are for your patient.
✓ Highlight "kardex" data that includes code status, primary physician/group, location of IVs and any infusions, new orders, activity, and labs to be drawn on next shift.
✓ Last set of vital signs and any clinical trends that may be significant. Identify patient norms for any vital signs that are outside textbook norms.

✓ Highlight head-to-toe nursing assessment with data that includes an emphasis on the most relevant body system based on the primary problem as well as abnormal assessment findings.

How to RECEIVE Report

When the nurse is leading the dance by giving report, there are principles that need to be followed to be a good receiver of report. Here are some guidelines to make receiving report easier and facilitate this important handoff.

- **Be aware of what your nonverbal behavior communicates.** Be friendly, pleasant and smile! When I am giving a nurse-to-nurse report, I can immediately sense how smoothly this is going to go based on the nonverbal behavior of the receiving nurse. When the receiving nurse is friendly, smiles, and greets you warmly with direct eye contact, you know report is going to go well. Conversely, when the nurse is abrupt, sour-faced, and does not acknowledge you as a person, this creates an atmosphere of increased stress that will likely make report more difficult.

- **Limit the number of questions you ask during report.** Remember how important it is to not interrupt a nurse when they are accessing medications because it could increase the risk of an error? Have the same attitude when receiving report. Because most nurses use a systematic approach to report as I shared earlier, when questions not directly related to the current topics are asked, this can get the nurse giving report off track. He may have difficulty remembering where he left off, possibly causing important aspects to be missed. If you have questions, save them until the nurse is done giving report.

- **Don't nitpick.** Some nurses receiving report seem to delight in pointing out details or aspects of care that you did not know or did not complete. Do not be that nurse! Be gracious and merciful to your colleagues because you have no idea how busy or difficult their shift was. There was likely a good reason why everything may not have gotten done. You must be empathetic toward a newer nurse. He/she needs your understanding, not your judgmental attitude if you tend to be a nurse who expects perfection. Just as empathy is essential to demonstrate toward your patients, it must also be given to your nurse colleagues.

How to Communicate Effectively with Primary Care Providers

In one survey of nurses who had recently graduated, one of the themes in this survey that were identified was that they were not well prepared to communicate with physicians and were uncomfortable doing so when they needed to communicate a concern (Neal-Boylan, 2013). Communicating effectively with interprofessional care providers such as physicians or nurse practitioners requires much more than knowing how to use the SBAR format of situation, background, assessment, and recommendation that are typically taught in nursing school.

In order to help new nurses effectively communicate with primary care providers, I went to the source and discussed this issue personally with physicians and nurse practitioners I currently work with. The insights I was able to obtain will help you understand their perspective and help bridge the gap that currently exists when communicating between the disciplines.

When I mentioned to a physician that nursing education does not prepare students to communicate effectively with physicians, he laughed and said that medical school does not prepare doctors to communicate effectively with nurses! Could this be part of the problem?

As I discussed this concern with other care providers, I was able to identify themes that will help any nurse, but especially new nurses, so that they can effectively and succinctly communicate a concern. The goal is to advance the plan of care, advocate for your patient, and avoid adverse outcomes when a possible change of status is detected by the nurse.

Principles to Prepare the Way

In order to communicate effectively with physicians, there must be an understanding of the lived reality of the one you are communicating with. The following insightful points were from a highly respected physician who stated what nurses need to keep in mind and remember when communicating with physicians:

- Most physicians are by nature very competitive. Do not challenge this competitive spirit by provoking them with a hint of/or obvious challenge. If this is sensed, the nurse will quickly lose.
- Physicians are extremely intelligent and as a result, some struggle to communicate effectively, or have difficulty communicating when stressed, so keep it simple and on point.
- Male physicians from the Middle East and other countries in the world do not consistently have a culturally high regard for women. If you are a woman communicating in this context, know that your perspective may not be valued or validated, but be persistent and diligent to advocate for your patient.

Time to Talk!

How to communicate a clinical concern in the middle of the night to a just awakened physician will give most new nurses sweaty palms and high levels of anxiety. But take a deep breath, and carefully consider the following principles that other physicians shared that will guide and increase your comfort level in communicating a concern:

General Principles

- Communicate a spirit of collaboration if a physician is being difficult. State your concern, but preface it with, "I need your help."
- Do not DEMAND your recommendation. If your patient needs additional pain medication do not state, "My patient is in severe pain and needs his morphine dose increased from 4 mg to 8 mg every four hours as needed." Instead, communicate your concern for more pain meds, recommend a higher dose, but then state, "What do you think?" This approach promotes collaboration and a team approach to meeting the needs of the patient.

Specific Points

- Dialogue and have a voice in any interaction. When requesting a pain medication and you suggest morphine and the physician agrees or suggests Dilaudid, but states a dose that is likely too low, don't be afraid to have a little give and take. Suggest a slightly higher dose range or more frequent prn schedule and you will likely get what your patient needs.
- If you do not understand the rationale for an order or medication the doctor wants to order, be humble and do not hesitate to ask for clarification. Don't fake it! Remember that this is also a patient safety issue.

- When calling because of a patient concern, make it a priority to give just enough information to allow the provider to visualize what is going on. Don't give too little information and don't give too much that is not directly relevant to the primary concern. Make it "just right"!
- If you have a serious concern, be specific with clinical data that supports your concern and if possible be clear on what you want.
- Know the patient's story well enough so that you are able to answer basic questions related to your clinical concern.
- If a physician is inappropriate, bullying, angry or harsh with you, call out this behavior before hanging up by simply stating in a calm respectful tone, "I called because I had a concern. Your tone of voice is needlessly harsh and I don't deserve to be treated like that."

Principles of Proper Delegation

You can't do it all in clinical practice, especially with large or heavy patient assignments. Safe and appropriate delegation of care to the appropriate member of the team is an important responsibility of the professional nurse. Providing care is a team effort and each member of the health care team has a part. Just because each player (nursing assistant, LPN, etc.) has differing levels of education, they must be treated with respect and as equally important. Do not let your new degree and status as a professional nurse go to your head! Continue to be a team player, and treat the members of your team the way you would want to be treated.

Prepare the Way for Effective Delegation

In order to successfully delegate, the following themes were identified by nursing assistants and LPN's I requested feedback from at the hospital where I work. Carefully consider their perspective to maintain a healthy working relationship among each member of the team.
- *"REQUEST, don't demand! Can you, will you instead of demanding, 'Get the patient in room 205 a blanket?'"*
- *"Delegate by using my name in the request. This communicates respect."*
- *"Be aware of what your nonverbals are communicating. Watch the tone of voice and attitude.*
- *Request politely, in a gentle tone of voice in a non-condescending manner."*

Many of those I interviewed experienced unprofessional behavior from nurses. This behavior also had the consequence of driving a wedge between team members because it communicated disrespect. Determine to NOT be that nurse who:
- Ignores call lights and continues to surf the web or talk at the desk with other nurses while waiting for the nursing assistant to answer the patient call light.
- Does not carry their load. Delegates tasks to others when they are not busy.

Principles of Professional Delegation

The following are principles of delegation that will prepare you for clinical practice as well as NCLEX questions that will assess this nurse responsibility:
- The essence of a task that can be safely delegated is that it is an intervention that is repetitive, requires little to no supervision, and not invasive for the patient.

- Examples of tasks that can be delegated to LPN:
  - ✓ Reinforcement of patient education
  - ✓ Medication administration (IV meds may not be allowed in some states)
  - ✓ Insertion of Foley catheter
  - ✓ Administer enteral tube feedings
  - ✓ Suctioning
  - ✓ Trach cares
- Examples of tasks that can be delegated to nursing assistant or assistive personnel (AP):
  - ✓ Vital signs on stable patients
  - ✓ Intake and output
  - ✓ Specimen collection
  - ✓ Activities of daily living including bathing, toileting, dressing, ambulating, feeding, positioning (Sommers et al., 2013).
- **Lead by example.** This communicates VALUE to the team. There is NOTHING that is beneath the nurse to provide care in the clinical setting. Make beds, answer call lights, and do whatever is needed when not busy.
- **Assist those you delegate to whenever possible**. If a patient needs to be cleaned up and requires two staff, offer to be the second if you are available.
- **Put yourself in the shoes of those to whom you delegate tasks.** If they are obviously busy, share the burden and offer to help. This will not be quickly forgotten and will build and maintain needed goodwill and teamwork.
- Delegate to the full scope of practice of what you have been trained to do and are capable of, but no more.

The Nurse Is a Leader

Every nurse is a leader. Remember that leadership is not always tied to a title or position of authority. Each nurse has the potential and responsibility to provide some form of leadership in your specific area of practice. Nurses should consider leadership as a skill, rather than as a role (Grossman & Valiga, 2013).Though it was once thought that great leaders are born that way, it has been shown that leadership skills can also be developed.

Florence Nightingale was a remarkable nurse leader whose example can still influence your nursing practice today. Her leadership model was based on a vision of health care improvement, nurses united in purpose, exercising authority influenced by their moral character, and being members of a mutually supportive profession. She also embraced the responsibility inherent as a nurse leader (Attewell, 2012).

In order to identify the passion and fire that led Nightingale to lead nursing out of the dark ages, the following quote can provide a guide to all who aspire to be leaders in nursing today (Attewell, 2012, p. 35):

> *"I have had a larger responsibility of human lives than ever man or woman had before. And I attribute my success to this: I never gave or took an excuse...when a disaster happens, I act and they make excuses."*

Do you see yourself as a leader or do you have a vision to become a leader once you become a nurse? A leader is one who has the ability to inspire others and present a vision of a desired goal.

Regardless of where you are on a leadership spectrum, it is imperative to embrace the role and responsibility of being a nurse leader after you graduate.

As a nurse who is also a leader, you must realize that you can't achieve positive outcomes for your patients alone. It is always a TEAM effort. You will achieve more when the entire unit functions well as a team. The nurse is the leader who sets the tone and culture of the unit. Value the importance of the role that every person has and draw upon the strengths of each staff member.

Regardless of your personality and communication style, you can be a leader. Can you live out by your example what a professional nurse looks like? Then you can be a leader! This is why the values and character traits discussed earlier are so important to practice. This is where every nurse can begin to exert her influence as a leader with co-workers. Your title as a nurse does not make you a leader. HOW you lead and your personal characteristics will earn the respect of others, and that makes the difference (Melnyk, Malloch, Gallagher-Ford, 2014).

Characteristics of Effective Leaders

Leadership is also a skill that can be improved through instruction. Use the following principles to improve and refine your leadership abilities.

- **Take initiative to get things done.** If a problem is present or you see how it could be improved, take initiative and responsibility to see it through.
- **Inspire others with a vision.** Present a vision of what could be to others and communicate this vision to achieve needed buy in.
- **Maintain a positive attitude.** Don't get bogged down by setbacks but see them as an opportunity!
- **Communicate effectively. Be direct, but t**reat others in a way that communicates RESPECT.
- Be committed to deliver quality patient care.
- Empathize and understand and value the perspective of others.
- Be insightful to the feelings of others.
- Encourage constructive criticism and is open to new ways of doing things.
- Don't make assumptions or judgments on emotionally charged issues until all the facts have been gathered and carefully considered (Sommers et al., 2013).
- Be passionate about the value of patient care and making a difference.

Take Charge!

I have observed in practice that most nurses have a love-hate relationship with assuming the leadership and responsibility of being charge nurse. It is either barely tolerated or embraced and enjoyed. Regardless of how you may feel, it is the most common leadership role that even new nurses may assume right after graduation. This is typical in a skilled care setting, where you may be the only professional nurse managing non-licensed nursing staff. Regardless of the clinical setting you may practice in, remember that the charge nurse is also a nurse leader and manager for the shift. You are ultimately responsible for the quality of care that each patient on the unit receives.

Preparing the Way: General Principles

Regardless of your leadership style, to assume this newfound responsibility with confidence, use the following principles to help guide you.

- Act with integrity in all that you do. The essence of integrity is that you are fully integrated. Your behavior and how you act does not change whether you are in public or behind closed doors.
- Set realistic goals for yourself and others.
- Communicate clearly and often with others on the team.
- Use the principles of effective delegation addressed earlier in this chapter.
- Encourage those you work with by recognizing them and verbalizing what they do well.
- Inspire others by your example to provide the best care possible (Nursing Leadership: Management & Leadership Styles, 2014).

The Seven Habits of Highly Successful Charge Nurses

To identify the habits and attitudes of successful charge nurses, I reflected on my own observations operating in this role in critical care as well in a busy emergency department. I also interviewed other charge nurses where I currently work in acute care. The following "pearls" will further guide you to be successful in this important role.

1. **Remember that you can't please everyone.** This does not give you permission to be a jerk, but is a reminder to lower your expectations of being liked by all of your staff. Patient care assignments can be a land mine where this truth will be realized almost every shift. Do your best to be fair with patient assignments and let the chips fall where they may. Whether you are assigning patients for other nurses or nursing assistants, I have found this to be a universal dilemma and occurrence.
2. **Get out from behind the desk or unit.** Make it a priority to circulate and round the unit throughout the shift. Patients can change status and develop potential problems at any time and the nurse responsible may need your help. Remember that "Jason" is still out there!
3. **Be a team player by serving others.** The best charge nurses are those who are aware of what is going on, recognize the need to help, and offer to do so!
4. **Be a resource.** Though you may feel that you don't know enough as a new nurse to be a resource, know where to go when a question arises. How do you access the policy and procedure manual for any clinical question that comes up? Be willing to assist your team to find the answer if they are too busy.
5. **Know your team and their weaknesses and strengths.** This will take time, but make a determined effort to know the clinical experience and length of time they have operated in their current role as well as personality dynamics. Learn how to navigate when there is conflict or other concerns.
6. **Be direct with your communication.** Leave nothing to chance by being ambiguous. Follow up with delegated tasks to ensure that they were done.
7. **Manage conflict.** Personality conflicts and performance concerns need to be addressed quickly, directly, and privately. Though most prefer to avoid conflict and confrontation at all costs, there are some things that cannot wait another day or be delegated to your manager. Though this is probably the most difficult aspect of being a charge nurse, it is typically not a daily occurrence.

Nightingale on Charge

The necessity of having a charge nurse goes all the way back to the beginning of the modern era with Florence Nightingale. Hospital ward care required a nurse to also take responsibility to ensure that patients were properly cared for in that era as well. Nightingale's insights, though over 140 years old, still speak today:

- *"To be 'in charge' is certainly not only to carry out the proper measures yourself but to see that everyone else does so too; to see that no one either willfully or ignorantly thwarts or prevents such measures. It is neither to do everything yourself, nor to appoint a number of people to each duty, but to ensure that each does that duty to which he is appointed. This is the meaning which must be attached to the word by those 'in charge'"* (Nightingale, 1860).
- *"A person in charge must be felt more than she is heard-not heard more than she is felt. She must fulfill her charge without noisy disputes, by the silent power of a consistent life, in which there is no seeming, and no hiding, but plenty of discretion. She must exercise authority without appearing to exercise it"* (Attewell, 2012, p. 41).

Be a Follower

If the idea of leadership still intimidates you, then consider the importance of being a good follower. Remember that leaders can be leaders only if they have followers. Being a good follower requires special talents and abilities just as being a good leader does. Many of these qualities are complementary and include the importance of being willing to take risks, challenge the status quo, and being passionate about a goal. Followers do so voluntarily, but without effective followers, leaders will be left without the needed support to realize the vision, make change, and positively impact the organization (Grossman & Valiga, 2013).

Traits of Successful Followers

If you want to be an effective follower, the following traits will help guide you in this important role.

- Be passionate about what you do as a nurse.
- Set high standards for yourself. Others will follow your example.
- Actively seek out mentors who can guide you.
- Develop positive relationships with colleagues and be a team player.
- Know your job and do it well by demonstrating excellence and competence in all that you do.
- Be enthusiastic and let this enthusiasm be contagious.
- Be involved in your practice setting and have a sense of ownership and investment.
- Be actively involved in professional organizations.
- Be willing to speak up and speak out so others can benefit from your perspective.
- Independently think and develop an advocate for new ideas (Grossman & Valiga, 2013).

- The nurse is an educator who is responsible for ensuring that both the patient and family understand the current plan of care.
- To educate effectively, the nurse must utilize the principles of keeping education simple and reinforcing what is taught.
- The nurse must delegate safely and appropriately by assigning a task that is repetitive, requires little to no supervision, and is not invasive for the patient.
- The nurse is also a leader who must lead by example as well as by recognizing that it is also a skill that can be learned.
- Characteristics of effective leaders include taking initiative to get things done, maintaining a positive attitude, communicating effectively, and feels passionate about the value of patient care and making a difference.
- The charge nurse role is the most common "official" leadership role of the registered nurse.
- To be effective as a charge nurse include the importance of being a resource, helping out your team as needed and able, and managing conflict whenever it presents itself.
- Remember that every leader also needs a good follower. Be a good follower by being passionate about what you do as a nurse. Maintain and set high standards and seek out those nurses who can mentor and guide you.

Additional Resources

- Book: *The New Leadership Challenge: Creating the Future of Nursing* (2013) by Sheila Grossman and Theresa Valiga
- Book: *Illuminating Florence: Finding Nightingale's Legacy in Your Practice* (2012) by Alex Attewell
- Book: *Nursing Assessment: Head-to-Toe Assessment in Pictures* (2015) by Jon Haws

Chapter Reflections

1. What did you learn from the review of head-to-toe assessment pearls?

2. What will you incorporate into your practice to strengthen this skill?

3. Do you embrace the responsibility of the nurse as an educator as a student?

4. What principles will you incorporate to help strengthen this aspect of your practice?

5. Do you have difficulty identifying clinical priorities and/or managing your time in the clinical setting? What principles can you incorporate to make this your strength?

6. Would you rather be a good follower or leader? Explain why.

7. What will be your philosophy of leadership once in practice? Write this out in your own words.

You know you're a nurse when...
you count going to the bathroom as taking a break.

Chapter 11

Mastering the ABC's

Tie It All Together with
Clinical Reasoning Case Studies

Thinking Is a Skill That Must Be Practiced

My son Levi is an amateur motocross racer. We have a small motocross track that has increased in size every spring. The problem is, the track was completely smooth afterwards. In order for it to be usable, DEEP and WIDE ruts in the dirt were required. It took numerous repetitions going round and round the track to establish these ruts that would be the basis for a safer and faster track.

This is also a metaphor that will help you understand the value of repetitive practice of any skill in nursing, including thinking! Just as my son established ruts in the dirt by going around over and over again, science has demonstrated that "neuronal ruts" are established in the brain. When anything is done repeatedly, it becomes ingrained, intuitive, and second nature over time. There is no substitute for clinical experience to acquire this salience that leads to increased confidence in the clinical setting as well as progression from a novice to expert nurse.

In order for any nursing student to become proficient with any clinical skill it must be practiced over and over again. When I taught fundamentals and the clinical skill of sterile technique/Foley catheterization was demonstrated, students immediately recognized their need to PRACTICE.

Most spent hours doing it over and over until they were confident they could pass the skills check-off. In the same way, nurse thinking must be practiced. My clinical reasoning case studies provide the opportunity to make this practice possible so that you can translate this thinking skill readily to the clinical setting.

Mastering the ABC's

Some of the most common medical problems that nurses see in clinical practice working with adults across most care settings are COPD/pneumonia, heart failure, and sepsis. These medical problems also represent the ABC's (airway/breathing/circulation) of priority setting. COPD/pneumonia is an airway/breathing priority problem, while heart failure and sepsis represent circulatory or problems of perfusion. Priority setting using the ABC's is foundational to practice as well as for the NCLEX® licensure examination.

To prepare you for the unique challenges of each of these illnesses and practice the thinking that is required to provide safe nursing care, I have created case studies that mirror themes seen in clinical practice. They emphasize clinical reasoning, which is the essence of thinking like a nurse. These three case studies are found in the attachments in the eBook and can be easily downloaded to print and then work through.

To provide the opportunity to strengthen your learning and to practice the nurse thinking of pneumonia/COPD, heart failure, and sepsis, I have included clinical reasoning case studies of these three problems derived from themes I have consistently seen in clinical practice. The case studies begin with a realistic clinical scenario and require identification of what clinical data is relevant and why. Then questions that follow provide a systematic template of nurse thinking discussed in chapter 9 that experienced nurses use every day in practice.

By working through each clinical reasoning case study, you will PRACTICE the nurse thinking skill of clinical reasoning. Other unique strengths of these case studies are that they emphasize the same key components that the NCLEX utilizes to assess student learning. If you have not taken the NCLEX, these case studies will COMPLEMENT any other review programs because they situate the following KEY NCLEX principles that are also relevant to clinical practice:

- APPLICATION of content/concepts to the bedside
- PRIORITY SETTING based on the unique scenario
- Clinical data RELEVANT to this scenario
- RATIONALE for nursing interventions and physician orders

Additional Resources

I have additional clinical reasoning case studies on a wide variety of topics as well as workbooks that have 12 case studies of the most important concepts seen in clinical practice.

- Clinical Reasoning case studies: http://www.keithrn.com/clinical-reasoning-case-studies/
- FUNDAMENTAL Reasoning workbook: http://www.keithrn.com/home/store/
- RAPID Reasoning case study workbook: http://www.keithrn.com/home/store/
- UNFOLDING Reasoning case study workbook: http://www.keithrn.com/home/store/

If you think doctors are smarter than nurses, ask yourself why patients need several different doctors while in the hospital, but just one nurse.

Part IV

GO!

Starting Your Nursing Career

As you approach graduation or if you have already successfully completed your education, the final four chapters will help you complete the final leg of your journey to become a nurse. In chapter 12, the NCLEX licensure examination is broken down into key components that it uses to assess each graduate nurse. The test blueprint is also included.

When you understand that the NCLEX is an examination that assesses the graduate nurse's ability to clinically reason by identifying relevant clinical data and establish and recognize the need to act based on a clinical scenario, this will help you see the importance and relevance of my earlier chapter on clinical reasoning. Use this content to help improve your chances to not only pass the NCLEX, but also to apply this knowledge to the bedside where it matters most!

Once you have passed the NCLEX, how can you put the odds in your favor that you will get the nursing position you apply for? In chapter 13, I discuss practical strategies to construct an effective cover letter, resume, letters of recommendation, as well as what to do and what not to do in your interview.

Once you begin your first position as a nurse, chapter 14 identifies final steps that will prepare and help you successfully transition in this new role including practical strategies to strengthen and communicate effectively with physicians and how to respectfully address incivility and bullying behaviors if they come your way.

In chapter 15, I asked experienced physicians, nurse practitioners, and staff nurses in practice in my clinical setting what "pearls" of advice they would offer a new nurse to get started on the right foot. Their collective wisdom will provide essential insight. In the final chapter, I share how you can really make a difference as you serve others in nursing that will put your journey in perspective. It is not about the nurse, but as you care and serve others, your life will leave a legacy that will far outweigh any financial compensation you will receive.

Chapter 12
Passing the NCLEX®

Pass NCLEX on the First Attempt

The NCLEX licensure examination is the final hurdle and examination you must pass to obtain your nursing license. A word to the wise, do not to plan any "celebratory" vacations or have the mindset that "school is over" after you graduate! The sooner you successfully pass NCLEX, the sooner you can start applying for RN positions or new nurse graduate residency programs. Take the time you need to be successful. Keep your focus on the next step of studying for, and passing the NCLEX.

You've come this far and you want to retain as much knowledge as you can to help you to pass the NCLEX. Some say that 1,000 NCLEX type questions should be completed with review of the rationale by the student prior to exam for success. If possible, I recommend that you wait no longer than six to eight weeks after graduation to take the test. Your goal is to pass the NCLEX the first time!

There are a variety of options to help you study and prepare for the NCLEX. You can obtain books for self-study or you can take a formal class online or face-to-face (i.e., Kaplan, ATI, etc.). There are advantages to each method and you need to decide which method is best for you. If you like learning using many approaches, you may enjoy a formal class where a facilitator will help with NCLEX question dissection, strategies for test taking specific to NCLEX and offer diagnostic exams to support you in remediation related to areas where you may need to refresh your knowledge.

If you prefer to read independently and perhaps supplement with computer-based NCLEX questions, then you might consider purchasing a book. One thing is important, no matter what method you choose, make sure you are prepared in each of the categories that NCLEX will test. To pass the NCLEX you must be above the "line of minimum competency" in each area by answering questions that are at the application/analysis level. Focus on remediation of your weaker areas and make them your strength!

It is helpful to remember that the NCLEX is essentially a multiple-choice test that is meant to ensure that the graduate nurse meets a basic minimal standard of safety and clinical decision making to provide autonomous patient care. But to demystify and understand the essence of the NCLEX, it is an examination that measures your ability to clinically reason.

Clinical Reasoning and the NCLEX

When clinical reasoning is deeply understood and practically applied, this essential nurse thinking skill will not only prepare you for real-world practice but the NCLEX as well. Following is a review of the most important principles that will directly correlate to NCLEX success because these are also the same priorities that the NCLEX assesses throughout the examination:

- Every question is a brief clinical scenario that is contextualized to the bedside.
- Emphasis is on SAFETY, primarily safe clinical judgments.
- There are no NANDA-I nursing diagnostic statements to identify nursing priorities on the NCLEX.
- Emphasis is on principles of clinical reasoning:
  - ✓ What is the best clinical judgment to make?
  - ✓ What is the nursing priority?
  - ✓ What is the rationale for every nursing intervention or physician order?
  - ✓ What is the expected outcome for any medication or physician order?
  - ✓ Within the context of the clinical scenario, what are significant and relevant clinical data?
  - ✓ What are the most common laboratory values and the nursing implications if they are abnormal?
  - ✓ Compare/contrast normal physical assessment findings with those that are abnormal, and then reflect and determine if these abnormal findings are clinically significant.
  - ✓ Compare/contrast normal vital sign findings with those that are abnormal, and then reflect and see if these abnormal findings are clinically significant.

NCLEX Test Plan

The NCLEX has a blueprint ("NCLEX-RN Test Plan," 2013) that consists of four major categories of client needs. It also has a predictable percentage of content for each category. Two of these major categories are divided for a total of six subcategories for a total of eight categories of content. This is the current NCLEX blueprint that includes the percentage of content, a brief definition, and the most common concepts that will be found in each category.

Safe and Effective Care Environment

16–22%–Management of Care
This is the highest weighted single category that emphasizes the ability to recognize clinical priorities. Providing and directing nursing care that enhances the care delivery setting to protect clients, family/significant others, and health care personnel are also situated:
- Establish priorities
- Collaboration w/treatment team
- Advocacy

8–14%–Safety and Infection Control
Protecting clients, families, and health care personnel from health and environmental hazards:
- Error prevention
- Safe use of equipment
- Injury prevention

Health Promotion and Maintenance (6–12%)

The nurse provides and directs nursing care of the client and family/significant others that incorporates knowledge of expected growth and development principles, prevention, and/or early detection of health problems, and strategies to achieve optimal health:

- Disease prevention
- Physical assessment
- Client education

Psychosocial Integrity (6–12%)

Nurse provides care that promotes and supports the emotional, mental, and social well-being of the patient and family who are experiencing stressful events:

- Coping mechanisms
- Therapeutic communication
- End of life care

Physiologic Integrity

6–12%–Basic Care and Comfort

Providing comfort and assistance in the performance of activities of daily living:

- Elimination
- Nutrition/oral hydration
- Mobility/immobility

13–19%–Pharmacological and Parenteral Therapies

This is the second highest weighted category, so be sure that you have a deep understanding of pharmacology! Remember that only generic names of all medications are used on the NCLEX. Emphasizes providing care related to the administration of medications and parenteral therapies:

- Expected actions, adverse/side effects
- Medication administration
- IV therapies
- Dosage calculation

10–16%–Reduction of Risk Potential

Reducing the likelihood that clients will develop complications or health problems related to existing conditions, treatments, or procedures

- Changes in VS
- Diagnostic tests
- Lab values
- System-specific assessments
- Potential for alterations in body systems

11–17%–Physiological Adaptation

Managing and providing care for clients with acute, chronic, or life-threatening health conditions. In other words, the ability of the nurse to "rescue" when there is a change in status. The following aspects are also emphasized:

- Pathophysiology
- F&E imbalances
- Medical emergencies

The percentages of each of the Client Need categories are NOT equally weighted. The following categories, though they comprise 50 percent of the categories, can be weighted from 50–74 percent or almost three quarters of the NCLEX if weighted on the high side. Though all NCLEX client need categories are relevant, these four are the most important!

1. Management of care (16–22%)
2. Medication/IV therapies (13–19%)
3. Physiologic adaptation (11–17%)
4. Reduction of risk (10–16%)

These four categories represent the importance of possessing a deep understanding of the applied sciences and nurse thinking that situates clinical reasoning. It emphasizes the need to recognize clinical priorities and identify relevant data that may suggest a need to rescue. These four categories also reflect the essence of and how important mastery of the advanced level of nursing education is to safe clinical practice.

In contrast, the remaining four Client Need categories of the NCLEX represent 26–50 percent or about a quarter of the NCLEX if weighted on the low end.

5. Safety/infection control (8–14%)
6. Basic cares/comfort (6–12%)
7. Health promotion/maintenance (6–12%)
8. Psychosocial integrity (6–12%)

These categories are primarily basic level content areas. This does not diminish the importance of these topics to nursing education, but it serves to illustrate the content areas that must be emphasized and DEEPLY understood by students to ensure passing the NCLEX the first time! To deepen your understanding of the NCLEX test blueprint and how the passing score is determined by the National Council of State Boards of Nursing (NCSBN) go to www.ncsbn.org.

Application/Analysis Knowledge Required!

Knowledge and comprehension are lower levels of thinking. Though this is important, if this is the highest level of knowledge you possess on content from nursing education, you will FAIL the NCLEX. You MUST be able to use and APPLY knowledge and analyze data to identify the correct nursing priority or nursing intervention. To compare and contrast these two levels of knowledge, here is an example of lower level knowledge/comprehension question:

1. What pharmacologic category does propranolol belong to?
    a. Calcium channel blocker
    b. ACE inhibitor
    c. Beta blocker
    d. Nitrates

If you chose (c.) beta blocker, you are correct! This was content knowledge, and probably too easy for most.

Let's look at the higher level thinking required to pass the NCLEX. Application is the ability to APPLY your knowledge to a clinical context. Analysis includes the ability to compare and contrast information and deduce the correct response. This is high level thinking that requires DEEP UNDERSTANDING of the content so you can readily apply it to the wide variety of clinical situations you will see in practice. This is the bar that must be met in order to pass the NCLEX. Let's do a test question using this level of knowledge and see if you find it a bit more difficult.

2. Your patient is receiving propranolol daily. What is the most important question that the nurse should ask?
    a. How have you been sleeping at night?
    b. Have you noticed a decrease in your urine output?
    c. How would you describe your ability to breathe?
    d. Have you been experiencing a dry cough?

In order to come to the correct response you must UNDERSTAND the mechanism of action and pathophysiology of a beta blocker. Knowing that propranolol is a nonselective beta blocker, how will this mechanism of action potentially affect the lungs? The nurse must relate pharmacology to practice by recognizing that blocking beta 2 receptors on the bronchioles has the potential to cause bronchoconstriction which would then lead to shortness of breath.

Therefore, the correct answer is c. How would you describe your ability to breathe? Remember that every NCLEX question is situated with a clinical scenario.

Are you overwhelmed yet? This is a high order of mastery for any new graduate! You may not feel you were adequately prepared for this level of knowledge and clinical practice. The clinical reasoning case studies I have constructed and included in this book reflect real-world practice and incorporate these key NCLEX objectives that correlate with an emphasis on clinical reasoning in practice.

If you make it a priority to APPLY and translate the content of your nursing program to the bedside, and if you work through the case studies that I have created and then carefully review the answer key that contains well-developed rationale, you are well on your way to being prepared not only for the NCLEX, but more importantly, the rigors of professional practice!

CHAPTER 12 HIGHLIGHTS

- The NCLEX licensure examination is essentially a test that assesses your ability to use knowledge, clinically reason, and make a correct clinical judgment.

- Principles of clinical reasoning that must be applied to bedside patient care include the ability of the graduate nurse to identify relevant clinical data, abnormal assessment and lab values, the rationale for nursing and medical interventions, and the correct clinical priority.

- Though there are eight client need categories of test questions on the NCLEX, they are not equally weighted. The top three categories that comprise the majority of NCLEX questions are: "Management of Care" that assesses your ability to establish the correct nursing priority, "Pharmacological and Parenteral Therapies" that is all about pharm and medication administration, and "Physiological Adaptation" that assesses your ability to use knowledge related to pathophysiology and fluids and electrolytes.

- In order to pass the NCLEX, it is not enough to know or memorize content. You must be able to APPLY knowledge to the clinical scenario on each test question.

Additional Resources

- *Saunders Comprehensive Review for the NCLEX-RN® Examination 6th ed.* by Linda Anne Silvestri
- *Saunders Comprehensive Review for the NCLEX-PN® Examination 5th ed.* by Linda Anne Silvestri
- Kaplan NCLEX Review program: http://www.kaptest.com/nursing/nclex-prep/
- Hurst NCLEX Review program: http://www.hurstreview.com/

Be nice to me...I may be your nurse someday!

Chapter 13
How to Get Your
First Nursing Position

"Your work is going to fill a large part of your life, and the only way to be truly satisfied is to do what you believe is great work. And the only way to do great work is to love what you do. If you haven't found it yet, keep looking. Don't settle."
–Steve Jobs, founder of Apple

You have graduated from nursing school. The next step is to pass the NCLEX and then obtain employment as a registered nurse. I'd like to share some practical strategies for helping you with this transition from student to employed registered nurse. Let's assume that you have passed the NCLEX and are now ready to attain your dream to become a professional nurse. You now need to get hired.

How do you practically and effectively make that positive impression that will set you apart from other applicants? In order to take the next step, you must:

- Know what to include in a cover letter
- Put together an effective resume
- Obtain references and letters of reference
- Nail your interview

Reach Your Dream

Though you may have a dream specialty clinical area, in most cases you would be better served and prepared if you first acquired some basic clinical experience in cardiac telemetry or med/surg if acute care is an option to lay a foundation to build your specialty experience upon. Your first year of nursing practice should be considered as your "finishing school" where your education and practice all come together. You want to be in a clinical environment where you will be well supported and not overwhelmed as a new nurse.

To obtain additional support that will smooth your transition to clinical practice, a new graduate nurse residency program should be pursued if acute care facilities in your community offer this option. Sometimes this is done more informally through an intensive orientation and mentoring program. Either way, you will need a supportive environment where you can continue to learn, grow, and ask questions as a new nurse. Another option to obtain additional support is to consider applying for positions in a teaching hospital. The distinctives of a teaching hospital include working alongside health care professionals who are immersed in an environment where students from different disciplines are actively learning. Many sets of eyes will be on your patient and everyone is trying to do their best as students. Questions are expected and are seen as a part of the care experience among colleagues.

If you know that you want to work in a specialty area of nursing such as critical care, obstetrics, pediatrics, or the emergency department, have a concrete plan that will make this possible. Review job postings for minimum requirements listed for the position you want to obtain and make plans to acquire those experiences and skills. However, while you are working toward gaining those valuable experiences, remain engaged and learn all that you can wherever you are.

Don't be tempted to feel any experience is "beneath" you. Maintain the attitude of a servant and practice humility. By doing so, you will learn throughout your professional career and add things to your "tool belt" which will make you a better nurse overall. Many organizations require one to two years of med/surg experience to move into any specialty area including ED and ICU. Any clinical experience is valuable regardless of the setting.

Consider each person that you encounter valuable in this learning journey – your colleagues (licensed and non-licensed), your patients, and the families. As you develop those relationships and show value to those people around you, the healing environment blossoms into a collaborative environment for the health and betterment of everyone you work with.

What Organization Would You Like to Work For?

This may seem like a simple question and you might be tempted to say, "Anywhere I can get a job" and "Does it matter?" The answer is yes, it does matter. You want to explore the organization's mission, vision, and value statements on its website. Do they align with your own personal values? Is this an environment where you can truly embrace and live out these carefully thought out statements? The organization where you are employed will expect this.

Knowing the mission statement will also help during your interview at that organization and in writing your cover letter for seeking employment. Look for areas where you have commonality and have already demonstrated that the values the organization holds match values you hold. You may have the opportunity to make a statement during the interview about how the organization's values align with your own. Be prepared for the follow-up question of "How do they align?" and think of examples ahead of time which speak to this.

One area where institutional values may collide with personal values is abortion. A nurse colleague found herself working at a public hospital and was told that she was required to participate in performing an abortion or lose her job. She was personally against abortion but did not understand this to be a requirement of her job. She chose to participate in this procedure to keep her job. Had she further evaluated the institution's mission and position on abortion, she could have sought employment at other institutions where abortions were not performed.

But this moral conflict did not have to happen. There are two broad categories in which nurses can conscientiously object to participate – based on provisions addressed in the ANA Code of Ethics. Nurses can refuse to participate in all instances of an intervention – such as an abortion or sexual reassignment surgery – based on religious or moral grounds. Nurses who hold these strong beliefs should make their objections to participate in these types of interventions or procedures known at the time of hiring ("Conscientious Objection," 2015).

In order for nurses to ethically and morally object to participating in an intervention, that intervention must challenge their moral integrity and must violate a deeply held conviction of what is right or wrong. The Code does not allow nurses to refuse care based on prejudice, discrimination, or dislike. For example, a nurse cannot refuse care because the patient abuses alcohol or is homosexual ("Conscientious Objection," 2015).

Constructing Your Cover Letter

A cover letter should be brief and consist of only three paragraphs. The introductory paragraph is used to introduce yourself and explain your interest in the specific position for which you are applying. State how you found this position and why you chose this particular hospital and would like to work for them.

The body or second paragraph (you may use bulleted phrases) serves to relate your specific skills and experiences to the specific position you are applying for. This is not a summary of your resume. Connect your experience to the position and how this makes you an outstanding candidate for this particular position.

The third or request paragraph is a short recap of your interest in the position, your strengths, and some general sentiments (e.g., "I look forward to discussing the position and my qualifications with you soon" or "Thank you for your time and consideration. I look forward to meeting you to discuss my qualifications in greater detail."

Before you send a cover letter with your resume to a potential employer, the following suggestions will increase your chances of making an impression that will lead to an invitation for an interview:

- Personalize your cover letter in a way that describes both the qualities and experience you would bring to the organization and how those align with the mission, vision and/or values of the organization.
- Address your cover letter to a person if you can find out the name of the person who will review your materials. Sometimes you can discover the name of the nurse recruiter in human resources with a phone call.
- Limit use of the word "I" in the start of your letter and as the first word of new paragraphs. Take time to read the position description and highlight the qualifications you have which match the position posting.
- Incorporate any awards the organization has received, if applicable. This will show that you have taken the time to get to know the hospital or care facility and understand the quality culture it seeks to maintain. You can usually find this on the hospital website.
- List skills that can be clearly measured. Remove nonmeasurable words such as "team player."
- If you don't hear anything within 10 days, follow up with a phone call or email in a polite and professional manner inquiring as to the status of your application and any time frame for decisions which might exist.

If you are applying to a large organization, computers may be used to pre-screen applications and your word choice is important. You want to match key words in the job description for minimum or even preferred qualifications so that your cover letter and resume "match" the position for which you are applying. This is not the time to be creative and use synonyms for keywords. If it says that it is preferred you have experience with an electronic medical records system called "EPIC," then be precise and use that term in your experience if you have it.

Constructing Your Resume

Just because you are entering a job market that may have numerous nursing positions available, do not assume that a properly constructed resume is not that important. You want to make an excellent first impression that conveys professionalism and communicates that you pursue excellence in all that you do.

Your resume speaks volumes about you, and your potential employer recognizes this. Put your best foot forward by following these practical strategies to construct a resume that will open the first door of your employment (Isaacs, 2015)!

- **Show your value to the organization.** Begin your resume with a qualifications summary that provides an overview of the value you bring to the organization. Paint a picture of what you have to offer by including a narrative statement of your goal, specialty area, level of experience, and any other credentials.
- **Add an expertise section.** Use a bulleted list of your proficiency areas and give hiring managers a snapshot of your capabilities. Your expertise could be a nursing specialty or unique skills.
- **Provide details of your nursing related experience.** Hiring managers want to understand the scope of your experience so they can see if you're a good match for the job opening. When describing your nursing or nurse-related experience, write about the type of facility and area of specialization. Graduate nurses with limited work experience should provide details of their unpaid work or clinical rotations.
- **Communicate that you are a top performer.** Think about how you went above and beyond your job duties to make a positive contribution to your employer, patients, families, and the community. Did you promote health and well-being by providing free community health care seminars or were you involved in any type of medical mission? By providing details about your accomplishments, you show potential employers that you would be a valuable asset to their organization.
- **Highlight your academic achievements.** In your Education section, mention any academic honors, scholarships, and fellowships. If you have been inducted into Sigma Theta Tau, the honor society of nursing, this must be included! Include your GPA (if 3.0 or greater) and related courses. Be sure to never round up your GPA!
- **Print your resume on quality parchment stock.** You have come this far by producing a top-notch resume. Do not print it on traditional white copy paper! Use a quality ivory linen or parchment paper that communicates quality and excellence.

I have included two excellent examples of actual graduate student resumes in the appendix.

Applications on the Organization's Website

Most organizations prefer that applications be made through their website or a third party vendor who screens applications for them. Be prepared to create usernames and passwords for each system. Keep careful track of these for later use. If you do come back to apply for a new or different position, make sure you always check which cover letter and resume they have archived for you and update each of these to match the new position you are applying for. Carefully read each required document you need for the complete application. If they ask for "transcripts, resume, cover letter, and three letters of recommendation" be sure that each of these items are included. If you do not submit one element, your application will be considered incomplete and you may not be passed through the screening process.

Pre-hire Testing and Screening

Before you are considered as a new hire, you may be required to pass a medication written exam, which may cover things such medication calculation, safe administration, rights of medication administration, and common side effects. Patient safety is foundational to nursing practice. Because errors in practice can impact patient outcomes and even result in patient deaths, as a soon-to-be professional nurse, you owe it to your patients and their families to do everything you can to demonstrate the highest levels of safety by passing any tests that a prospective employer may use.

You may also be required to pass a pre-employment physical exam. This may be done by your own health care provider or one the employer uses. Their objective is to make sure you are able to perform the duties of the job safely, to support your own health and well-being, and to contribute to safe patient care. This process usually involves a drug and alcohol screening. Expect background checks. Some states require registration and screening by state care services background entities. There may be other tests or screenings, depending on the organization. If you are required to fill out any disclosure forms, always be sure that you are completely honest and ethical in your responses.

You will also be required to provide proof of immunizations or be prepared to have titers drawn so that you are not a facilitator of communicable diseases to the patient population. If you are not fully immunized because you conscientiously object to immunizations, you will not be allowed to work in a hospital with patients who are immunocompromised.

References and Letters of Recommendation

If you are asked to provide references, it is important that you ask those individuals if they are willing to be a reference for you ahead of time. If possible, give them a copy of the job description and the cover letter, which highlights how you are uniquely qualified for this position. Ask your reference to clarify how they want their name and credentials listed as well as which contact methods you may provide to potential employers. You do not want to provide personal cell phone numbers if your reference has not given that permission. If you ask a former faculty member for a reference, there is often a release form you are required to fill out for the school so this can be done.

In addition to references, some employers may want you to provide letters of recommendation. This can also be done by those who are willing to be your reference. If possible, get this letter on the letterhead of the organization where they work as this lends to credibility of their position. If this is not allowed, then a personal stationary recommendation is fine. But ask them to provide their complete credentials after their name and contact methods for any follow-up questions. You may be asked to draft a letter of recommendation that describes how you are prepared for the position you are applying for.

This letter of recommendation should include your skills, education, and experience. Allow the person writing the letter to be flexible and adjust the letter to fit their writing style. Be honest and do not exaggerate what they know about you and then ask them to sign it. Allow them to have liberty to edit the letter to accurately represent their knowledge and recommendation of you.

Practical Professionalism

Professionalism starts from the first encounter you have with the organization, whether in writing or in person. The person at the front door matters. How you treat each person shows how you will treat each patient, their family, coworkers, and others in the organization. Each person matters and is valuable. You may find yourself riding in the elevator with the person who will interview you. Smile, be friendly, professional, and authentic.

Be sure to follow up with a thank you card for in-person interviews that are sent to each person you met with. Take time to write down their names or better yet, ask for their business card if they have one. This card gives their email address, the correct spelling of their name, and their title. If you forget, go online or call the organization and explain that you are writing a thank-you letter and would like to verify spelling of names and titles. Often the person who answers the phone can provide this basic information.

When you write your thank-you note, keep it short but relevant to your interview. Thank them for their time and one specific thing you learned from them about the position or organization. State that you feel you would be a good fit for the job/organization and that it would be a privilege to work there or be part of the team. Close with something which indicates that you look forward to the next steps in the process (if there are next steps). Choose a clean-lined and simple, gender-neutral, plain white or off-white, and professional pack of note cards. Avoid thank-you cards that are bought individually as they tend to be less professional.

If you send an email which is becoming more acceptable, keep the same professional approach. If you currently have an email address that is less than professional, please consider starting a new account that is more professional in your address. For instance if your email address is "crazypartyanimal@anydomain.com," how would this reflect on your character to those who do not know you?

If you participate in social media such as Facebook, clean it up! Do not post pictures of yourself in situations that would be less than professional and do not accept tags of others that do not put you in the best possible light. Do not be surprised if someone in the hiring process will unofficially search for how you represent yourself on the World Wide Web.

Nail Your Interview!

Be prepared! Use the career service office at your college for guidance. Be sure to research and practice interview questions you may be asked that will require forethought to make a favorable impression. How would you answer the following questions below? Review and reflect upon the following questions that you may be asked in an interview (Anonymous, 2003):

1. Where do you see yourself in three years?
2. What do you bring to this position? How do you stand out from the other applicants?
3. What attracts you to this facility? To this position? What do you hope to get out of the experience?
4. How would you describe your ideal job? Your ideal work environment?
5. Who are your career role models and why?
6. What are the most important lessons you've learned in your career?
7. How much supervision do you want or need?
8. What professional organizations do you belong to?
9. How have you participated in the professional organizations you belong to?
10. What nursing publications do you subscribe to?

Make sure that how you dress is professional during all encounters. This includes visiting the organization to pick up brochures or inquire about applications. You may be remembered for either good or bad first impressions. Sometimes those screening or making decisions are in view or earshot of the front desk where you may be. Professional dress is generally accepted as business wear. This does not mean evening wear or casual wear. Dress in comfortably fitting clothes. If you have clothes that do not fit well, it will be noticed and you will be uncomfortable. Wear shoes that you will be able to walk around for extensive impromptu tours of the facility. Be prepared to take the stairs instead of the elevator – avoid high heels.

Women, dress slacks are appropriate as part of a suit, but if you wear a skirt or dress, keep it professional. Do not dress as if you were going out for the evening. Ensure it that your clothing does not reveal cleavage. A skirt should go to the bottom of your knee so that when you sit down it does not ride up too high, or if you cross your legs, everything remains covered. If you do need to cross your legs when sitting, consider crossing your ankles only. This presents a more polished look and avoids any gaps.

Do not wear excessive jewelry. Keep earrings to a single hole (posts are preferred) for each ear only. Take out any facial piercings. Make sure any tattoos are covered by your clothing as much as possible. Keep makeup simple and minimal. Keep rings and wrist jewelry to a minimum, such as a wedding ring and a watch. If you wear a necklace, keep it simple. You want to be remembered for who you are and not any over-the-top accessories or dress.

For men, dress pants that are pleated and fit well with a belt that matches dress shoes always looks good. A dress shirt with buttons and a professional tie is the essence of what is needed. It is not necessary to wear a three-piece suit or a suit coat unless you feel comfortable in this attire. If you tend to get nervous and perspire, a suit coat can cover this up and make you less self-conscious.

If your interview is after a meal, be sure to brush your teeth and check your smile. When people are nervous they can get a dry mouth and a lozenge may help. Avoid bold colored lozenges so your tongue and teeth do not become discolored. Use lozenges only if you can do it with no one present and if you can tuck it in your cheek and keep it there and it is NOT noticeable when you are talking. Never move the lozenge in your mouth; this will be distracting.

Never come to an interview chewing gum. During the interview, bring a clean notepad for taking notes, or better yet a portfolio case with additional copies of your resume, paper, and pen. Write down important points as others share them and also keywords for questions you are asked. Sometimes when you are answering questions, it is easy to wander away from the original question. This notepad will help you to quickly look down to stay on track.

At the end of an answer to a complex question, it is okay to follow up by stating, "Does that answer your question?" (or a variation thereof). This provides an opportunity for positive affirmation from the interviewer and also a window if they would like different or more information. Print out and bring a copy of the organization's mission, vision, and values statements. You may be able to refer to these as common touch points during your interview but keep it simple and don't overdo it.

Always bring professional hard copies of your resume to an interview. Do not assume they will have it or sometimes they ask another person to come into the interview at the last minute and copies have not been made. This is your opportunity to look well prepared. You want to bring at least three copies of your resume to an interview if you know one person will be interviewing you. By having a copy of your resume with you it can also help you to quickly glance at your qualifications to go into more detail as needed.

At the end of the interview, ask about the timeline for the decision-making process and any next steps there may be. Thank the interviewer for their time and state that you look forward to hearing from them. If they do not initiate any discussion on validation for parking, do not ask for this. Be prepared ahead of time to pay for your own parking.

But most importantly during the entire interview process, be your kind, authentic self!

CHAPTER 13 HIGHLIGHTS
• In order to obtain your first position as a professional nurse, you need to do more than apply and show up. You must make a professional and positive first impression by crafting a professional resume and cover letter.
• Begin to compile a list of references and letters of recommendation from current employers or nursing faculty from your program that you can use when you begin to apply for open nursing positions.
• Maintain a positive first impression and professionalism in your interview with appropriate dress and being relaxed and confident, maintaining appropriate eye contact.

Chapter Reflections

1. What organization/facility would you like to work for after graduation?

2. What is its mission statement and other relevant facts you would need to know to plan for an interview?

3. What student organizations are you currently involved in that would benefit you when included on your resume?

    If you are not currently involved, what could you become involved in before graduation?

4. If you are in your final year of nursing school, begin to create a draft of a cover letter and resume so you can get the input of others, including nursing faculty.

5. Construct a series of possible questions that you may be asked by a prospective employer for an interview. Practice your answers with another student for feedback, then switch places!

> *Knock, Knock!*
> *–Who's there?*
> *HIPAA!*
> *–HIPAA who?*
> *I can't tell you that.*

Chapter 14
Practical Principles for Professional Preparation

You have accepted your first nursing position and are now entering clinical practice. Congratulations! Do not be overwhelmed with what you don't know. Instead, remember that you passed nursing school as well as the NCLEX. Maintain a positive attitude regarding your capabilities to successfully transition to autonomous professional practice. You are now opening a new chapter in your life's journey that will also bring new challenges. In my journey over the past 30 years in clinical practice, I have lived out as well as observed several principles that will help guide you to fulfill your potential as a professional nurse.

These practical principles include:

- Transitioning from nursing student to licensed nurse
- Identifying your best fit
- Progressing and becoming an expert nurse
- Knowing the importance of being certified
- Being a life-long learner
- Strategizing to transition successfully

Transitioning from Nursing Student to Licensed Nurse

Reality Shock

The differences between your academic environment and the values you were taught may collide with the clinical culture in which you will practice. Reality shock can be described as your lived experience when you enter the nursing profession but find yourself feeling unprepared. You will soon see the differences between what you learned in school and what is current clinical reality and practice.

It is important to recognize your limitations and need for time and clinical experience to fully develop as a nurse in practice. Benner's highly acclaimed model of nurse development has demonstrated that it requires at least two to three years of clinical experience to advance from your current level as an advanced beginner nurse to the next stage of competence (Benner, 1982). I will discuss Benner's model in detail later in this chapter.

The education-practice gap is an ongoing problem in nursing education and directly affects students who graduate from even the best programs. Simply stated, the gap is the gulf between how students are taught and what they will experience in real-world clinical practice. For example, in the clinical setting after graduation you will no longer have one or two patients as you did in nursing school clinical, but will be responsible for four to eight patients in an acute care setting, and double this in transitional or skilled care setting. If you are not well prepared to multitask and priority set for this reality it inevitably causes a high degree of stress and "reality shock."

You will be torn at times regarding which set of values you are supposed to embrace – the ones that you learned in school or the ones you see every other nurse on your unit using. As you experience this tension and feelings of unpreparedness, your attitude is essential. Despite what you are feeling, you must convince yourself that you have made it this far and that you truly do have what it takes to be a nurse. As you acquire experience, things will begin to become easier and you will begin to find your stride in just a matter of time!

But some nurses are casualties of reality shock. Unfortunately, many new graduate nurses leave the profession in the first year because of job stress, lack of organizational support, poor nurse-physician relations, unreasonable workloads, uncivil work environments, and difficulty transitioning to practice (Clark & Springer, 2012).

Knowing that reality shock is a documented phenomenon, I want you to expect this reality, but more importantly, be prepared when it comes your way. When you recognize that the feelings of fear, anxiety, and lack of feeling prepared are normal, this knowledge will hopefully help you weather this storm.

What Am I Feeling?

You don't need to know everything as a new grad! Now is the time to develop realistic expectations for yourself. Remember that it will take at least a year to learn and grow in your new role. When I recently asked many of the new nurses in our hospital their feelings as they started their first position, would it surprise you that they all shared similar feelings of:

- Being overwhelmed
- Anxious
- Fearful
- Thankful at the end of the shift that they did not harm or kill their patients!

If you can identify with these feelings, know that you are not alone! Because of a lack of clinical experience, the full force of reality shock will intensify the normal stress and anxiety that any person experiences when starting a new job.

These same nurses admitted that their feelings of anxiety and fear were a daily occurrence for at least the first six months of clinical practice. After six months they began to turn a corner and began to feel more comfortable and confident in their skills and abilities as a nurse. That is why it is so important to hang in there and persevere regardless of the storm that feels like it is going to take you under. Think of each shift as a clinical day. As you acquire additional clinical experience, it will prepare you for the next day as you translate your knowledge and what you have learned from each shift you work to the next.

How to Cope

It is one thing to experience the painful feelings that accompany reality shock; it is another to cope and to overcome them. The following are some practical strategies that you can incorporate to help you cope and overcome this experience as a new nurse.

- Develop relationships with your preceptor and new co-workers. Find a new or best friend at work as well as a mentor!
- Share your struggles and feelings with a trusted nurse colleague or mentor. This is another reason to establish meaningful relationships with others on your unit.
- Know where to access need-to-know resources as well as nurses who are your best guides and resources.
- It is normal to experience some dissatisfaction with your new role and work environment. Have realistic expectations and be kind to yourself!
- Learn and pattern your practice after nurses who are excellent role models. Just because you see poor examples of nurses does NOT give you permission to lower your practice to their level!
- Use reflection to identify what is going well and what can be improved. Celebrate and acknowledge what you are doing well and do not focus on the negative!
- Keep a journal so you can reflect on your practice and acknowledge your feelings. This will help you to see the progress you are making on your journey!
- Identify and manage conflicts as they arise. Be direct with your communication. Do not allow inevitable conflict with co-workers to steal your joy and exacerbate reality shock (Ferris, 2012).

Patient Complexity

A weakness of textbook learning is that it does not take into context how patients typically present in the clinical setting. Each patient is unique and the way that they can present with their primary problem can be different from the textbook norms of illness presentation. For example, it is not uncommon for patients to present with a myocardial infarction not with chest pain but only with referred pain such as to the jaw or arm. Expect these deviations and recognize the importance of not being focused on the concrete norms and content that are in the textbook.

As a novice nurse who tends to be a concrete textbook learner, you must work to recognize your reliance on textbook norms and realize that clinical practice will be ambiguous and not always consistent with what is taught in your textbook. Your goal is to learn what the common unique deviations from textbook content may be for each illness and then make that part of your knowledge base for practice. This is how clinical experience over time is your best preparation for ongoing clinical practice!

Another weakness of textbook learning is that it can only present one topic at a time, discuss it in depth, and then go to the next related topic in the chapter. In clinical practice most patients do not have just a single problem. They have multiple problems that influence their current presentation in the clinical setting.

It is not uncommon for patients to have two, three, or even more illnesses or disease processes that influence the current chief complaint. The ability to recognize these clinical relationships of disease processes is a challenge that will contribute to your reality shock. I recently cared for a patient with shortness of breath who had a diagnosis of sepsis, but also had a history of COPD, heart failure, fluid overload, and anxiety. Any of these other problems can also cause SOB and must be considered. Expect this level of complexity in your patients, especially in the acute care setting.

That is why it is so important to have a deep understanding of pathophysiology. Recognizing the relationships of pathophysiology will help demystify patient complexity. When you understand how other illnesses develop and are influenced by diabetes, for example, the resultant hyperlipidemia that can lead to coronary artery disease and myocardial infarction that can cause ischemic cardiomyopathy, which influences the development of renal failure, will begin to be understood and expected.

Navigating the Matrix of Hospital/Unit Politics

A nurse mentor is an essential guide, like Yoda in the Star Wars trilogy, to reveal the unseen matrix of hospital/unit politics that though not visible are clearly present and must be uncovered in order to successfully navigate a new setting. The matrix of unit politics is revealed through the unspoken culture and unofficial leaders in the clinical setting. It is also revealed by the way that nurses and the team work together. Is this unit a healthy culture were teamwork is the norm? Or is it defined by its animosity and incivility and lack of respect towards one another?

The clinical setting can consist of landmines that one can step on and not realize until it is too late that you could have avoided that blowup! The matrix includes the nuances of primary care providers and how to communicate with each one effectively based on what other nurses know from their experience working with these individuals. Use a trusted mentor to ask questions regarding these unspoken assumptions and aspects of communicating with other members of the team so that you can make your best first impression possible.

How to Progress and Become an Expert Nurse

Patricia Benner, whom this book is dedicated to and whose work is widely cited in this text, is best known for her early nursing research that led to her book *From Novice to Expert: Clinical Excellence and Power in Clinical Practice.* This work detailed how nurses progress, develop skills and understanding of patient care over time.

The five levels of nurse proficiency in nursing practice that Benner identified are:

1. Novice
2. Advanced beginner
3. Competent
4. Proficient
5. Expert

Summary of Novice to Expert

The relevance of Benner's framework now that you have graduated is that it defines the definite levels of clinical progression and the characteristics of nursing practice at each level. The following is a summary of her theory:

Novice

- First-year nursing student with no experience
- Taught and uses general textbook rules to help perform tasks
- Rules of clinical practice are related to textbook learning, independent of specific cases, and applied universally because of a lack of clinical experience
- Concrete (textbook) learner whose thinking is limited and inflexible
- Task oriented

Advanced Beginner

- Graduating nursing student who demonstrates basic level of performance
- Because of limited prior experience in clinical settings, is able to recognize patterns

- Does not consistently recognize clinical priorities

Competent

- Typically requires two to three years of clinical experience after graduating from nursing school
- Gains perspective from planning nursing actions based on conscious, abstract, and analytical thinking and helps to achieve greater efficiency and organization
- Recognizes clinical priorities

Proficient

- Begins to see abstract situations as a whole
- Holistic understanding improves decision making
- Learns from prior experiences and what to expect in certain situations and how to modify plan of care

Expert

- No longer relies as heavily on principles, rules, or guidelines to put the clinical picture together and guide interventions
- Has intuitive grasp of clinical situations
- Performance is fluid, flexible, and highly proficient (Benner, 1984)

To place these five distinct levels of nursing progression in context, you began nursing school as a "novice," which is the first level of Benner's framework. Because you had no prior clinical experience as a nurse, you were unable to recognize relevant clinical data and when an exception to standards of care was in order (Benner, 1982).

For example, knowing that normal O2 saturation is >95% and your patient with end-stage COPD has O2 saturation of 90%, which is likely their normal, you may not recognize this exception because of the lack of clinical context and inflexible, rule-governed behavior. As a graduate nurse you are now on the second level of proficiency which is "advanced beginner." You will tend to be strongly TASK oriented, and will not readily recognize priorities and what task is most important to do first (Benner, 1982).

To progress and become "competent," which is the third level of proficiency typically requires two to three years of experience in the same clinical area (Benner, 1982). At this level, the nurse knows what needs to be done and is able to set needed priorities to efficiently organize and manage the day.

Centrality of Caring to Progression

Caring remains central for the nurse to progress and develop to become an expert practitioner. The heightened level of INVOLVEMENT that caring represents is foundational to expert nursing practice (Benner & Wrubel). CARING is what makes the nurse notice what interventions are most effective and identify subtle signs of improvement or deterioration.

Benner studied the characteristics that made expert nurses effective in practice. She identified that knowledge and technique were not enough; caring is an essential component that will lay the foundation to becoming an expert in nursing practice (Benner, Hooper-Kyriakidis, & Stannard, 2011).

Progression vs. Regression

An important point to consider as you examine each of these levels of proficiency is to realize that they are not static, but you can progress or regress over time. If the nurse is engaged and motivated in practice, she will progress with time and experience to an expert level. But what happens if that same nurse experiences depression, stress of a divorce, or burnout? Is it realistic to maintain the same level of motivation and engagement under these circumstances? For most it is not and regression to a lower level of proficiency is inevitable.

This is why the professional discipline and habit of reflection is so important. It is possible to regress and not realize it. Form meaningful relationships with your colleagues that you can be honest about the difficulties you are experiencing and draw upon them for needed support.

At a minimum, the nurse must uphold and perform the standards of safe practice. To progress through these stages requires time in clinical practice. There is no substitute for clinical experience! But time alone will not make you an expert clinician.

To progress to be an expert nurse, you must be motivated and guided by the DESIRE to be excellent in what you do in practice. Excellent practice at its very root is SELF-MOTIVATING (Benner, Hooper-Kyriakidis, & Stannard, 2011). Pursuing certification in your desired nursing specialty, even if it is not required, is an example of self-motivated professional growth that will likely lead to expert practice over time.

Identify Your Best Fit

Each one of us is unique. Regardless of your disposition and temperament, there is a place for you in nursing! Did you know that there are 104 clinical nursing areas in which to specialize? Identify what specialties interest you, acquire relevant information, and determine the education and clinical experience that is needed. Johnson & Johnson has provided all this essential information in one place on its website, "Explore Specialties." Be sure to check it out! (http://www.discovernursing.com/explore-specialties#categories=management).

Research numerous nursing specialties using the Johnson & Johnson link above. Reflect and journal on the nursing specialty explored and why this area is of interest to you. This will help you to consider the wide range of other possibilities in nursing of which you may have not been aware.

Another approach that you can consider to guide you in exploring nursing specialties is to identify your basic temperament. Gather more information on areas that are a best "fit" with your personality and temperament so that you have a good idea of what areas of practice you want to pursue after graduation. From the four basic temperaments listed below (Richards, n.d.), see which one aptly describes the essence of who you are:

Sanguine

- Impulsive and pleasure-seeking
- Chronically late, and tend to be forgetful
- Sociable and charismatic
- People persons who enjoy talking, social gatherings and making new friends
- Enjoy time alone
- Sensitive, compassionate and thoughtful
- Struggle with following tasks all the way through
- Confident

Nursing roles to consider:
- Floor nursing of any kind
- Skilled care/transitional care units

Choleric
- Ambitious and leader-like, assertive
- Lots of energy, and/or passion, and try to instill it in others
- Like to be in charge of everything
- Either highly disorganized or highly organized
- Struggle with balance. One extreme to another
- Prone to mood swings.

Nursing roles to consider:
- Intensive care (ICU)
- Emergency department (ED)
- Rapid response team
- Operating room (OR)
- Mental health
- Nurse anesthetist
- Nurse practitioner
- Nursing leadership

Melancholic
- Introverted and thoughtful
- Pondering and considerate
- Highly creative
- Perfectionists
- Self-reliant and independent
- Get so involved in what they are doing they forget to think of others

Nursing roles to consider:
- Home health care
- Critical care (ICU)
- Emergency department (ED)
- Operating room (OR)
- Nursing education

Phlegmatic
- Relaxed and quiet
- Content with themselves, kind
- Accepting and affectionate
- Prefer stability to uncertainty and change

- Consistent, relaxed, calm, rational, curious, and observant
- Passive-aggressive

Nursing roles to consider:
- Home health care
- Skilled care/transitional care units
- Nursing administration

Non-bedside Nursing Options

Though most nursing positions involve direct patient care, here are settings that are either indirect or non-patient care that you may want to consider depending on your temperament:

1. Physician clinic
2. Nursing case manager
3. Nursing informatics
4. School nurse
5. Legal nursing consultant
6. Nursing research
7. Diabetic nurse educator
8. Cruise ship nurse
9. Camp nurse

Advanced Practice Positions

If you want to pursue an advanced practice degree in nursing, this is currently a master's level of preparation or about two years of college education after you have a baccalaureate degree. The education required to become a nurse practitioner and nurse anesthetist are moving toward a doctorate level of education that will require an additional year to complete, though this is not currently the standard. The following are the most common advanced nurse practice specialties you may want to consider and pursue after acquiring relevant clinical experience:

- Nurse Practitioner
- Nurse Anesthetist
- Nurse Midwife
- Clinical nurse specialist
- Nurse Educator
- Nursing Leadership and Administration
- Nursing Informatics

Get Certified

Once you have settled into a clinical area that is a good fit for you and you plan on staying in this specialty area, make it a priority to pursue your certification in that specific specialty. The essence of being certified in any nursing specialty is that it validates your knowledge and expertise in that specialty setting. Nursing certification recognizes the unique knowledge, skills, and abilities needed beyond the scope of RN licensure.

In order to become certified, the nurse must pass a difficult examination. To pass this examination requires mastery of content unique to this specialty setting as well as clinical experience. It is like taking the NCLEX, but with all questions derived from the clinical area in which you seek certification. Study manuals to prepare for the certification examination typically include need-to-know content with numerous practice questions with rationale.

Most clinical areas provide nursing certification but most require at least one to two years of clinical experience in that setting before you can take the certification examination.

Some of the most common nursing certifications and abbreviations you may see on a nurses name badge include the following:

- CCRN: Certification in Acute/Critical Care Nursing
- CEN: Certified Emergency Nurse
- RN-BC: Board Certified Psychiatric-Mental Health Nurse
- PCCN: Certified Progressive Care Nurse
- CHPN: Certified Hospice and Palliative Nurse
- CNOR: Certified Nurse, Operating Room
- CRNL: Certified Registered Nurse, Long-term care
- CVN: Certified Vascular Nurse
- CHN: Certified Community Health Nurse

I am currently certified in the two specialty areas that I practice in, emergency department (CEN) as well as critical care (CCRN). Once I had the required clinical experience, I recognized the value and desired to be certified in these clinical areas to be the best possible nurse I could be and to validate my expertise with certification. Studying for certification strengthened and developed the critical thinking and made me a better caregiver as a result.

Though it may look like I have alphabet soup behind my name, it is not what motivated me. But when families or your patient notice the additional letters behind RN on your name badge, when you briefly explain what it means, they value and appreciate a caregiver who has demonstrated their knowledge and expertise with certification. Certification validates specialty knowledge, experience, and clinical judgment.

According to one study, nurses whose clinical judgment has been validated through certification believe that they make decisions with greater confidence. This study also found that certified nurses felt that certification enabled them to feel more satisfied as a nurse in practice. Because it is voluntary, specialty certification makes it evident that they have a commitment to progress as a professional and are dedicated to be the best nurse possible, particularly in a constantly changing health care environment (AACN, 2015).

Be a Lifelong Learner

Mandates in the Nurse Practice Act make it clear that you must stay current in practice. When one of the reviewers of this book was interning at the Maryland Board of Nursing, she witnessed many nurses who were being investigated by the Board for practice concerns who could not identify any formal ongoing learning since they became a nurse. This lack of ongoing growth and development as a nurse clearly contributed to their deficient clinical practice. Decide right now to NOT be that nurse!

Your journey of learning to become a nurse does not end by successfully completing nursing school. It has only begun. You must have a thirst and desire to learn and grow as a health care professional throughout your career in order to provide the best current and evidence-based care your patients deserve. Health care and nursing are continually developing based on new research and standards of care, and change is a given.

To keep abreast of change requires continual learning. Technology changes. Treatments and nursing procedures change with evidence-based practice findings. Embrace this reality, but when you enjoy the journey you will have the aptitude that will lead to your ongoing success and professional development as a nurse. After graduation make it a priority to subscribe to relevant nursing journals that will keep you abreast of current research findings and feed your knowledge as a lifelong learner.

Nurse.com (http://www.nurse.com/) is an excellent web-based resource to keep abreast of regional and national news relevant to nursing and much more. Micromedex is a common pharmaceutical database with thorough content on the mechanism of action. My personal favorite database for understanding the pathophysiology of disease processes is http://emedicine.medscape.com/. Do NOT sell all your textbooks after graduation. You will need and refer to those relevant to your clinical setting as you transition into practice.

Incorporating Evidence-Based Practices into Your Practice

As a nursing student you most likely completed an evidence-based practice assignment. The importance of evidence-based nursing practice is not just a one-time project to complete in nursing school but an ongoing endeavor that the professional nurse must embrace as long as you are in clinical practice. The only way that you will be able to keep abreast of changes and opportunities to incorporate evidence-based practice is by reading appropriate and relevant nursing journals.

There are many excellent nursing journals for every clinical specialty. The American Journal of Nursing (AJN) is an excellent resource that is relevant for all practice settings. Make it a priority to subscribe to these relevant nursing journals in your specialty as well as be familiar with the electronic resources in your practice setting. This will allow you to be not only on the cutting edge of what is current and best practice but also be a leader for needed change in your clinical setting!

Teamwork Made Practical

You are part of a team when providing patient care and are never alone. As I observe new nurses in clinical practice they tend to operate in a silo mentality and some do not even acknowledge that there are other nurses they are working with. Recognize your limitations and do not go all the way under before you ask another nurse for help! If you need help from another colleague, most nurses are more than willing to help if they are asked.

I find the following principles helpful to create a team-oriented culture whenever or wherever you work:

- **Introduce yourself to the nurses in your work area.** Though you may know all your co-workers, if there is a float nurse or a newer nurse, be sure to take this first step. This is especially important with those nurses who are proximal to your assignment. Though this is basic professional courtesy, from my own experience, some nurses do not make this effort to introduce themselves. As a float pool nurse, I am not as well-known as core staff nurses. I consistently introduce myself and let them know that I am in the float pool. This simple gesture builds a bridge of collaboration that starts the shift off on the right foot!

- **Convey availability to your colleagues at the beginning of the shift.** Conveying availability is a caring intervention that communicates caring to patients. In a similar way, conveying availability communicates teamwork and caring to your colleagues. Some nurses hesitate to reach out when they are struggling. Knowing that you have taken the first step to reach out and are available is comforting and appreciated!

- **Provide help to a nurse who asks as soon as you are able.** It is important to follow through with a smile whenever someone takes you up on an offer for help. Be aware of nonverbal communication. I have observed in my own practice that when I have asked for help with some nurses, their nonverbal communication of eye rolling, deep sigh, or irritated facial expression make it all too apparent that I am inconveniencing them. Make it a priority to not be that nurse!

- **Remember that you are one unit and one nurse.** Nightingale communicated to new nurse graduates the truth that *"we are all one nurse"* (Attewell, 2012, p. 76). Live this out by making yourself available to assist as needed with other nurses or answering call lights for people who are not your patients. Though you may have offered help to your colleagues at the beginning of the shift, whenever you have a moment and have completed all of your necessary responsibilities, round on the unit and touch base with each nurse you see to offer any help. Your example of professional and collegial teamwork is truly contagious and will be reciprocated!

Ready to Launch

Following are a number of practical "pearls" that will help you successfully launch your nursing career.

Tools of the Trade

- **Purchase a quality stethoscope!** My son recently graduated from a diesel mechanic program. Over two years of school, he was required to purchase over $10,000 worth of tools. In comparison, a nurse needs only a few tools and the most expensive is a quality stethoscope. Quality does matter and you will notice the difference. If you got through nursing school with an inexpensive model because of your budget, it is now time to upgrade. A friend of mine told me that it is not the cost of the stethoscope that matters; it is what is between the ears of the person using it! Though there is no substitute for a thinking nurse, for less than $100, I recommend the following models that I have used in practice:
  - ✓ ADC Adscope 600 Platinum Edition Ultimate Acoustic Cardiology
    - It has excellent acoustics, and priced around $95.
    - The ADC is half the price of a comparable Littman cardiology stethoscope, but I can tell no appreciable difference in quality or acoustics
  - ✓ Littman II SE
    - This is an all-around workhorse and can be used in all clinical areas. It has slightly less quality in acoustics than a cardiology stethoscope, but the difference is negligible. Priced around $70.
- **Use a stethoscope belt clip to carry your stethoscope with you always.** Wherever you go, your stethoscope must be with you. You never know when your patient may suddenly change

and your stethoscope is nowhere to be found. If you find it uncomfortable having the weight of your stethoscope around your neck, then purchase a stethoscope belt clip for just a few dollars and you can easily carry your stethoscope on your hip instead.

     ✓ **Be sure to disinfect/clean this stethoscope as well as all tools of the trade between patient rooms.** In one study, almost half of all stethoscopes cultured were contaminated with 50 potentially pathogenic microorganisms. The most common organism (86%) was Staphylococcus aureus, and 42% of these staph organisms were methicillin-resistant S. aureus or MRSA (Campos-Murguia, Leon-Lara, Munoz, & Macias, 2013).

- **Always carry a small LED flashlight.** Since I work nights, having a small, flat LED flashlight is priceless when making rounds. You can unobtrusively check your patient's IV site or IV pump without having to turn on the lights in the room. It also can be used to assess pupillary response with neuro checks. They are typically 1" x 2" and ¼" deep. They can be purchased at any hardware store for less than $5.

- **Always carry a scissors, forceps, and medical tape with you.** You can carry these essential tools with you at all times. Taking a forceps, thread the tip through your roll of tape and attach the forceps to the side of your pants at the belt loop level. Then take a bandage scissors and place in the center of the tape hole. You now have all three pieces of equipment in one place and all together at your side when you need them!

- **Use a smart phone holster that has small built-in pockets.** I use a Night Ize smart phone hip holster. In addition to holding my smart phone, it has built-in loops to securely carry a carpuject for IV/IM medications, as well as small pockets to hold a small, flat LED flashlight, and safety pins (always handy to secure an NG tube to a gown to prevent needless tugging).

- **Always carry a pocket full of alcohol wipes before you start your clinical shift.** You will use them for numerous purposes such as preparing the skin for any injections and cleansing the hub of IV tubing before administering medications.

In the Trenches

- **Do what is needed to get adequate rest.** This can be difficult if you work rotating shifts, but make it a priority. Your patients will thank you!

- **Use the ride in to work to mentally prepare.** Use rituals that are meaningful to you, such as prayer or meditation to prepare for the demands of patient care.

- **Arrive at least ten minutes before your shift begins.** This will give you time to prepare mentally and establish a sense of calm, before the storm begins! Being on time is also a professional behavior that your colleagues will appreciate!

- **Mentally prepare for a difficult shift.** Then when it does not materialize, you were prepared and can be thankful for a better than expected shift!

- **Pack a nutritious meal or snack.** Don't graze on junk food on the unit in case you have little time to eat. Have a protein-rich snack such as a protein shake, yogurt smoothie, or protein bar that will give you fuel in the tank in case you don't have time for a full meal break

- **Write down all important phone numbers to communicate with the team in your facility.** Respiratory therapy, pharmacy, and physician practice groups are NEED-to-know contacts. Place on the back of your name badge or make a memo list on your smart phone.

- **Label syringes with IV medication vial.** It is essential to label all syringes that you have drawn up and will take into the patient's room to administer. One quick and easy way to do this is to take a piece of tape and attach the neck of the IV bottle to the cap of the needle on the syringe. This accomplishes two things: It identifies the syringe, and you can easily scan the medication if your institution uses bedside scanning.

- **The environment matters.** Do all that you can to create a healing environment that is as quiet, dimly lit as needed, and as clean as possible. Don't forget that Nightingale also was a nursing theorist who recognized that a clean and healing environment improved patient outcomes. She wrote in her first textbook of nursing: *"Unnecessary noise, or noise that creates an expectation in the mind, is that which hurts a patient"* (Nightingale, 1860).

- **No task is beneath you as a nurse.** Though you have a degree, continue to serve others with humility and do whatever is needed to provide patient care. Cleaning rooms or helping to clean up a soiled patient is not only the responsibility of the nursing assistants or housekeepers. Nightingale also made this point clear in her probationer address to newly graduated nurses. *"And don't despise what some of you call housemaids work"* (Attewell, 2012, p. 74).

- **Know your limitations.** This includes being honest and aware of what you do not understand. Be humble enough to recognize when you don't understand, and know when you are in over your head and the need the help of other nurses. If you are not aware of your limitations and when you need help, you will be unsafe and will likely harm your patients!

  Do not hesitate to ask questions at any time if you are unsure about anything in practice. Be honest in accepting your limitations if you have not done a skill that you are expected to do as a nurse. It is not uncommon to have not performed a Foley catheter insertion or naso-gastric tube insertion as a student. If you have not performed these skills, embrace the learning opportunity, but let your nurse colleagues know that you need their backup and have them accompany you to be safe and ensure best practice.

- **Give yourself grace to be a new nurse.** Just as it is essential to give yourself grace to be a student learner, this applies once you are in practice as well. Remember that it takes at least two years to be competent and comfortable in practice (Benner, 1982). There is no substitute for clinical experience. Early on in your career, you will struggle to put the clinical picture together and remain focused on the tasks. But in time this will change, and your proficiency will increase with clinical experience!

- **Assume the best of your colleagues.** Be slow to make judgments about other nurses. If the room is messy, supplies are missing, or other are aspects not up to your standards, assume they had a busy and difficult shift. If patterns become apparent, they need to be directly addressed.

- **Get a thick skin.** You will work with colleagues and primary care providers who will irritate you and may rub you the wrong way. Don't take every interaction personally and give grace to others for being stressed, tired and not always being kind and gracious with every interaction they have with you. Remember that you, too, will need this same grace extended to you at times as well!

- **Know how to access essential nursing information.** How do you access the hospital policies related to any procedure that you are not familiar with? How do you fill out an incident report online? Where can you access Micromedex and other online nursing resources that your facility provides? Be sure that you can access this information and know where it is found before you are off orientation. This will facilitate your transition to a new setting because you will always have questions. You just need to know where to find the answers!

Practical Principles to Transition Successfully

Though you are early in your journey, I would like to share a few closing thoughts that will help you successfully transition to professional practice after you graduate (Neal-Boylan, 2013).

- **Get a mentor.** Make this priority one when you enter into clinical practice! Identify nurses with whom you work who are excellent, experienced, and model the essence of the professional nurse you aspire to be. Your mentor can be official or unofficial, depending on where you work and the orientation process. A good mentor will imprint the intangibles of nursing that will positively influence your professional development.
- **Ask questions.** Never fake it! You could put your patient's life at risk. If you have a question, use your resources. If you are still not able to find what you need, ask your nurse colleagues. One experienced nurse said it beautifully but bluntly: "A good nurse is always willing to ask questions even if it makes them look stupid. It is better to be willing to appear stupid than be dangerous to your patients."
- **Be humble.** Although you have learned much in nursing education, you are still a novice nurse. Demonstrate a hunger and desire to learn as much as you can from those more experienced.
- **Show respect.** Respect the knowledge and experience of the nurses you work with. Even if your personalities may not mesh, look beyond this and respect their knowledge and learn as much as you can from them.
- **Network with other nurses and find a solid support system.** A healthy unit is comprised of positive and meaningful relationships with your colleagues. Make it a priority to engage with your colleagues and take advantage of opportunities to go out after work or any outside activities planned by other staff. These will allow you to get to relate to your staff and see them in a different light. Not all nurses can be approached to ask a question. Identify those who are "safe" and will support you as a new nurse so you can share your thoughts, feelings, and struggles as a nurse transitioning from school to practice.
- **Take care of yourself.** Self-care was addressed earlier but is worth repeating. Take time for adequate rest and use the vacation days you have acquired. Do not feel guilty if you need to call in sick. By being proactive, you will be less likely to burn out and will persistently carry the passion of caregiving as you care for others.

CHAPTER 14 HIGHLIGHTS

- There are numerous ways to serve as a nurse. Depending on your personality, some positions will be a better "fit" than others.
- There are five distinct stages of professional nurse development that require clinical experience and nurse engagement to progress through. There are no shortcuts!
- A new graduate nurse is in the second stage of "advanced beginner." It will take two to three years of experience to advance to the next stage of "competent." Do not take this to mean that you are not competent as a new graduate nurse. It takes time to develop confidence and comfort in the clinical setting that as a new graduate you will not possess.
- Becoming certified in your clinical specialty is a practical way to demonstrate your commitment to excellence and develop your knowledge.
- Utilize techniques that emphasize collaboration and teamwork to effectively communicate with primary care providers.
- Commit to the highest levels of professionalism and create a culture of civility wherever you practice.
- Stand up for the absent colleague and use cognitive rehearsal to directly and respectfully address incivility when it comes your way.

Additional Resources

- Book: *A Nurse's Step-By-Step Guide to Transitioning to the Professional Nurse Role* (2015) by Cynthia Thomas, Constance McIntosh & Jennifer Mensik
- Book (complete PDF!): *From Surviving to Thriving: Navigating the First Year of Professional Practice* (2012) by Judy Boychuk Duchscher
- Book: *A Daybook for Beginning Nurses* (2009) by Donna Wilk Cardillo
- Book: *Your First Year As a Nurse, Making the Transition from Total Novice to Successful Professional*, 2nd edition (2010) by Donna Wilk Cardillo

Chapter Reflections

1. Review websites for information on Benner's Novice to Expert theory. Compare and contrast the characteristics of a novice, advanced beginner, and competent levels of practice to your current level.

2. What is similar and how does your practice differ from your current level?

3. What aspects of your practice do you need to strengthen in order to progress to the next level?

4. What clinical specialty are you currently most interested in pursuing after graduation?

5. What is the nursing certification for this specialty and what are the requirements to apply for certification?

6. What nursing journals do you currently or plan to subscribe to after graduation?

7. What aspects of communicating with a primary care provider cause you the most anxiety?

8. What can you do to prepare to discuss a patient concern? Consider role-playing this interaction with another student, then reverse roles!

9. How will you be the needed change in nursing by addressing incivility respectfully?

> *Every time I write RN after my name,*
> *I still do a little happy dance in my head!*

Chapter 15
Words of Wisdom from Health care Professionals

"It is not how much you do, but how much love you put in the doing."
"Unless life is lived for others, it is not worthwhile."
–Mother Teresa

I have captured the clinical wisdom and encouragement from experienced physicians, nurse practitioners, and nurses, some old and some new, whom I respect and have been blessed to work with in clinical practice. Their insights have been tested, tried, and refined through their clinical experience. If you note any recurrent themes of wisdom from these responses, recognize that this point is especially relevant for you to consider!

Words of Wisdom

Primary Care Providers

"When calling to provide an update or clinical concern, make the following a priority:

- *Be clear on what you want*
- *Know the patient's story well enough so that you are able to answer basic questions related to your clinical concern.*
- *Give just enough information to allow the provider to visualize in my head what is going on. Don't give too little information and don't give too much that is not directly relevant to the primary concern. Make it "just right!"*

–Elice Tiegs, RN, CNP

"Take the responsibility of the professional nurse seriously! Embrace the ownership of your patient that includes the need to assess the response to physician orders and treatments, know what to expect and anticipate, and when the expected response does not materialize communicate this promptly. Reassess vital signs and relevant nursing physical assessments consistently!"

–Warren Kearney, MD

"When performing an assessment and you are delineating the primary chief complaint, identify the body system that corresponds with this complaint. If there is more than one complaint, continue this line of thinking with each aspect of the complaint that is different from the prior. This will guide you to do a

thorough assessment of that body system to identify a potential problem. Though the complaints may be different, use your knowledge to see if there is a relationship between the different complaints or not."

–Suzanne MacDonald, MD

"Anticipate potential needs for your patients and call SOONER not later. This is appreciated when a call can be avoided in the middle of the night. Before you make that call, review the chart to know the patient's story and to ensure that the physician has not addressed the concern in the most recent progress note or prior order. Then when you call, know specifically what the current problem is, what clinical data supports the problem, and what you want or think your patient needs."

–Dan O'Laughlin, MD

"If you as the primary nurse are concerned about abnormal lab results or other clinical data you have collected and feel that it warrants a call to the physician, don't just call and report the data you are concerned about; that is passing the buck. Do your best to interpret the data, identify the specific or problem that this data could represent, and do your best to make a clinical judgment. Then when you call, report both the data and your clinical judgment. That helps me to have a clearer picture of what the clinical problem may be and then I can determine if I need to do something about it or not."

–Susan Seatter, MD

"Maintain an open line of communication that lets me know any changes for better or for worse as soon as possible. Err on the side of communicating too much, not too little."

–Phillip Mumm, MD

Registered Nurses

"Pay attention to the PATIENT because it is so easy to miss something. I recently had a patient who was lethargic and I was not clear as to why. By asking myself "WHY IS THIS?" I had an ABG done and the CO_2 was >100; he needed to be intubated. Also pay attention to the LITTLE THINGS. Check IV tubing and all connections on your patient to prevent problems before they start. Some days you will make a mistake and feel like quitting. It is easy to think it would be better somewhere else, but you need to have the courage to keep coming back."

–Pam, RN, 30 years/ICU

"Know your medications! The time-action-profile found in nursing drug handbooks is essential to know so you know when to follow up and assess the response to what you gave to see if it is working. As a newer nurse, identify the best and most approachable nurses on your floor so they can be a real world resource as well as an example to model your nursing practice by."

–Andrew, RN, 1 year/med-surg

"Never be afraid to ask questions. You will get yourself into trouble if you don't, and you will learn a lot more if you do!"

–Melissa, RN, 3 years/ICU

"Lean heavily on experienced nurses; not those who eat their young, but those that are safe to ask questions."

–Mike, RN, 16 years/ICU

"Have a willingness to put your ego aside and do not feel that you have to prove yourself and show that you know it all. Remain teachable."

–Eric, RN, 8 years ED/ICU

"Give it a year to become comfortable in practice. I was ready to quit after six months because I was unsure of myself in practice. I was worried that I was going to harm my patients. Also do not be afraid to ask questions! I am always concerned about a new nurse who appears to know it all."

–Brant, RN, 10 years/ICU

"Time management. Be ready to multitask with at least three to four patients. Focus on patient care, NOT on charting."

–Jay, RN, 3 months/ED

"Treat your patients like you would want your family members to be treated."

–Jill, RN, 20 years/ED

"Be prepared to make mistakes because you are still human."

–Darcy, RN, 10 years/ED

"Forgive yourself when you make mistakes or when you do not know what you think you should know."

–Tracy, RN, 22 years/ED

"You don't know what you don't know. The only dumb question is the one not asked."

–Mandy, RN, 6 years/ED

"Ask questions. Expect to flounder the first six months. Treat your patients like family members."

–Rana, RN, 9 years/ED

"Trust your gut. You know more than you think you do. Give yourself credit for what you already know."

–Rachel, RN 5 years/Float Pool

"Give yourself at least one year to get comfortable in practice. Learn to set priorities as this is the foundation to practice. Know what you can change and what you cannot. Also ask, ask, ask! There is so much that you don't know, that you don't even know it."

–Gayle, RN, 40 years/Float Pool

"Accept your limitations. Know when to ask for help."

–Mellina, RN, 17 years/Float Pool

"A good nurse is always willing to ask questions even if it makes them look stupid. It is better to be willing to appear stupid than be dangerous to your patients."

–David, RN, 17 years/ Rapid Response Team (RRT)

"Don't be afraid to step back from a stressful situation and take a deep breath when you are feeling overwhelmed. Get your priorities straight and do not miss the big picture."

– Justin, RN, 1 year/ED

"Time management is key. Know who your priority is and see those patients first because things can change so quickly."

– Michelle, RN, 5 years/Float Pool

"You will not spend hours obsessing over care plans as you do in nursing school. In practice you need to identify what is your care priority and what will you do to advance the plan of care. It is that simple."

–Kate, RN, 10 years/Float Pool

"Look at the BIG PICTURE with every patient. Do not focus on the tasks, but look at the patient and see how they look and how they are doing."

–Becky, RN, 25 years/med-surg

"Watch your patient closely and stay in tune with your patient. Then you will be able to identify when something changes. Though you may not be able to identify specifically what you are assessing, you will know that it is different from their baseline and will recognize the need to do something."

–Alice, RN, 20 years/ICU

"Use your eyes, ears, and really look and listen to your patient. Be thorough and be vigilant. Remember that there is no such thing as a routine assessment!"

–Carrie-RN, 6 years/Float Pool

"Trust your intuition, even if the doctor says not to worry about it! If you sense that something is wrong in your gut, don't ignore it because it is almost always right."

–Marcia, RN, 7 years/PACU

"It's OK to be scared. It's OK to ask questions. It's OK to delegate, to give some of your work away. Recognize your limitations knowing that you can't do it all."

–Shawn, RN, 15 years/Float Pool

"Know who your resources are every shift such as your charge nurse and colleagues that you trust. To effectively communicate with the physician when you call know three things: what is your concern, what is your assessment data to validate the concern, and know what you want! (Remember the R of SBAR?) If the physician becomes upset or short with you, don't let it affect you. Be a turtle and let it roll off your back knowing that you are advocating for your patient."

–Louellen, RN, 27 years/Float Pool

"Learn to be kind. Not only for your patients but for yourself. Be true to yourself but hold back the biting words. Think before you speak then follow your gut."

–Kari, RN, 30 years, Rapid Response Team (RRT)

"Instead of complaining about what a horrible day it is or will be because of... Embrace adversity and the daily challenges that are not uncommon in clinical practice. If you see adversity as a challenge to OVERCOME instead of something to ENDURE, you will thrive instead of merely surviving!"

–Keith, RN, 30 years/Float Pool

"Be honest in all interactions with patients, family members, colleagues, and providers. Always look at your patient. Pay attention to your patient and what they are saying. Hold your nursing ethics close to your heart and your clinical practice!"

–Georgia, RN, 29 years, Surgery Nurse

Why yes, my friends and I will ruin a perfectly good conversation
with gross stories from clinical.
You should be used to it by now.

Chapter 16

Make a Difference

"To know even one life has breathed easier because you have lived,
that is to have succeeded."
–Ralph Waldo Emerson

"One whose life makes a great difference for all:
All are better off than if he had not lived."
–Florence Nightingale, 1820–1910

As a nurse you will be in a unique position to make a difference in the lives of your patients and their families. You will have access to patients and their families in the best of times and the worst of times. Times of joy and celebration with the delivery of a new life into the world, and times of sorrow as families say goodbye to a loved one who is dying.

My Journey

As I reflect on my journey in nursing over the past three decades, the desire to make a difference has been the unifying thread of my story. It motivates all that I do as a nurse and nurse educator. This desire to make a difference has also influenced my desire to serve the poor through medical missions in Honduras and Haiti. On one recent medical mission trip to Haiti, I had no idea how my skills as a nurse would be used to benefit one elderly woman in a life-threatening crisis.

As our team was conducting a community outreach clinic at a church in Port-au-Prince, an elderly woman had a syncopal episode and collapsed on the street in front of the church. She was severely dehydrated as a result of vomiting and diarrhea secondary to cholera. Her presenting BP was 60/30. We were able to establish an IV, gave 2 liters of 0.9% NS, and she was transported by a family member to a cholera hospital in Port-au-Prince. I found out on our next trip that she had survived. She likely would have died without these immediate interventions. This was a graphic reminder how serving others with a desire to make a difference can impact others and even save a life!

In Closing

Taking the time to share my observations and reflections on what it takes to be a nurse was hard work, but well worth it knowing that it will make a difference. I hope that you were able to use this resource to strengthen and embrace what is required by one who desires to become a professional nurse.

May you, too, embrace the responsibility to make a difference in your attitude and the value you place on being a professional nurse. Though serving as a nurse is challenging, difficult, and at times thankless, because you are caring for human life of infinite value and worth, you will leave your mark on the hearts and lives of those you serve. Florence Nightingale poured herself out in her calling and realized her personal vision of a life well lived.

I want to encourage you to have this same sense of vision and purpose as you begin your career as a nurse. Nightingale had no idea that she would transform the nursing profession by caring for the sick as she began her nurse training, but she did. In the same way, health care today is ever changing and visionary leadership is needed to transform our profession as well as nursing education.

Will you be willing to embrace not only the responsibility of being a caregiver and pursue nursing with a passion to make a difference not only with each patient you care for, but use your unique abilities to possibly make lasting contributions to the profession?

Like Florence, you, too, are unique and have God-given talents that you have a responsibility to steward. Will you take the hard, but narrow, path to use what you have been given to serve others and make a difference by pursuing excellence in all that you do as a nurse, or will you take the broader path that many pursue by doing only what is needed and be content to be average in practice?

We have one chance at this life. It is imperative not to waste it. May the lives of Florence Nightingale, Mother Teresa, and other unsung caregivers who sacrificially served and cared for others inspire you to pour yourself out for broken humanity here and in other countries of the world where the need is so great.

Isabel Hampton Robb (1900), an influential American nurse educator, recognized not only the value, but also the eternal significance of caring for others. May her timeless vision and perspective inspire and influence you to embrace this same ethic in your practice:

> *"The spirit in which she does her work makes all the difference. Invested as she should with the dignity of her profession and the cloak of love for suffering humanity, she can ennoble anything her hand may be called upon to do, and for work done in this spirit there will ever come to her a recompense far outweighing that of silver and gold."*

Chapter Reflections

1. How do you want to make a difference as a nurse?

2. What "bigger picture" vision or purpose would you like to see realized through your career as a nurse?

3. What would it look like for you to look back and reflect on your years of service as a nurse and be able to say, "Well done"?

Acknowledgements

This second edition was extensive and could not have been accomplished without the guidance and feedback of many nurse educator colleagues.

One of my first workshop presentations was at California State University, Chico, where Carol Huston, MSN, MPA, DPA, FAAN was the dean. I want to thank you Carol not only for your initial support, but for your willingness to provide global edits and content structure revisions to improve the flow of my manuscript.

I want to thank Karla Larson, PhD, MSN, RN for her willingness to take time out of her busy schedule as a full-time nurse educator to review this manuscript and make meaningful contributions to this text. You took some of the rough edges off my 25 reflection questions in chapter 1, and made the questions and reflections so much better. Your contributions of constructing a cover letter, resume, and effective interviewing were needed and appreciated!

As a nurse educator who has been lacking for a mentor to guide me as an inexperienced but passionate nurse educator, I want to thank Barb Hill, RN, MSN, CNE, CMSRN for recognizing the value of my work early on and making the time to provide needed support, encouragement, but most importantly guidance. Your decades in nursing education has provided you with many stories and lived wisdom that has made me a better nurse educator.

I will never forget my very first full-time nursing position. It was there that I met a kindred spirit who was also immersed in clinical practice as an educator who helped me navigate a difficult and toxic academic culture. Thank you Georgie Dinndorf-Hogenson, PhD, RN, CNOR for your support and encouragement. Though our paths have gone in different directions over the last several years, you took the time to review this manuscript and provided that final polish.

At the last minute Catherine Griswold, EdD, MSN, RN, CLNC, CNE offered to share her expertise as a faculty reviewer of other textbooks of nursing and review my manuscript despite her busy academic load. Thank you Cathy for living out the highest levels of professional behavior and kindness, but also for providing a scholarly influence that strengthened and supported my manuscript.

Thank you Dean Arnott, RN, BSN, MA, LICSW for taking time out of your schedule that includes being a clinical adjunct as well as fellow colleague in the critical care float pool to review my manuscript. Your lens of clinical practice to validate and add to my content was needed and appreciated.

It goes without being said that behind every good man is a better woman, and that woman is my wife, Rhonda. I am so thankful for your practical day to day support and willingness to sacrifice so that I could complete my masters in nursing education and pursue my passion as a nurse educator. Without your support this book and all that I have been able to do as a nurse educator to transform nursing education would not have been possible.

Finally, I must humbly acknowledge my dependence upon God and my savior, Jesus Christ, who has forgiven, redeemed, and restored my life. By your grace you have given me a talent to teach. This book and all that I have been able to accomplish is a testimony to your love and grace.

References

Aiken, L. H., Clarke, S. P., Sloane, D. M., Sochalski, J. A., Busse, H., Clarke, H., . . . Shamian, J. (2001). Nurses' reports on hospital care in five countries. *Health Affairs, 20*, 43–53.

Alexander, L. L. (2012). Burnout–impact on nursing. Retrieved from http://www.netce.com/coursecontent.php?courseid=827

Alfaro-LeFevre, R. (2013). *Critical thinking, clinical reasoning, and clinical judgment: A practical approach.* (5th ed.). St. Louis, MO: Elsevier–Saunders.

American Association of Colleges of Nursing (AACN). (2014). Nursing shortage. Retrieved from http://www.aacn.nche.edu/media-relations/fact-sheets/nursing-shortage

American Nurses Association (ANA). (2001). Code of ethics for nurses with interpretive statements. Retrieved from http://www.nursingworld.org/MainMenuCategories/EthicsStandards/ CodeofEthicsforNurses/Code-of-Ethics.pdf

American Nurses Association. (2015). *Code of ethics for nurses with interpretive statements.* Silver Spring, MD: Author. Retrieved from http://www.nursingworld.org/codeofethics

Amiodarone. Micromedex. (2014). Retrieved from http://www.micromedexsolutions.com/ micromedex2/librarian/ND_T/evidencexpert/ND_PR/evidencexpert/CS/D1F681/ND_AppProduct/e videncexpert/DUPLICATIONSHIELDSYNC/CE977D/ND_PG/evidencexpert/ND_B/evidencexpert /ND_P/evidencexpert/PFActionId/evidencexpert.DisplayDrugpointDocument?docId=025645&conte ntSetId=100&title=Amiodarone+Hydrochloride&servicesTitle= Amiodarone+Hydrochloride&topicId=mechanismOfActionPharmacokineticsSection&subtopicId=null

Anonymous (2003). 65 Interview questions for nurses. *Nursing 2003, 33*(1), 38-40.

Anthony, A. S. (2004). Gender bias and discrimination in nursing education: Can we change it? *Nurse Educator, 29*, 121–125.

Atenolol. Micromedex. (2014). Retrieved from http://www.micromedexsolutions.com/micromedex2/ librarian/ND_T/evidencexpert/ND_PR/evidencexpert/CS/039F3A/ND_AppProduct/evidencexpert/D UPLICATIONSHIELDSYNC/BD9C5B/ND_PG/evidencexpert/ND_B/evidencexpert/ND_P/eviden cexpert/PFActionId/evidencexpert.DisplayDrugpointDocument?docId=048215&contentSetId=100& title=Atenolol&servicesTitle=Atenolol&topicId=mechanismOfActionPharmacokineticsSection&sub topicId=null

Attewell, A. (2012). *Illuminating Florence: Finding Nightingale's legacy in your practice.* Indianapolis, IN: Sigma Theta Tau International.

Ajzen, I. (2011). The theory of planned behaviour: Reactions and reflections. *Psychology and Health, 28*(9), 1113–1127.

Baldacchino, D. R., & Galea, P. (2012). Student nurses' personality traits and the nursing profession: part 1. *British Journal of Nursing, 21*(7), 419-425.

Bandura, A. (1994). Self-efficacy. In V. S. Ramachaudran (Ed.), *Encyclopedia of Human Behavior* (p. 71-81). New York, NY: Academic Press.

Bartholomew, K., (2006), *Ending nurse to nurse hostility: Why nurses eat their young and each other.* Marblehead, MA: HCPro Incorporated.

Bartholomew, K. (2007). A study of nurse-to-nurse hostility: Why nurses eat their young. Proceedings for the 18th international nursing research congress focusing on evidence-based practice. Vienna, Austria: Medscape Nurses. http://dx.doi.org/doi:http://dx.doi.org/10.5480/1536-5026-32.6.362

Behaviors that undermine a culture of safety [Sentinel event alert]. (2008). Retrieved from http://www.jointcommission.org/sentinel_event_alert_issue_40_behaviors _that_undermine_a_culture_of_safety/

Bell-Scriber, M. J. (2008). Warming the nursing education climate for traditional-age learners who are male. *Nursing Education Research, (29)*3, 143–150.

Benner, P. (1982). From novice to expert. *American Journal of Nursing, 82*(3), 402–407.

Benner, P. (1984). *From novice to expert: Excellence and power in clinical nursing practice.* Upper Saddle River, NJ: Prentice Hall

Benner, P. (2012). International Nurses Christian Fellowship speech.

Benner, P. (2013). Teacher curiosity, passion, engagement and self-cultivation–Essential for transformative education. Retrieved from http://www.educatingnurses.com/articles/teacher-curiosity-passion-engagement-and-self-cultivation-essential-for-transformative-education/

Benner, P. & Wrubel, J. (1988). Caring comes first. *American Journal of Nursing, 88*(8), 1073–1075.

Benner, P. & Wrubel, J. (1989). *Primacy of caring: Stress and coping in health and illness.* Menlo Park, CA: Addison-Wesley Publishing Company.

Benner, P., Tanner, C., & Chesla, C. (1996). *Expertise in nursing practice.* New York: Springer.

Benner, P., Hooper-Kyriakidis, P., & Stannard, D. (2011). *Clinical wisdom and interventions in acute and critical care: A thinking-in-action approach.* (2nd ed.). New York, NY: Springer.

Benner, P., Hughes, R.G., & Sutphen, M. (2008). Clinical reasoning, decisionmaking, and action: Thinking critically and clinically. Retrieved from http://www.ncbi.nlm.nih.gov/books/NBK2643/

Benner, P., Sutphen, M., Leonard, V., & Day, L. (2010). *Educating nurses: A call for radical transformation.* San Francisco, CA: Jossey-Bass.

Bensley, R. (1991)Defining spiritual health: A review of the literature. *Journal of Health Education, 22*(5), 287-290.

Berman, A. & Snyder, S. (2012). *Fundamentals of nursing.* (10 th ed.). Upper Saddle River, NJ: Prentice Hall.

Berman, A., Snyder, S. & Frandsen, G. (2016). *Fundamentals of nursing.* (9th ed.). Upper Saddle River, NJ: Prentice Hall.

Bittner, N. & Tobin, E. (1998). Critical thinking: Strategies for clinical practice. *Journal for Nurses in Staff Development, 14,* 267–72.

Blainey, G. (2011). *A short history of Christianity.* Penguin Viking.

Boychuk Duchscher, J.E. (2009). Transition shock: The initial stage of role adaptation for newly graduated Registered Nurses. *Journal of Advanced Nursing, 65,* 1103–13.

Brady, M. S., & Sherrod, D. R. (2003). Retaining men in nursing programs designed for women. *Journal of Nursing Education, 42*(4), 159–162.

Brown, B. (2000). Men in nursing: Ambivalence in care, gender and masculinity. *International History of Nursing Journal, 5,* 4–13.

Bullough, B. & Bullough, V. (1987). Our roots: What we should know about Christian pioneers. *Journal of Christian Nursing,* p.12.

Bush, E. (2001). The use of human touch to improve the well-being of older adults: A holistic nursing intervention. *Journal of Holistic Nursing, (19)*3, 256-270.

Campos-Murguia, A., Leon-Lara, X., Munoz, J.M., & Macias, A.E. (2014). Stethoscopes as potential intrahospital carriers of pathogenic microorganisms. *American Journal of Infection Control, 42*(1), 82-83. Retrieved from http://www.ajicjournal.org/article/S0196-6553%2813%2901095-X/fulltext

Cappelletti, A., Engel, J.C., & Prentice, D. (2014). Systematic review of clinical judgment and reasoning in nursing. *Journal of Nursing Education, (53)*8, 458.

Caputi, L. (2011). Critical thinking skills and strategies. Retrieved from http://www.lindacaputi.com/userfiles/Thinking_Skills_Explained(1).pdf

Carnahan, B. (1988). A gentle touch: Massage therapy for the chronically and terminally ill. *Massage Magazine, 14,* 18-45.

Carol, R. (2006). Discrimination in nursing school: Thing of the past or alive and well? *Minority Nurse,* 56–62.

Cavendish, R., Konecny, L., Mitzeliotis, C., Russo, D., Kraynyak Luise, B., Lanza, M., et al. (2003). Spiritual care activities of nurses using nursing interventions classifications (NIC) labels. *International Journal of Nursing Terminology Classifications, 16,* 120–121.

Cho, J., Laschinger, H.K.S., & Wong, C. (2006). Workplace empowerment, work engagement and organizational commitment of new graduate nurses, Nursing Leadership, 19(3), 43-62.

Clark, C. M. (2008). The dance of incivility in nursing education as described by nursing faculty and students. *Advances in Nursing Science, 31,* E37–E54.

Clark, C. M. (2011). Pursuing a culture of civility: An intervention study of one program of nursing, *Nurse Educator, 36*(3), 98–102.

Clark, C. M. (2013). National study on faculty-to-faculty incivility: Strategies to foster collegiality and civility. *Nurse Educator, 38*(3), 98–102.

Clark, C. M. & Carnosso, J. (2008). Civility: A concept analysis. *Journal of Theory Construction & Testing, 12,* 11–15.

Clark, C. M. & Springer, P.J. (2010). Academic nurse leaders' role in fostering a culture of civility in nursing education, *Journal of Nursing Education, 49*(6), 319–325.

Clark, C.M., & Springer, P.J. (2012). Nurse residents' firsthand accounts on transition to practice. *Nursing Outlook, 60*(4), E2-E8.

Clark, C. M., Olender, L., Kenski, D., & Cardoni, C. (2013). Exploring and addressing faculty-to-faculty incivility: A national perspective and literature review. *Journal of Nursing Education, 52*(4), 211–218.

Clarke, S.P. & Aiken, L.H. (2003). Failure to rescue. *American Journal of Nursing, 103,* 42-47.

Conscientious Objection (2015). The American Nurse. Retrieved from http://www.theamericannurse.org/index.php/2014/09/02/conscientious-objection/

Conco, D. (1995). Christian parents' views of spiritual care. *Western Journal of Nursing Research,* 17(3), 266-276.

Cooper, J., Walker, J., Winters, K., Williams, P., Askew, R., & Robinson, J. (2009). Nursing students' perceptions of bullying behaviors by classmates. *Issues in Education Research, 19,* 212-226.

Core Competencies of Nurse Educators with Task Statements (2005). Retrieved from http://www.nln.org/docs/default-source/default-document-library/core-competencies-of-nurse-educators-with-task-statements.pdf?sfvrsn=0

Core Concepts of Jean Watson's Theory of Human Caring/Caring Science (2010). Retrieved from http://watsoncaringscience.org/files/Cohort%206/watsons-theory-of-human-caring-core-concepts-and-evolution-to-caritas-processes-handout.pdf

Coursey, J. H., Rodriguez, R.E., Dieckmann, L.S., & Austin, P.N. (2013). Successful implementation of policies addressing lateral violence. *AORN Journal, 97*(3), 101–109.

Cronin, S., & Harrison, B. (1998). Importance of nurse caring behaviors as perceived by patients after myocardial infarction. *Heart & Lung, 17,* 374–381.

del Bueno, D. (2005). A crisis in critical thinking. *Nursing Education Perspectives, 26*(5), 278–282.

Dellasega, C. A. (2009). Bullying among nurses. *American Journal of Nursing, 109,* 52–58.

DeWit, S. (2009). *Fundamental concepts and skills for nursing.* St. Louis, MO: Saunders Elsevier.

Dinndorf-Hogenson, G.A. (2015). Moral courage in practice: Implications for patient safety. *Journal of Nursing Regulation, (6)*2, 10-16.

Dolan, J., Fitzpatrick, L., & Krohn Herrmann, E. (1983). *Nursing in society: A historical perspective.* 15th ed. Philadelphia: W.B. Saunders, p.43.

Dossey, B. et al. (1995*). Holistic nursing: A handbook for practice.* Rockville, MD: Aspen.

Dyck, J. M., Oliffe, J., Phinney, A., & Garrett, B. (2009). Nursing instructors' and male students' perceptions of undergraduate, classroom nursing education. *Nurse Education Today, 29,* 649–653.

Dossey, B. M. (1999). *Florence Nightingale: Mystic, visionary, healer.* Springhouse, PA: Springhouse Corporation.

Edelwich J. & Brodsky, A. (1980). *Burn-out: Stages of Disillusionment in the Helping Professions.* New York, NY: Springer.

Eldredge, J. (2001). *Wild at heart: Discovering the secret of a man's soul.* Nashville, TN: Thomas Nelson.

Eraut, M. (1994). *Developing professional knowledge and competence.* Washington, DC: Falmer Press.

Evans, J. (1997). Men in nursing: Issues of gender segregation and hidden advantage. *Journal of Advanced Nursing, 26,* 226–231.

Evans, J. (2004). Men nurses: A historical and feminist perspective. *Journal of Advanced Nursing, 47,* 321–328.

Evans, J. A. (2002). Cautious caregivers: Gender stereotypes and the sexualization of men nurses' touch. *Journal of Advanced Nursing, (40)*4, 441–448.

Faas, A. I. (2004). The intimacy of dying: An act of presence. *Dimensions of Critical Care Nursing, 23*(1), 76–78.

Ferns, T. & Meerabeau, E. (2009). Reporting behaviours of nursing students who have experienced verbal abuse. *Journal of Advanced Nursing, 65,* 2678–2688.

Ferris, T. (2012). Reality shock. Retrieved from http://newgraduatenurses.weebly.com/reality-shock.html

Figley, C.R. (1995). *Compassion fatigue: Coping with secondary traumatic stress in those who treat the traumatized.* New York, NY: Brunner Mazel Inc.

Fish, S. & Shelly, J. (1983). *Spiritual care.* (2nd ed.). Downers Grove, IL:InterVarsity.

Frankyl, V. (1978). *The unheard cry for meaning: Psychotherapy and Humanism.* New York: Simon & Schuster.

Freda, M. (2004). Issues in patient education. *Journal of Midwifery & Woman's Health,* retrieved from http://www.medscape.com/viewarticle/478283_3

Galbraith, N. D., Brown, K. E., & Clifton, E. (2014). A Survey of Student Nurses' Attitudes Toward Help Seeking for Stress. *Nursing Forum, 49*(3), 171-181.

Giddens, J. (2013). *Concepts for nursing practice.* St. Louis, MO: Elsevier.

Gorman, D. (2003). A nurse by any other name...*Nursing Spectrum, 7*(10), 10 [northeast edition.]

Griffin, M. (2004). Teaching cognitive rehearsal as a shield for lateral violence: An intervention for newly licensed nurses. *The Journal of Continuing Education in Nursing, 35*, 257–263.

Griswold, C. M. (2014). Understanding causes of attrition of 1st- and 2nd-year nursing students (Doctoral dissertation Walden University).

Grossman, S.C. & Valiga, T.M. (2013). *The new leadership challenge: Creating the future of nursing.* (4th ed.) Philadelphia, PA: F. A. Davis Company.

Grover, S.M. (2005). Shaping effective communication skills and therapeutic relationships at work. *Journal of American Association of Occupational Health Nursing, 53*(4), 177-182.

Halter, M. J. (2004). Stigma and help seeking related to depression: A study of nursing students. *Journal of Psychosocial Nursing and Mental Health Services, 42*(2), 42–51.

Hampton Robb, E. (1900). *Nursing ethics.* Cleveland, OH: E.C. Koeckert.

Harding, T. (2009). Swimming against the malestream: Men choosing nursing as a career. *Nursing Praxix in New Zealand, 25*(3), 4–16.

Harding, T., North, N., & Perkins, R. (2008). Sexualizing men's touch: Male nurses and the use of intimate touch in clinical practice. *Research and Theory for Nursing Practice: An International Journal, 22*(2), 88–101.

Hardy, H. (1979). *The spiritual nature of man.* Oxford: Clarendon Press.

Hatmaker, D.M., Park, H.H., & Rethemeyer, R.K. (2011). Learning the ropes: communities of practice and social networks in the public sector. *International Public Management Journal 14*, 395–419.

Heinrich, K.T. (2010). An optimist's guide for cultivating civility among academic nurses. *Journal of Professional Nursing, 26*(6), 325–331.

Henderson, M. (2009). Hostility and violence in the nursing profession. Retrieved from http://www.suite101.com/content/hostility-and-violence-in-the-nursing-profession-a149150

Henderson, V. (1991). *The nature of nursing: Reflections after 25 years.* New York: National League for Nursing Press.

Highland, M. & Cason, C. (1983). Spiritual needs of patients: are they recognized? *Cancer Nursing.*

Hoel, H., Giga, S.I. & Davidson, M.J.(2007). Expectations and realities of student nurses' experiences of negative behaviour and bullying in clinical placement and the influences of socialization processes. *Health Services Management Research, 20*, 270–278.

Honesty/Ethica in Professions. (2015). Gallup. Retrieved from http://www.gallup.com/poll/1654/honesty-ethics-professions.aspx

Hummel, C. (1967). Tyranny of the urgent. Retrieved from http://www.my279days.com/wp-content/uploads/2010/08/Tyranny-of-the-Urgent.pdf

Incivility, Bullying, and Workplace Violence (2015). Retrieved from http://www.nursingworld.org/Bullying-Workplace-Violence

Isaacs, K. (2015). 7 best resume tips for nurses, Retrieved from http://allhealthcare.monster.com/careers/articles/3843-7-best-resume-tips-for-nurses?page=4

Jackson, D., Hutchinson, M., Everett, B., Mannix, J., Peters, K., Weaver, R., et al. (2011). Struggling for legitimacy: nursing students' stories of organisational aggression, resilience and resistance. *Nursing Inquiry, 18*(2), 102-110.

Jaslow, R. (2013). Number of male U.S. nurses triple since 1970. Retrieved from http://www.cbsnews.com/news/number-of-male-us-nurses-triple-since-1970/

Johnson, S. J. & Rea, R. E. (2009). Workplace bullying: Concerns for nurse leaders. *The Journal of Nursing Administration, 39*(2), 84–90.

Jones, M. C., & Johnston, D. W. (1997). Distress, stress and coping in first-year student nurses. *Journal of Advanced Nursing, 26*, 475–482.

Kautz, D.D., Kuiper, R., Pesut, D.J., & Williams, R.L. (2006). Using NANDA, NIC, and NOC (NNN) language for clinical reasoning with the outcome-present state-test (OPT) Model. *International Journal of Nursing Terminologies and Classifications, (17)*3, 129-138.

Kidder, R. M. (2005). Moral courage, digital distrust: Ethics in a troubled world. *Business & Society Review, 110*(4), 485–505.

Knight, K. (2012). Catholic Encylopedia: Hospital, retrieved from http://www.newadvent.org/cathen/07480a.htm

Koharchik, L., Caputi, L., Robb, M., & Culleiton, A.L. (2015). *American Journal of Nursing, (115)*1, 58-61.

Kothari, R. U., Pancioli, A., Liu, T., Brott, T., & Broderick, J. (1999) Cincinnati prehospital stroke scale: Reproducibility and validity. *Annals of Emergency Medicine, 33*, 373–378.

Kouta, C. & Kaite, C. P. (2011). Gender discrimination and nursing: A review of the literature. *Journal of Professional Nursing, (27)*1, 59–63.

Kubler-Ross, E. (1970). *On death and dying.* London: Tavistock.

Labrague, L. J., McEnroe-Petitte, D. M., Papathanasiou, I. V., Edet, O. B., & Arulappan, J. (2015). Impact of Instructors' Caring on Students' Perceptions of Their Own Caring Behaviors. *Journal of Nursing Scholarship, 47*(4), 338-346.

Leininger, M. (1988). Leininger's theory of nursing: Cultural care diversity and university. *Nursing Science Quarterly, 1*, 152–160.

Leininger, M. (1991). *Culture care diversity and universality: A theory of nursing.* New York, NY: National League for Nursing.

Levett-Jones, T., Hoffman, K., Dempsey, J., Yeun-Sim Jeong, S., Noble, D., Norton, C. Hickey, N. (2010). The 'five rights' of clinical reasoning: An educational model to enhance nursing students' ability to identify and manage clinically 'at risk' patients. *Nurse Education Today, 30*, 515–520.

Lewis Coakley, M. (1990). The faith behind the famous: Florence Nightingale: Christian history sampler. *Christianitytoday*.com. Retrieved from http://www.christianitytoday.com/ch/1990/issue25/2537.html?start=1

McAllister, M., & Lowe, J. B. (2011). *The resilient nurse: Empowering your practice.* New York: Springer.

McClellan, J. & Dorn, H. (2006). *Science and technology in world history: An introduction.* Baltimore, MD: The John Hopkins University Press.

McDonald, L. (1999). Nightingale's spirituality: The faith of Florence Nightingale. Retrieved from http://www.uoguelph.ca/~cwfn/spirituality/spirituality.html.

McLaughlin, K., Muldoon, O.T., & Moutray, M. (2010). Gender, gender roles and completion of nursing education: A longitudinal study. *Nurse Education Today, 30,* 303–307.

Mackintosh, C. (1997). A historical study of men in nursing. *Journal of Advanced Nursing, 26*, 232–236.

Macrae, J. (1995). Nightingale's spiritual philosophy and its significance for modern nursing. *Image Journal of Nursing Scholarship, 27*(8), 8-10.

Managers note less professionalism among nurses (2013). *Bold Voices, 5*(7), 6.

Maxwell, J.C. (1999). *The 21 indispensable qualities of a leader: Becoming the person others will follow.* Nashville, TN: Thomas Nelson.

Meadus, R. J. & Twomey, J. C. (2011). Men student nurses: The nursing education experience. *Nursing Forum, 46,* 269–279.

Moral Distress in Academia (2015). Retrieved from http://www.nursingworld.org/MainMenuCategories/EthicsStandards/Courage-and-Distress/Moral-Distress-in-Academia.html

Mother Teresa – Biographical. Retrieved from http://www.nobelprize.org/nobel_prizes/peace/laureates/1979/teresa-bio.html

Murphy, L. S., & Walker, M. S. (2013). Spirit-guided care: Christian nursing for the whole person. *Journal of Christian Nursing, 30*(3), 144–152.

Murray, J. S. (2008). No more nurse abuse. *American Nurse Today,* 17–19.

NCLEX-RN Examination-Test Plan for the National Council Licensure Examination for Registered Nurses. (2013). Retrieved from https://www.ncsbn.org/2013_NCLEX_RN_Test_Plan.pdf

Neal-Boylan, L. (2013). *The nurse's reality gap.* Indianapolis, IN: Sigma Theta Tau International.

Niebuhr, R. (1942). The serenity prayer. Retrieved from http://en.wikiquote.org/wiki/Reinhold_Niebuhr

Nightingale, F. (1860). *Notes on nursing: What it is and what it is not.* London: Harrison.

Nurse Certification Benefits Patients, Employers and Nurses (2015). Retrieved from http://www.aacn.org/wd/certifications/content/benefitstoptempnrs.pcms?menu=certification

Nursing Leadership: Management & Leadership Styles (2014). Retrieved from http://www.aanac.org/docs/white-papers/2013-nursing-leadership-management-leadership-styles.pdf?sfvrsn=6

Nurturing Cultural Competence in Nursing (2010). Retrieved from http://www.oregoncf.org/Templates/media/files/reports/nccn_program_2010.pdf

O'Lynn,, C. (2003). *Defining male friendliness in nursing education programs: Tool development.* Unpublished dissertation, Kennedy-Western University, Cheyenne, WY.

O'Lynn, C. (2012). *A man's guide to a nursing career.* New York, NY: Springer Publishing Company

O'Lynn, C. E. (2004). Gender based barriers for male students in nursing education programs: Prevalence and perceived importance. *Journal of Nursing Education, 43*(5), 229–236..

O'Lynn, C. E. & Tranbarger, R. E. (2007). *Men in nursing: History, challenges, and opportunities.* New York, NY: Springer Publishing Company.

Orlick, S. & Benner, P. (1988). The primacy of caring. *American Journal of Nursing, 88*(3). 318–319.

Ornstein, J. (2007). Dennis Quaid files suit over drug mishap. Retrieved from http://www.latimes.com/entertainment/gossip/la-me-quaid5dec05-story.html

Our Mission (2014). Retrieved from http://www.allinahealth.org/uploadedFiles/Content/Allina-Health-mission-vision-values-promise.pdf

Pai, H,. Eng, C., & Ko, H. (2013). Effect of caring behavior on disposition toward critical thinking of nursing students. *Journal of Professional Nursing, 29*(6), 423-429.

Paterson, B. L., Tschikota, S., Crawford, M., Saydak, M., Venkatesh, P., & Aronowitz, T. (1996). Learning to care: Gender issues for male nursing students. *Canadian Journal of Nursing Research, 28*(1), 25–39.

Lifelong Learning (2014). Retrieved from http://magazine.nursing.jhu.edu/2012/11/lifelong-learning/

Pavey, A. E. (1952). *The story of the growth of nursing.* London: Faber and Faber Ltd.

Pearcey, P.A . & Elliott, B.E.(2004). Student impressions of clinical nursing. *Nurse Education Today, 24,* 382–387.

Peplau, H. (1988). The art and science of nursing: Similarities, differences, and relationships. *Nursing Science Quarterly, 1*(1), 8-15.

Pesut, D.J. & Herman, J. (1998). OPT: Transformation of nursing process for contemporary practice. *Nursing Outlook, 46,* 29-36.

Pesut, D.J. & Herman, J. (1999). *Clinical reasoning: The art and science of critical & creative thinking.* Albany, NY: Delmar Publishers.

Pines, E. W., Rauschhuber, M. L., Norgan, G. H., Cook, J. D., Canchola, L., Richardson, C., et al. (2012). Stress resiliency, psychological empowerment and conflict management styles among baccalaureate nursing students. *Journal of Advanced Nursing, 68*(7), 1482-1493.

Porter-O'Grady, T. (2010). Nurses as knowledge workers. In L. Caputi, *Teaching nursing: The art and science, Vol.2.* Glen Ellyn, IL: College of DuPage Press.

Potter, P. A. & Perry, A. G. (2004). *Fundamentals of nursing.* (6th ed.). St. Louis, MO: Mosby.

Potter, P. A. & Perry, A. G. (2009). *Fundamentals of nursing.* (7th ed.). St. Louis, MO: Mosby–Elsevier.

Potter, P. A. & Perry, A. G. (2012). *Fundamentals of nursing.* (8th ed.). St. Louis, MO: Mosby–Elsevier.

Pre-Licensure KSAS. (2014). QSEN.com. Retrieved from http://qsen.org/competencies/pre-licensure-ksas/#patient-centered_care

Pulidio-Martos, M., Augusto-Landa, J.M., & Lopez-Zafra, E.(2011). Sources of stress in nursing students: A systematic review of quantitative studies. *International Nursing Review, (59)*1, 15-25.

Randle, J. (2003). Bullying in the nursing profession. *Journal of Advanced Nursing, 43,* 395–401.

Ranse, K. & Grealish, L. (2007). Nursing students' perceptions of learning in the clinical setting of the dedicated education unit. *Journal of Advanced Nursing 52,* 171–179.

Registered Nurses. (2014). Bureau of Labor Statistics/Occupational Outlook Handbook. Retrieved from: http://www.bls.gov/ooh/healthcare/registered-nurses.htm

Rex-Smith, A. (2007). Something more than presence. *Journal of Christian Nursing, 24*(2), 82–87.

Rhodes, J. (1990). A philosophical study of the art of nursing explored within a metatheoretical framework of philosophy of art and aesthetics. Ph. D. dissertation, University of South Carolina.

Richards, D.J. (n.d.). The four temperaments. Retrieved from http://www.odportal.com/personality/four-temperaments.htm

Rischer, K. (2013). Think like a Nurse! Practical preparation for professional practice. Minneapolis, MN.

Roberts, D. (2009). Friendship fosters learning: the importance of friendship in clinical practice. *Nurse Education in Practice. 9,* 367–371.

Roth, J. E., & Coleman, C. L. (2008). Perceived and real barriers for men entering nursing: Implications for gender diversity. *Journal of Cultural Diversity, 15*(3), 148–152.

Sacco, T.L., Ciurzynski, S.M., Harvey, M.E., & Ingersoll, G.L. (2015). Compassion satisfaction and compassion fatigue among critical care nurses. *Critical Care Nurse, (35)*4, p. 32-41.

Schmukle, S. C., & Egloff, B. (2008). Validity of the five-factor model for the implicit self-concept of personality. *European Journal of Psychological Assessment, 24*(4), 263-272.

Scott, B.A. (2009). *Thinking as a nurse.* Bloomington, IN: iUniverse.

Sengstock, B. (2008). A grounded theory study of nursing students' (Doctoral dissertation). Retrieved from http://eprints.qut.edu.au/30282/1/c30282.pdf

Shelly, J.A. & Miller, A.B. (2006). *Called to care: A Christian worldview for nursing.* Downers Grove, IL: InterVarsity Press.

Simoni P., Larrabee J., Birkhimer T., Mott C. & Gladden S. (2004). Influence of interpretative styles of stress resiliency on registered nurse empowerment. *Nursing Administration Quarterly* 28(3), 221–224.

Smucker, C. (1996). A phenomenological description of the experience of spiritual distress. *Nursing Diagnosis, 7*(2), 81-91.

Sommers, S., Johnson, J., Roberts, K., Redding, S., & Churchill, L. (2013). *Nursing leadership and management review module edition 6.0.*

Spot a Stroke. American Stroke Association. Retrieved from http://strokeassociation.org/STROKEORG/

Stagg, S. J., Sheridan, D., Jones, R., & Gabel Speroni, K. (2011). Evaluation of a workplace bullying cognitive rehearsal program in a hospital setting. *The Journal of Continuing Education, 12*(9), 395–401.

Stewart-Brown, S., Evans, J., Patterson, J., Petersen, S., Doll,

H., Balding, J. et al. (2000). The health of students in institutes of higher education: An important and neglected public health problem? *Journal of Public Health Medicine, 22,* 492–498.

Stamm, B.H. (2002). Measuring compassion satisfaction as well as fatigue: Development and history of the compassion fatigue test. *Treating compassion fatigue.* New York, NY: Brunner-Routledge.

Stephens, T. M. (2013). Nursing Student Resilience: A Concept Clarification. *Nursing Forum, 48*(2), 125-133.

Stocker, S. (1995). Pretty scary stuff. *The American Nurse,* p.6.

Stott, A. (2007). Exploring factors affecting attrition of male students from an undergraduate nursing course: A qualitative study. *Nurse Education Today, (27)*4, 325–332.

Swanson, K. M. (1991). Empirical development of a middle range theory of caring. *Nursing Research, 40*(3), 161–166.

Swanson, K. M. (1999). *What is known about caring in nursing: A literary meta-analysis.* In A.S. Hinshaw, S.L. Feetham, & J.L.F. Shaver, eds. *Handbook of clinical nursing research.* Thousand Oaks, CA: Sage Publications.

Sweeney, C. (2012). *160 ways to empathize.*

Swenson, R. (2004). *Margin: Restoring emotional, physical, financial, and time reserves to overloaded lives.* Colorado Springs, CO: NavPress.

Szutenbach, M. (2013). Bullying in nursing: Roots, rationales, and remedies. *Journal of Christian Nursing, 30*(1), 16–23.

Tanner, C. A. (1990). Clinical education, circa 2010. *Journal of Nursing Education, 41*(2), 51–52

Tanner, C. A. (1990). Caring as a value in nursing education. *Nursing Outlook, 38*(2), 70–72.

Tanner, C. A. (2004). The meaning of curriculum: Content to be covered or stories to be heard? *Journal of Nursing Education, 43*(1), 3–4.

Tanner, C. A. (2006). Thinking like a nurse: A research-based model of clinical judgment in nursing. *Journal of Nursing Education, 45*(6), 204–211.

Taylor, H., & Reyes, H. (2012). Self-Efficacy and Resilience in Baccalaureate Nursing Students. *International Journal of Nursing Education Scholarship, 9*(1), 1-13.

Thomas, S.P. & Burk, R. (2009). Junior nursing students' experiences of vertical violence during clinical rotations. *Nursing Outlook, 57,* 226–231.

Thompson, C., Cullum, N., McCaughan, D., Sheldon, T., Raynor, P. (2004). Nurses, information use, and clinical decision making: The real potential for evidence-based decisions in nursing. *Evidence-Based Nursing, 7*(3), 69–72.

Thompson, C., Dalgleish, L., Bucknall, T., Estabrooks, C., Hutchinson, A., Fraser, K., deVos, R., Binnekade, J., Barrett, G., Saunders, J. (2008). The effects of time pressure and experience on nurses' risk assessment decisions: A signal detection analysis. *Nursing Research, 57*(5), 302–311.

Thompson, E. H. (2002). What's unique about men's caregiving? In B. J. Kramer & E. H. Thompson (Eds.), *Men as caregivers: Theory, research, and service implications* (pp. 20–50). New York: Springer.

Tillman Harris, C. (2011). Incivility in nursing. Retrieved from Tips to improve patient education skills (2015). *Bold Voices, (7)*8, 14.

Vallant, S. & Neville, S. (2006). The relationship between student nurse and nurse clinician: Impact on student learning. *Nursing Praxis in New Zealand*, 22, 23–33.

Vallerand, A.H., Sanoski, C.A., & Deglin, J.H. (2013) *Davis's drug guide for nurses.* (13th ed.). Philadelphia, PA: F.A. Davis Company.

Van Leeuwen, A. & Poelhuis-Leth, D. J. (2009). *Davis's comprehensive handbook of laboratory and diagnostic tests with nursing implication*s. (3rd ed.). Philadelphia, PA: F.A. Davis Company.

Walsh, J. J. (1929). *The history of nursing.* New York, NY: Kennedy & Sons.

Videbeck, S. (2007). *In psychiatric mental health nursing* (5th ed.). Philadelphia, Baltimore, New York, London: Wolters, Kluwer, Lippincott, Williams, and Wilkins.

Walton, A.G. (2015). Too much praise can turn kids into narcissists, study suggests. Retrieved from http://www.forbes.com/sites/alicegwalton/2015/03/09/parents-stop-overvaluing-your-kid-you-may-create-a-future-narcissist-study-says/

Ward, J. (2012). 5 strategies for a culturally competent patient care. Retrieved from http://www.nursetogether.com/5-strategies-culturally-competent-patient-care#sthash.BroQf68H.dpuf

Watson, J. (1995). Nursings caring-healing paradigm as exemplar for alternative medicine? *Alternative Therapies,* p.67.

Weiss, S.J. (1990). Effects of differential touch on nervous system arousal of patients recovering from cardiac disease. *Heart & Lung, 19*(5). 474-480.

Widerquist, J.G. (1992). The spirituality of florence nightingale. *Nursing Research, (41)*1, 51.

Wilkinson, J. M. & Treas, L. S. (2011). *Fundamentals of nursing. (*2nd ed.). Philadelphia, PA: F.A. Davis Company.

Wilt, D.L. & Smucker, C.J. (2001). *Nursing the spirit: The art and science of applying spiritual care.* Washington, D.C.: American Nurses Publishing.

Woodham-Smith, C. (1951). *Florence Nightingale.* New York, NY: McGraw-Hill.

Appendix A

Warming the Climate for Men in Nursing Education

Men have no place in nursing *"except where physical strength was needed."*
–Florence Nightingale

Quantitative research has shown that the barriers men face in nursing education
are *"pervasive, consistent, and have changed little over time."*
–Chad O'Lynn, RN, PhD

The male experience in nursing and nursing education has been very different from that of women in the modern era since the reforms initiated by Florence Nightingale. Don't believe me? Then let me ask a series of questions that will put this in perspective.

If you are a woman who chose to become a nurse:

- Was it suggested you may be a lesbian, or was your femininity questioned because you chose to enter the nursing profession?
- Were you cautious in how you touched male patients while caring for them because it could be interpreted as sexual?
- Did you feel uncomfortable and vulnerable while caring for women on a postpartum unit?
- Did you experience isolation and loneliness because in clinical and in practice there were so few women in the program?
- Did you feel especially visible as a student because you "stood out" and felt that the faculty singled you out in class or clinical?

As a woman this was likely NOT your experience. Yet, if you are a man who chose to enter nursing, you can readily identify and have likely experienced many of these barriers as a student and then in practice (Meadus & Creina Twomey, 2011). Was it coincidental that the blockbuster comedy *Meet the Parents* was hugely successful in part because it played off the gender stereotypes of men in nursing by the lead character GAYlord Focker?

Would it surprise you to realize that the earliest recorded caregivers were men and that men have a rich legacy of caregiving throughout world history? Let's take a brief walk through history, starting with the BC era, which will take us from the past to the present to put today's low male participation in perspective.

The following topics in this chapter include:

- Historical Legacy of Men as Caregivers
- Nightingale and the Modern Era
- Social/Cultural Barriers
- Educational Barriers

Historical Legacy of Men as Caregivers

Nursing has not always been primarily a woman's profession. From the beginning of recorded history, caring for the sick was primarily the responsibility of male caregivers. In the BC era, the following are historical examples:

- 400 BC: In Hippocratic writings in ancient Greece, public nursing care was provided by men (Brown, 2000).
- 400 BC: In ancient Rome, the best possible care was provided to soldiers in military hospitals by male caregivers called "*nosocomi*" (O'Lynn & Tranbarger, 2007). Unfortunately, this legacy has been tarnished because it is also the root word for "hospital" or "nosocomial" —acquired infection!
- 250 BC: In India, the first public hospitals were developed where only men were taught and trained as primary caregivers (O'Lynn & Tranbarger, 2007).

In the AD era, this historical trend continued as caring for the sick became a ministry of the early Christian church. Both men and women served as caregivers in this era. Examples of the ongoing legacy of male caregivers include the following:

- AD 100: Male deacons as well as female deaconesses were responsible for ministering and caring for those who were ill (Anthony, 2004).
- AD 100–476: Roman Empire–Men continued to serve as *nosocomi* in military hospitals until the fall of the Roman Empire in AD 476.
- AD 300: In early Christian Greece and Rome, orders of monks known as Parabolani sacrificially cared for victims of the plagues. As a result, many monks lost their lives (Anthony, 2004).
- AD 324–1453: Byzantine period in Eastern Europe. Both men and women were caregivers in the hospitals that provided care (O'Lynn & Tranbarger, 2007).
- AD 400–1600: Historical accounts of the monastic movement show that men were responsible for the nursing care of the sick, wounded, and dying (O'Lynn & Tranbarger, 2007).
- AD 1100: Brothers of St. Anthony developed hospitals in France, Spain, and Italy (O'Lynn & Tranbarger, 2007).
- AD 1400: Alexian Brothers cared for victims of the plague and buried the dead. They became a religious community that continues to serve the needs of the sick today (O'Lynn & Tranbarger, 2007).
- AD 1500: St. Camillus de Lellis, a Franciscan monk who founded the male caregiving order of the Camellians, created the symbol of the red cross that remains the universal symbol of health care. His order remains today and serves in 35 countries (O'Lynn & Tranbarger, 2007).

- AD 1600: Men also participated in nonmilitary orders during this time up until the sixteenth century when monastery orders were dissolved (Evans, 2004).

Nightingale and the Modern Era

Despite the rich historical legacy that men have experienced as caregivers, why are there so few men in nursing today? Men currently comprise 9.6% of registered nurses and 8.1% of licensed vocational nurses (Jaslow, 2013). In order to put the currently low participation rates of men in nursing in perspective, we have to go back only 150 years. Though I admire Nightingale for her passion and vision to pioneer the modern era of nursing, she had a philosophical worldview regarding men in nursing that continues to influence the present.

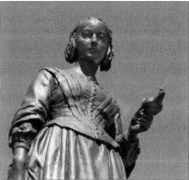

"No one individual was more responsible for ushering in a period of female domination of nursing than Nightingale" (O'Lynn & Tranbarger, 2007, p. 323). When Nightingale instituted the modern era of nursing, she chose to firmly establish it as a woman's occupation. To her, *"every woman was a nurse,"* and a woman who entered nurse training was doing only what came naturally (Evans, 2004). European religious sisterhoods also embraced Nightingale's reforms, which by their very nature were exclusive to women (Anthony, 2004).

Nightingale believed that men have no place in nursing *"except where physical strength was needed"* (Villeneuve, 1994) and that men's *"hard and horny"* hands were not fit to touch, bathe, and dress wounded limbs, however gentle their hearts may be (Brown, 2000). In England during the late 1800s, men who remained in nursing were excluded from general nursing practice as well as Nightingale's schools of nursing.

The only practice environment available to men was in the insane asylums where men were needed because of their superior strength to restrain violent patients. The psychiatric education of men was considered inferior in length and quality in comparison to the women who attended Nightingale's schools of nursing. If a man wanted to expand his learning to include obstetrics and maternal-child nursing, he was perceived as a pervert and threatened with expulsion (Evans, 2004).

There were also other social and cultural forces in the mid-1800s that contributed to the lack of men who chose to enter the nursing profession. These social forces included the decline of male monastic orders that began in the 1500s with the Protestant Reformation, the increase in the number of convents and female nursing orders, and the Industrial Revolution of the 1800s that attracted men for its higher pay and no demand for formal education (O'Lynn & Tranbarger, 2007).

Institutional/Educational Bias

Because men were not allowed to be trained as general nurses, by 1900, general hospitals in England were dominated by female nurses. By 1919, the General Nursing Council (the equivalent of our current state boards of nursing) offered full membership only to women who were "general trained." Since most men were not able to be admitted to these schools, nursing consolidated its position as the first self-determining female profession (Mackintosh, 1997). Men comprised only 0.004 percent of nurses in England from 1921–1938 until the laws were changed to allow general nursing schools to accept men in 1947 (Mackintosh, 1997).

In the United States, men in nursing were excluded from membership in professional organizations such as the American Nurses Association (ANA) that was founded in 1897 by Isabel Hampton Robb. African-American nurses faced no similar bias. Men continued to be barred from the ANA until 1930 when the official position of the ANA was changed to strongly support men in nursing (O'Lynn & Tranbarger, 2007). National laws that were in place between 1901 and 1955 prevented men from serving as nurses in the United States Army Nurse Corps. It was only after the Korean War that this policy was changed. This continued to lower male participation in nursing in the United States so that by 1930, less than 1 percent of nurses were men (Anthony, 2004).

Men in Nursing: By the Decades

In order to put past gender bias and discrimination that men have experienced in historical context, the small but incremental increases over the decades validates the early struggles that men experienced in the modern era and suggest the power of ongoing social, cultural, and educational barriers that persist today.

- 1950: 1%
- 1960: 1%
- 1970: 2.7%
- 1980: 4.1%
- 1990: 5.7%
- 2000: 7.6%
- 2011: 9.6%

In comparison, it is ironic to witness the monumental gains of female participation in the once male-dominated profession of medicine. The percentage of female residents has now surpassed that of men. But it wasn't always that way. Women had comparably low percentages of participation in the 1950s but achieved gender parity with dramatic increases in the last twenty years.

- 1950: 5.7%
- 1970: 9.4%
- 1980: 28.2%
- 1990: 39.2%
- 2005: 51%
- 2011: 46%

Lingering Bias

Though gender bias and discrimination toward men in nursing was evident in the past, is this bias still evident today and are there examples that demonstrate that it may still linger? Would it surprise you to know that up until the 1960s only 15 percent of public nursing schools were willing to admit men into their program? As recent as 1981, a public school of nursing continued to exclude men because of their gender (Jaslow, 2013).

As recently as 2004, a hospital in West Virginia had a policy that prevented qualified male nurses from working in obstetrics due to concerns of patient privacy. This case was appealed all the way to Supreme Court (Kouta & Kaite, 2011). It is ironic that male obstetricians are widely accepted in this clinical area, but male nurses typically are not. A male nurse colleague who previously worked in labor and delivery reported to me that though he was a clinical expert in this specialty, he was consistently met with verbal and nonverbal derision by female colleagues who openly questioned his motives for working in this setting.

Social/Cultural Barriers

Though the discriminatory policies of the past have been a contributing factor to the low participation rates of men in nursing, why don't more men seriously consider entering the nursing profession today? Numerous studies have addressed this topic and some of the barriers that men most commonly identified include (Roth & Coleman, 2008):

Traditional Feminine Image of Nursing

- Because nursing remains a female-dominated profession, the perception that nursing is "women's work" is not inherently attractive to most men. Combine this perception with an adolescent male who may be struggling to establish a sense of gender identity and what it means to be a man, and nursing will not be seriously considered as an option.

Gender Role Strain

- Masculine role strain can be defined as the tension that is experienced when a man chooses to pursue a gender role that is perceived as being incompatible with being a man. This ties in closely with the first social barrier of nursing being a woman's profession.
- Depending on the degree of social support that a male student receives, if strong social support is not present, this will influence whether he will complete the program.

Lack of Male Role Models/Mentors

- Because the current participation of men in nursing remains less than 10 percent, men who decide to become a nurse have few if any male role models in the nursing profession. This influence is taken for granted by women who have mothers or other family members who are nurses and can look to them for guidance and affirmation in pursuing nursing as a career option.
- Consider the influence of media. What examples of men in nursing are positive role models that men can aspire to be like? Not many. Remember *Meet the Parents*? Though this movie was at times very funny, it did nothing to attract men to the nursing profession and reinforced the majority of negative stereotypes of men who choose to enter nursing.

The Name of the Profession...NURSE!

- Words do have power and carry strong associations. In one study of 100 male high school students, the number of male students who would consider nursing increased from 6 to 21 when nursing was renamed by the gender neutral title "registered clinician" (Gorman, 2003).
- The airline industry changed the name of the overtly feminine title "stewardess" to the inclusive and gender-neutral title of "flight attendant" when men began to enter this female-dominated profession.

- Professions that were once male dominated have changed their name to be gender-inclusive. For example, when women began to enter male-dominated occupations such as police and fire protection, the prior title of policeMAN and fireMAN were replaced with the gender-neutral titles of police OFFICER and fireFIGHTER.

Stereotypes

Stereotypes in nursing have the power to distort reality about what is true about those who comprise the profession. The power of distorted assumptions cuts both ways for men and women in nursing. For women, the most common stereotype is the "naughty nurse" who uses her position to seduce and meet the sexual needs of her male patients. The end result of this stereotype is that it demeans and degrades women as well as the nursing profession.

Unfortunately, the stereotypes that men experience are just as prevalent and just as powerful to distort reality (McLaughlin, Muldoon, & Moutray, 2010). Listed below are the most common assumptions and stereotypes that men encounter if they choose to enter the nursing profession.

- Homosexual
- Effeminate
- Underachievers–not smart enough for medical school
- Sexual predators
- Not as caring/compassionate

Was it just a coincidence that the lead character from *Meet the Parents* was named GAYlord (emphasis mine) Focker and played off the top three stereotypes that men in nursing are homosexual, effeminate, and not smart enough for medical school?

Educational Barriers

Male nursing students have some of the highest failure-to-complete nursing education rates of any demographic in nursing education today. In one study, the failure to complete rate for men was almost 30 percent; in comparison, women had a 10 percent failure to complete rate. The statistical relationship of gender and course completion in this same study was $p=0.009$ (McLaughlin, Muldoon, & Moutray, 2010)! These findings have been replicated where male failure to complete rates remain as high as 40–50 percent in some programs. Why do men in nursing education fail to complete what they begin? What can be done in nursing education to promote the retention of men?

Though nursing education has little control over the broader social/cultural barriers of men who enter the nursing profession experience, it does have control over its academic culture. Unfortunately, nursing educational barriers continue to exist to this day that directly impact the success of men in academia. Quantitative research has shown that the barriers men face in nursing education have not changed over time (O'Lynn, 2004). Though overt bias is rare, covert discrimination is much more common.

One way this more subtle form of discrimination manifests itself is the feminine emphasis on how to provide care. The underlying message to male students is that in order to be a nurse, you have to behave like a woman (Carol, 2006). In addition, fundamental nursing textbooks have limited or excluded historical male contributions to nursing while emphasizing those of women. This revision of nursing history perpetuates the myth that nursing has always been a female-dominated profession (Anthony, 2004).

Nursing faculty may also be inadvertently part of the problem. Men perceive an inherent bias in nursing education with feelings of isolation and loneliness exacerbated by the lack of male faculty who serve as role models, as well as the use of the pronoun "she" and assumption that nursing is a feminine profession. In addition, the pedagogies used in education emphasize feminine learning styles, communication strategies, personal reflection, and methods of caring (Dyck, Oliffe, Phinney, & Garrett, 2009).

Male students quickly realize that if they are assertive or question faculty (traditional masculine traits) they are stigmatized. As a result, men learn to temper their masculine behavior and act more feminine to "fit in." Though there is an assumption by some faculty that men who enter nursing are doing so primarily for financial gain, the motivation for men to enter nursing is similar to women: the desire to help others, a sense of calling, and job security (Harding, 2009).

A National League for Nursing (NLN) core competency for nurse educators is the need to create an environment that facilitates student learning. This is done by recognizing the influence of gender, experience, and other factors to learning ("Core Competencies of Nurse Educators with Task Statements," 2005). In essence, the NLN holds every nurse educator to a standard that breaks down perceived or actual barriers to learning. Therefore, every nurse educator has a responsibility to directly address and confront the educational barriers toward men that continue to persist in nursing education today.

Based on the literature, the following themes are the most significant barriers that persist in nursing education that may influence the ability of men to successfully complete nursing education:

1. No history of men in nursing (McLaughlin, Muldoon, & Moutray, 2010)
2. No guidance on masculine styles of caring (O'Lynn, 2003)
3. No guidance on "intimate touch" (Harding, North, & Perkins, 2008)
4. No guidance on differences of gender communication (O'Lynn, 2004)
5. "Chilly" classroom climate (Bell-Scriber, 2008)
6. Exclusive use of lecture in classroom (O'Lynn, 2004)
7. Feelings of isolation/loneliness (Stott, 2007)
8. Lack of male mentoring/role modeling (O'Lynn, 2004)

1. No History of Men in Nursing

If men have no knowledge of their historical legacy and identity as caregivers and have an inaccurate perception that nursing has always been "women's work," this may dissuade some men from considering the nursing profession and persevering in nursing education. Most fundamental nursing textbooks continue to limit or exclude the male contributions to nursing while emphasizing those of women (McLaughlin, Muldoon, & Moutray, 2010). This revision of nursing history perpetuates the myth that nursing has always been a female-dominated profession (O'Lynn & Tranbarger, 2007). If the historical legacy of men as caregivers was clearly presented in textbooks and widely known by nurse educators, this barrier could be eliminated immediately!

This obstacle is one of the most important barriers to bring down and also potentially the easiest. Faculty who recognize the need to make this legacy known can easily present this content in their classroom or create a handout for their students to address the current gap in nursing education regardless of what textbook publishers choose to publish.

I have been impressed with the accuracy and extensive inclusion of men in nursing history found in Kozier & Erb's *Fundamentals of Nursing* (2015). Unfortunately, this textbook is the exception. The following are examples of bias and even revision of nursing history in others:

- In a former edition of a top-selling fundamental textbook, the "Milestones in Nursing History" table begins with this entry: "AD 400, entry of women into nursing." They were off by almost 1,000 years and cited the wrong gender (Potter & Perry, 2004)!

- A recent edition of this fundamental textbook begins nursing history with Florence Nightingale, ignoring over 2,000 years of caregiving that I have included in the beginning of this chapter (Potter & Perry, 2012).

2. No Guidance on Masculine Styles of Caring

Certain masculine traits have been perceived as not being compatible with caring behaviors. This has led to a historical bias against men in nursing. Even Florence Nightingale thought that men were incapable of caring and advocated for the removal of men from direct patient care (Dossey, 1999). This assumption has been reinforced and strengthened by modern feminists including Gilligan and Chodorow, who have tied caring behaviors as belonging exclusively to woman (Thompson, 2002).

As a male member of the nursing profession, I can attest that men do care and are fully capable of caring behaviors. But just as there are distinct gender styles related to communication, there are also masculine styles of caring. In one qualitative study of male nursing students, Patterson et al. (1996) identified masculine caring by establishing a rapport with patients that was akin to friendship that was not dependent on the use of touch. In another study, men consistently used humor in their interactions with patients to develop a caring rapport.

Thompson (2002) has observed that men tend to provide care from an emotionally safe distance. Men also are more likely to adopt a "professional model" of caregiving that equates nursing care as work and emphasizes task-completion and problem solving to meet patient needs.

Women are much more likely to utilize physical touch. Since most nurse educators are women, they emphasize a feminine style of caring as the standard (O'Lynn, 2003) of evaluation for both men and women. In one quantitative study (O'Lynn, 2003), 30.9 percent of men reported that nursing faculty emphasized feminine styles of caring, while 53.6 percent reported that they had received no guidance or instruction regarding masculine caring styles.

3. No Guidance on "Intimate Touch"

Generally speaking, when men use touch with a woman, it can be interpreted as potentially sexual. When women use touch, it is generally seen as an act of caring. The use of physical touch for men who enter nursing becomes a potential concern when men perform intimate cares or procedures on women. In addition to the general unease and awkwardness that intimate touch inherently presents for men in the patient care setting, the other aspect that makes this stressful for men is the vulnerability they may experience if they have to defend themselves in the no–win situation of "my word against hers" should an allegation of inappropriate touch be made, even if the patient is confused.

Because most nurse educators are women, this perspective is typically not recognized or considered, but it is clearly documented in the literature (Evans, 2002). This important aspect of patient care is not addressed in most fundamental textbooks. Therefore, it is imperative to have a crucial conversation with all students but directed toward men when intimate procedures such as Foley catheterizations are taught and practiced. But more importantly, provide male students with practical strategies that will DECREASE stress and provide a sense of safety when providing intimate care in the clinical setting.

Male students need to know the importance of building a trust relationship with their patient and to be professional in all aspects of patient care. This will decrease the likelihood of any need for intimate touch to be misinterpreted. If an intimate procedure such as a Foley catheterization needs to be done on a woman, the following are the best practice recommendations from the literature (Harding, North, & Perkins, 2008) to decrease stress and vulnerability in nursing education as well as in practice:

Communicate and explain everything that you will do ahead of time and while you are doing it.
- This will decrease the likelihood of any touch being misinterpreted, especially when the labia are being cleansed and separated to prepare for insertion of the catheter.

Obtain permission to do intimate care/procedure
- This is something I routinely do for any intimate procedure, especially with younger women. It also communicates professionalism and respect for the feelings of a woman who may not say no unless she is given the opportunity to do so.
- If a woman gives me permission, I do NOT use a female chaperone.

Female chaperones when there's potential for being vulnerable
- The most common example of this intervention is when a female patient is confused.

Delegate intimate care to women
- If a female patient prefers a woman to do any intimate care, offer to do something that the female nurse needs done so that she does not get behind when intimate care is delegated.

Modify techniques to limit exposure
- Limiting exposure will allow the woman to feel safe, respected, and will likely not misinterpret intimate touch.
- A common example of limiting exposure that I use in the ED is when I need to place EKG electrodes on a female patient. With men I will take off their shirt, place the electrodes on their bare chest, and then put on the gown. For women, this would be obviously inappropriate. I allow her to place the gown on. I place the top three electrodes from the top of the gown and the lower two electrodes that go on the abdomen by going underneath the gown, never having to expose her breasts.

4. No Guidance on Differences of Gender Communication

Men and women are different. One area that these gender differences is how men and women communicate. This awareness will lead to understanding as well as more effective communication between men and women. O'Lynn (2004) identified that current barriers men in nursing education experience is a lack of preparation to work with women and instruction on communicating more effectively with women.

Women emphasize the relational nature of communication using verbal and nonverbal communication to establish "rapport talk" to connect with others. This may include sharing information about their family, children, significant others, or more intimate details of their life. In comparison, men emphasize the content aspects of communication that tend to focus on "just the facts" to accomplish needed tasks. The implication of this lived reality is that men tend to wonder when female nurses will get to the point, and women may make the inaccurate assumption that men are unfriendly or withdrawn because they do not reciprocate with "rapport talk" (O'Lynn & Tranbarger, 2007).

Another way that men and women communicate differently is how they give and receive praise. Women tend to liberally give and receive praise regularly to others. Praise communicates that their efforts are appreciated and noticed.

The norms of masculine communication emphasize goals and getting things done. Men tend to give praise in response to something that was significant or done very well, not routinely. This can lead to misunderstanding in the workplace by the male nurse who receives praise from women and may think that he is above average. Conversely, because men do not tend to offer praise for ordinary efforts, a woman may feel that he does not value or appreciate her efforts and make the assumption that he is cold or arrogant as a result (O'Lynn & Tranbarger, 2007).

Men and women tend to make judgments differently. While women tend to be nonjudgmental, men are more likely to rush to judgment and reach a decision more quickly. This has important implications in clinical practice, where men may be more likely to make premature clinical judgments. Clinical educators need to be aware of this tendency and model critical thinking that ensures that male students have addressed and examined all alternatives before making a decision (Brady & Sherrod, 2003).

5. "Chilly" Classroom Climate

"Chilly" can be defined by the degree of support that students experience in nursing education. According to the literature, men in nursing often do not feel supported, but singled out and held to a different standard because of their gender (Bell-Scriber, 2008).

In one study, researchers observed faculty interactions with students in a nursing program over an entire semester and then interviewed both men and women students. Male students reported the following behaviors of nurse educators:

- Faculty were harsh. "It's not the words they say; it is how they say it."
- Men observed that faculty spent more time with female students in clinical.
- Men experienced prejudicial comments from faculty such as, "Men are going into nursing for the wrong reason. They only want to be a CRNA."

When researchers asked, "Describe an experience that was personally meaningful to you as a student," ALL of the men reported an experience that they had with a PATIENT in the clinical setting. In comparison, 75 percent of female students described an experience with nursing FACULTY (Bell-Scriber, 2008).

6. Exclusive Use of Lecture in Classroom

Just as there are individual differences in learning styles, there are also unique gender distinctives between men and women and how they most effectively learn and process new information. For example, women tend to have a preference for auditory learning and prefer a more traditional learning environment that includes a formal classroom. In comparison, men tend to be visual as well as kinesthetic learners who prefer a more informal classroom that emphasizes active and applied learning strategies. Male nursing students prefer to be independent and self-directed in their learning (Brady & Sherrod, 2003). Men also prefer to have reading assignments as well as lecture content kept to a minimum with examples and application to real-world practice.

O'Lynn (2004) identified that one of the most frequent barriers that male students identified was a lecture-only format in the classroom. Men also have a preference and gain mastery of content when the technical aspects of nursing are emphasized (Stott, 2007).

7. Feelings of Isolation/Loneliness

Because men are currently a minority in nursing education, male camaraderie and support is limited. The consequence of this reality is that over time men experience isolation and feelings of loneliness in nursing education. Over time, men become ambivalent about becoming a nurse and as a result, begin to openly question their desire and motivation to complete nursing education (Stott, 2007).

The isolation that men experience is a clear contributing factor to the high failure to complete rates in nursing education. This finding reinforces the need of placing male students together in the same clinical group to decrease feelings of isolation and provide needed support (Meadus & Twomey, 2011).

8. Lack of Male Mentoring/Role Modeling

Male nursing students need a role model with whom they can identify and validate their decision to enter the nursing profession. Because there are currently so few men in nursing education, this support is lacking in most departments of nursing. Therefore, clinical nurse educators must make it a priority to identify if there are any male nurses who can be assigned to a male student on clinical days (Meadus & Twomey, 2011). This is a simple but effective strategy that will provide male students with a role model and needed support.

How's the Climate Today?

Though these barriers have been documented in the literature for years, is the current climate warmer toward male students in nursing education? It depends on the program. Incivility thrives where it is tolerated and becomes an accepted unit or academic norm. Gender bias and treating men differently because of their gender can also become an accepted norm that can adversely impact male students in that setting. When a culture of bias is present, the "hidden curriculum" (Tanner, 1990) of nursing education communicates to students that faculty bias against men is acceptable and female students can be influenced as a result. One educator's recent personal observations in his department highlights this reality:

> One female educator openly said in our department, "Men have no place in nursing." This attitude impacts male students who are perceived by female educators as troublemakers or difficult because they are willing to challenge faculty on areas they feel are incorrect. As a result, male students report being singled out, targeted, and not feeling supported. One male student told me he keeps his head down just so he can survive and get through the program. Other male students have considered leaving as a result of perceived differential treatment. Female students have observed and noticed that male students are also treated differently. When male students answer questions in class or make suggestions, some female students have been seen to roll their eyes and say things such as, "Why does it matter to you. You're a guy, why do you want to be a nurse anyway?"

Men Have a Place

I strongly encourage my male students to persevere in nursing education because of the wide variety of clinical opportunities that are an excellent fit for men. Though men practice in almost every clinical area, the highest concentration of male participation is found in the ED, critical care, and nurse anesthetists. Though men make up only 9.6 percent of registered nurses in the United States, they comprise 41 percent of nurse anesthetists (Jaslow, 2013)!

What do these three clinical areas have in common? There is a lack of association with feminine nursing traits, such as touch and the delivery of intimate nursing care. They are HIGH tech, LOW touch specialties. In these clinical areas men tend to create "islands of masculinity" within the profession (Evans, 1997). Another theme of these clinical areas is that they have high degrees of technology, adversity, autonomy, and high levels of acuity where the nurse can make a difference and literally save a life. Deep in the male psyche is the need to have a battle to fight and an adventure to live by (Eldredge, 2001), which each of these clinical areas represent.

Following are some general principles that I have found beneficial as a male member of the profession to engage and welcome men to a work culture that is predominantly female:

Find Common Ground with the Women You Work With

- Though you may not be able to identify with some of the intimate, personal things that women often share with one another and you will likely overhear, be intentional to find what you do have in common. You will be tempted at times to disengage because your female colleagues do not show an interest in sports, hunting, or fishing. But if you have children or pets, these topics are common ground that you can steer the conversation toward. Build bridges whenever possible.

Be a Team Player

- This is another way to intentionally engage with female co-workers. Make yourself consistently available by offering help of any kind whenever you have time. Though men sometimes get asked to literally do the "heavy lifting" on the unit, this assistance is always appreciated and is a practical way to build a bridge with the women you work with.

Celebrate Diversity!

- This cuts both ways for men and women. Much of the incivility in nursing is a result of not valuing and respecting the unique gender differences of men and women. The direct communication styles of men may create an offense to some women. Accept the gender distinctives of the opposite sex. Do not be critical of women because they are not more like men, and vice versa!

HIGHLIGHTS

- Men were the earliest recorded caregivers going back almost 2,500 years to the BCE era of ancient Greece and Rome.
- Though men were caregivers throughout the AD era, Florence Nightingale chose to establish the modern era of nursing as a woman's occupation where men were not permitted to attend the Nightingale schools of nursing.
- Men were relegated to practice in the insane asylums where their "physical strength was needed."
- Numerous social/cultural barriers to men in nursing include the traditional feminine image of nursing, gender role strain, and stereotypes that portray men in nursing as effeminate, homosexual, and not smart enough for medical school.
- In nursing education, men continue to experience ongoing barriers that include no history of men in nursing, lack of male mentoring/role modeling, feelings of isolation/loneliness, and no guidance on "intimate touch."

Additional Resources

- Book: *A Man's Guide to a Nursing Career* (2012) by Chad O'Lynn
- Book: *MAN UP! A Practical Guide for Men in Nursing* (2013) by Christopher Lance Coleman
- Website: American Assembly for Men in Nursing: http://aamn.org/
- Website: Men in Nursing/KeithRN.com: http://www.keithrn.com/men-in-nursing/

Reflections

1. If you are a male student, what stereotypes have you most commonly experienced?

   What did you do to overcome them?

2. Have you experienced any of the educational barriers identified in the literature?

   If so, which ones?

   How did you overcome them?

3. Have you felt that you were treated differently in your program because you were male?

4. What strategies have you found helpful to get through your nursing program?

Appendix B

Serving the Poor through Medical Missions

To put the needs of the developing world in context, if 100 jetliners crashed today killing 26,500 people, it would get the world's attention. If this happened day after day, you would demand that something be done to stop this ongoing loss of human life! But a tragedy of this scope occurs every day in the developing world. Every day, 26,500 children die of preventable causes related to their poverty. Over one year, this equates to 10,000,000 lives lost (Shah, 2013).

After the massive earthquake struck Haiti in January, 2010, I felt powerless and helpless yet wanted to do something to help with my ED background. The news reports dramatically witnessed the urgency of the medical needs of so many thousands dead and wounded with minimal resources to care for the suffering. I was able to go as part of a medical mission team through our church in May 2010. Though the critically wounded were by then cared for, our team was able to provide much-needed routine clinic care for many living in the tent cities in Port-au-Prince. When we left Haiti after a week, there was no coordination of other health care providers to take our place.

I have been back since then, including a team comprised of my second-year nursing students who were forever changed by their ability to make a difference in the developing world where the needs are great and ongoing. Though our team accomplishments may seem small and a proverbial "drop in the bucket," the "drop" matters, because every person matters to God and each of us have equal worth as we are created in His image.

Haiti has the highest rates of infant, under-age-5, and maternal mortality in the Western Hemisphere. The infant mortality rate is 57 per 1,000 in 2007; in the U.S., it is 6.7 deaths per 1,000. Maternal mortality is 523 deaths per 100,000 births in Haiti, compared with 13 per 100,000 in the U.S. Diarrhea, respiratory infections, malaria, tuberculosis, and HIV/AIDS are the leading causes of death. Not coincidentally, Haiti has the lowest number of nurses/1000 population in the world: 0.11 nurses/1000.

Though we lament the nursing shortage here in the U.S. (16th in the world at 9.37/1000), nothing compares to this! As a nurse, you have a skill that can serve others wherever you choose to practice. Based on my own personal observations and the feedback and reflections of my nursing students, even a one-week service trip can minister to the needs of the poor, possibly save a life, and give you a new lens to see the world by.

Haiti Nursing Foundation

Though serving the poor through medical missions in other countries is good, I believe that another and ultimately better way to make an impact to provide needed health care is to partner with nursing education in the developing world to improve the quality of nursing education. Most of the nurses who graduate from such a program will stay in their country to serve.

One excellent model of this approach is the Faculty of Nursing Science (FSIL) of the Episcopal University in Leogane, Haiti. This university is located less than an hour from Port-au-Prince, I recently had the opportunity to teach nursing students and assist in clinical at this university. It was a life-changing experience for me. I left Haiti hopeful, knowing that the quality of the baccalaureate education these students were receiving would prepare them to not only be exceptional care providers, but leaders who will influence the quality of nursing and healthcare wherever they serve in Haiti.

One practical way that anyone can make a difference is to sponsor or partially sponsor the cost of a nursing student's education, which is about $4,000 annually for tuition, room and board. Contact http://haitinursing.org/ for more information on how you can help.

Don't Waste Your Life

One book that continually challenges me is *Don't Waste Your Life* by John Piper. Each one of us has a finite amount of time to live our life for what really matters. The greatest tragedy is to come to the end of your days realizing that you wasted the one life you have been given on this earth. In addition to not wasting my life, I also do not want to waste this opportunity to encourage anyone who is reading this book to impact those in the developing world with a variety of ways to serve.

I have listed organizations that specialize in short-term medical mission outreach in the developing world. I also have a medical missions tab on my website that has numerous resources for those who may be interested in serving in this context as well.

Though the needs of the poor in the developing world are profound, there are people in your community that you can also serve through medical mission. Though it takes time, energy, and financial resources to go to another country, you can make a difference right in your own community. Partner with ministries that serve the homeless, or the poor in free medical clinics. There is no shortage of work to be done. Just open your eyes to see how you can be used to make a difference wherever you decide to serve.

Don't Sell Your Textbooks! Give Them to Liberian Nursing Students

Liberia, an English-speaking West African country is in desperate need of nursing textbooks because of a prolonged civil war that has devastated the country. It is not uncommon to have an entire nursing class of 80 students have just a few textbooks that are shared by all. A nurse colleague who is native to Liberia has an organization, Liberian Health Initiative, that coordinates shipments of nursing textbooks and other needed supplies for nursing education in Liberia. If you are a student who has textbooks you know you will never open after graduation, or an educator who has older editions of textbooks gathering dust, please send them directly to:

Liberian Health Initiative
P.O. Box 29628
Minneapolis, MN 55429

Additional Resources
Medical Missions
- Bulk Medications for Medical Ministry: Blessings International: http://www.blessing.org/
- Medical Mission Outreach: Medical Teams International: http://www.medicalteams.org/
- Medical Mission Outreach: Global Health Outreach: http://cmda.org/missions/detail/global-health-outreach
- Mercy Ships/Youth With a Mission: http://www.mercyships.org/
- Nursing Education: Haiti Nursing Foundation: http://haitinursing.org/
- Medical Missions: Liberian Health Initiative: http://www.liberianhealthinitiative.org/
- Book: *When Helping Hurts: Alleviating Poverty Without Hurting the Poor. . .and Yourself* (2012) by Steve Corbett & Brian Fikkert
- Book: *Let the Nations Be Glad 3rd ed.* by John Piper

Faith Based
- Nurses Christian Fellowship: http://ncf-jcn.org/
- Book: *Called to Care: A Christian Worldview for Nursing* by Judith Allen Shelly & Arlene B. Miller
- Book: *The Nurse with an Alabaster Jar: A Biblical Approach to Nursing* by Mary Elizabeth O'Brien & Judith Allen Shelly
- Journal: Journal of Christian Nursing (JCN)
- Book (free PDF download!): *Don't Waste Your Life* by John Piper: http://www.desiringgod.org/books/dont-waste-your-life
- Booklet: "For Your Joy" by John Piper: http://www.desiringgod.org/books/for-your-joy

Reflections

1. Do you have a desire to serve others through medical missions? If so, what country are you drawn to?

2. What ministries serve the poor in your community where you could serve others?

3. What can you do today to educate yourself on what is required to serve effectively in the country you are interested in?

Alexandra P. Mareck

808 27th Avenue ~ St. Cloud, MN 56301 ~ 320-***-*** ~ apmareck@email.edu

Dedicated, caring and hardworking individual
Proven leader abilities in volunteer, work, and school activities.

Nursing License	State of Minnesota	License: R******

Education

College of Saint Benedict, St. Joseph, MN — **May 2015**
Bachelor of Science in Nursing — **Cum GPA:** 3.75
Nursing Immersion Experience: South Africa Study abroad: provided care for underserved communities
Senior Capstone: Family Birthing Center, St. Cloud Hospital and the Good Shepherd Community, Sauk Rapids, MN

Evidence-Based Practice

St. Cloud Hospital

Evidence-based: to assess current ambulation practices in surgical patients. Performed chart audits; literature review of evidence-based findings of patient mobility progression; practice change recommendations presented to practice committee.

Good Shepherd Community

Quality improvement project: to assist the facility in preparing for Minnesota Department of Health visit. Conducted mock audits and provided evidence-based feedback to the interdisciplinary team.

Related Work Experience

Nursing Teaching Assistant, *College of Saint Benedict (CSB),* St. Joseph, MN — August 2014 – May 2015
Assisted and organized simulation labs, mentoring and assessment of skills
Mentored students requiring special assistance with assignments and nursing skills
Resource for students and faculty during St. Cloud Hospital clinical practice rotations

Pharmacy Assistant, *Apothecary Pharmacy,* Sartell, MN — August 2014 – May 2015
Provided customer service: office phones and assisting clients with products
Assisted pharmacists refilling and mailing out prescriptions

Valor Internship: Surgical & Specialty Care, *VA Medical Center,* St. Cloud, MN — June 2014 – August 2014
Provided care in a clinic assisting minor surgeries, procedures, ENT, podiatry and orthopedics
Gained independence in PACU upon being assigned a personal patient load

Voyageur Guide, *Les Voyageurs, Inc.,* Sartell, MN — May – August 2013
Guided 7 high school students through the Canadian Wilderness
Coordinated and provided care for a student who fractured ankle on trip

Global Activity, Mission Trip, Guatemala, Mexico — March 2011
Co-leader for Mission Trip

Professional Organizations

Sigma Theta Tau International Member Inducted — November 2014
Minnesota Student Nurses Association MSNA — January 2013- May 2015

Awards and Certificates

Outstanding Nursing Student EBP Award, St. Cloud Hospital — May 2015
President's Scholarship — August 2010-May 2015
Dean's List — Fall 2014
Public Health Nursing Certification — May 2015
American Red Cross Disaster Preparedness Certification — December 2014
Wilderness Advanced First Aid — June 2013

Interests and Activities

Mission Trip Co-leader to Guatemala and New Mexico (March 2012), Orientation Leader, Zumba Instructor, Boys and Girls Club, Benedictine Friends, Joint Events Council,

Mitchell W. McGraw

320-***-****   114 S. Swift Avenue
mmcgraw@email.edu   Anytown, MN 553**

OBJECTIVE: To obtain a nursing internship in the summer of 2014

EDUCATION:
Bachelor of Science   Anticipated: May 2015
St. John's University, Collegeville, MN   Major: Nursing   GPA: 3.84/4.0

Honors: Regents' Scholarship (academics & leadership), Graduated from Anytown High School in 2011
    with high honors
Professional Organization: Inducted Sigma Theta Tau International   November 2014-Present

RELEVANT EXPERIENCE:
Personal Care Attendant   July 2008-Present
Meeker County Community Homes, Any town, MN
- Perform daily cares for mentally disabled men
- Administer oral medications to residents
- Cook for and assist residents with meals

Nurse's Assistant   August 2011-Present
St. Raphael's Hall Nursing Home, St. John's Abbey, Collegeville, MN
- Help residents with getting ready for bed
- Ambulate residents daily
- Communicate with patients to keep them company
- Assist residents with dining

ADDITIONAL EXPERIENCE:
Hockey Referee   November 2003-Present
District 5 Youth Hockey
- Learned how to communicate in a calm manner with angered coaches
- Gained ability to express thoughts on a play that occurred
- Manages a busy schedule between school and games

Community Service
- Volunteered at Anytown Middle School to educate students in math
- Addressed students on the importance of performing well in school and ways to form study habits
- Voluntarily coach players in football and hockey in grades six through nine
- Helped raise money for St. Jude's Children Hospital in an on campus event called Up 'Til Dawn
- Volunteering for the Central Minnesota Boys and Girls Club

Leadership Experience
- Mentor and teach inexperienced hockey referees
- Lead high school football team as a captain during senior year
- Created a project for FCCLA (Family, Career, Community, Leaders of America) that attempted to improve middle school MCA math scores
- Member of National Honor Society

Awards and Recognition
- Graduated in the top ten of class at Anytown High School
- Received the Scholar Athlete Award at Anytown
- Was an All-Conference football player during senior year of high school
- Lettered in football, hockey, and tennis throughout high school

Appendix D

A Nurse's Prayer

Lord, let me bring your presence into my practice.

I acknowledge my need for your strength, patience, and perseverance today.

Help me to see those I care for through your heart and eyes.

Help me to be moved with your heart of love and compassion for humanity.

Help me to see your presence in every person I care for.

Help me to remember that when I touch and care for my patient in your name, I am caring and touching you.

Thank you for this day and the opportunities I will have to serve my patients.

Help me to remember that as I care and serve others in your name, I am making a difference and leaving a lasting legacy of your love.

Appendix E
Student Toolbox of Clinical Reasoning Resources

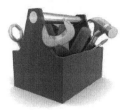

As a nurse educator, I have responded to the needs of my students to help them understand and master difficult but essential content. The following student handouts have been "field tested" and have been found beneficial to strengthen student learning.

WORKSHEET: Medications That Must Be Mastered
To strengthen your knowledge and understanding of the most commonly used medications, use this worksheet that incorporates the foundational five medications to make any medications that may be a weakness your strength.

HANDOUT: Most Commonly Used Categories of Medications
With over 5,000 meds used in clinical practice, this handout simplifies medication knowledge by grouping the most commonly used meds by pharmacologic classifications. The categories, most common side effects, and relevant nursing implications are listed for each pharmacologic classification.

WORKSHEET: Lab Planning
To strengthen your knowledge and understanding of lab values and relevant nursing assessments for an abnormal lab, use this worksheet with any labs that are currently a weakness to make them your strength.

HANDOUT: Clinical Lab Values and Nursing Responsibilities
This handout simplifies NEED TO KNOW knowledge and helps build a plan of care around abnormal, relevant lab values. This is a concise summary of the most important labs. Based on abnormal lab findings, what are the essential nursing assessments that need to be implemented so you can begin to do "lab planning"? This worksheet was referenced in Chapter 6.

HANDOUT: Clinical Reasoning Questions to Develop Nurse Thinking
My unique template breaks down clinical reasoning sequentially step-by-step. Eight PRE-clinical questions and four DURING-clinical questions to develop nurse thinking. This worksheet was referenced in Chapter 9.

WORKSHEET: Patient Preparation
If you have yet to develop your own personal patient prep worksheet to use in practice, I have used a similar worksheet for years and found it to work well to schedule my day, capture trends and patient care priorities. It compares most recent VS and assessment findings and has a second page with clinical reasoning questions to help establish nursing priorities and plan of care. This worksheet was referenced in Chapter 14.

Medications That Must Be Mastered Worksheet

Name	Dose: High-low-avg.?	Pharm. Class	Therapeutic Use/Mechanism of Action	Adverse Actions (most common SE)	Nsg. Considerations (what must be known before)

Most Commonly Used Categories of Drugs in the Clinical Setting

Category	Class	Body System Impacted	Generic Name	Brand Name	Most Common Side Effects (italics) SEVERE	Nursing Considerations and Vital Assessments
BP Agents	ACE Inhibitors	CV	Captopril Enalapril Lisinopril	Capoten Vasotec Prinivil	*Cough hypotension* **angioedema** <u>**agranulocytosis**</u>	*Obtain BP before administering-hold typically if SBP <90 *Change position slowly-especially with elderly to prevent orthostatic changes *Monitor for decreased WBC count, hyperkalemia, liver function, and GFR/creatinine (metabolized by liver-excreted by kidneys)
	Beta blockers	CV	Atenolol Metoprolol Propranolol	Tenormin Lopressor Inderal	*Fatigue, weakness,* <u>**bradycardia, CHF, pulmonary edema**</u>	*Obtain BP and HR before administering-hold typically if SBP <90. HR <60 *Change position slowly-especially with elderly to prevent orthostatic changes *Contraindicated in worsening CHF, bradycardia of heart block…use with caution in diabetes, liver disease
	Calcium Channel Blockers	CV	Amlodipine Diltiazem Nifedipine Verapamil	Norvasc Cardizem Procardia Calan	*Peripheral edema,* <u>**Cardiac arrythmias, CHF**</u>	*Obtain BP and HR before administering-hold typically if SBP <90. HR <60 *Change position slowly-especially with elderly to prevent orthostatic changes *Measure I&O closely and fluid status due to potential for edema *Monitor liver and kidney function (metabolized in liver-excreted by kidneys)

Category	Class	Body System Impacted	Generic Name	Brand Name	Most Common Side Effects (italics) SEVERE	Nursing Considerations and Vital Assessments
	Vaso-dilators	CV	Hydralazine Isosorbide Nitroglycerine	Apresoline Isordil Tridil	*Dizziness, headache, hypotension, tachycardia*	*Obtain BP before administering-hold typically if SBP <90 *Tolerance common and serious problem with long acting nitrates. Nitrates lose their effectiveness if transdermal patches remain on continually. Patches must be taken off at night and then reapplied in the morning *Contraindicated if client taking any erectile dysfunction meds as these are a similar nitrate that improves blood circulation to the penis-synergistic effect can cause dramatic hypotension
Cholesterol Binding Agents	Statins	CV	Lovastatin Rosuvastatin Simvastin Atorvastatin	Mevacor Crestor Zocor Lipitor	*Abd. Cramps, constipation, diarrhea, heartburn, rashes* **Rhabdomyolosis**	*Can cause liver injury/damage-watch ALT/AST/alk phos/bili levels closely *Can cause muscle injury/damage. If CPK elevated DC use
Heart Rhythm Stabilizers	Class III Antiarryth.	CV	Amiodarone	Cordorone	*Dizziness, fatigue, malaise, ataxia, bradycardia* **Pulmonary fibrosis**	*Assess for QT prolongation-can lead to VT/VF with IV administration *Assess HR before giving-hold if <60 with IV administration *Can cause pulmonary toxicity with chronic use-assess for crackles, diminished breath sounds, fatigue, pleuritic chest pain *Assess for neurotoxicity (ataxia, muscle weakness, tingling in fingers/toes, tremors) *Assess for signs of thyroid dysfunction (lethargy, weight gain, edema...HYPOTHYROIDISM or tachycardia, weight loss, nervousness-HYPERTHYROIDISM) *Monitor liver labs (AST-ALT-bili) and throid labs (T3-T4)

Category	Class	Body System Impacted	Generic Name	Brand Name	Most Common Side Effects (italics) SEVERE	Nursing Considerations and Vital Assessments
	Digitalis	CV	Digoxin	Lanoxin	*Fatigue, bradycardia, anorexia, N&V* **arrythmias**	*Assess apical pulse for 1 minute before giving-hold if <60 *Increases fall risk for elderly-assess closely *Monitor K+, Mg+, Ca+ levels closely-if these are low more likely to become dig. toxic. Elderly also more likely to be dig. toxic *Assess serum levels of digoxin (norm 0.5-2.0 ng/ml) **Assess for toxicity: abd. pain, anorexia, N&V, bradycardia, visual changes**
Diuretics	Loop	CV	Furosemide	Lasix	*Dehydration, hypovolemia, hypokalemia, hyponatremia, hypomagnesemia*	*Obtain BP before administering-hold typically if SBP <90 *Change position slowly-especially with elderly to prevent orthostatic changes *Monitor sodium and K+ levels closely as well as Mg+, GFR and creatinine *assess for signs of hypokalemia (weakness-fatigue-increased PVC's on cardiac monitor). Potassium is the lyte that will be most quickly depleted in most pts
	K+ sparing		Spironolactone	Aldactone	*Hyperkalemia*	*Aldactone and ACE inhibitors can cause resultant hyperkalemia *If on Aldactone-make sure does not use potassium based salt substitutes or foods rich in K+
	Thiazides		Hydrochlorothiazide	HCTZ	*Hypokalemia*	*Monitor BP, I&O, daily weight and for presence of edema **If on digoxin, assess closely for signs of dig. toxicity since they are at higher risk of developing because of the K+ depleting effects of the diuretic** Monitor K+, Na+, Mg+, and creatinine levels closely

Category	Class	Body System Impacted	Generic Name	Brand Name	Most Common Side Effects (italics)	Nursing Considerations and Vital Assessments
Anti-Coagulants	Anti-Coagulant	Blood	Warfarin	Coumadin	**Bleeding (GI) most common** (SEVERE)	*Assess for bleeding: tarry black, or maroon stools, nosebleeds, bruising, or hematuria** *Monitor Hgb, INR (therapeutic range is 2-3 for anticoagulation) *Excreted by liver-assess AST/ALT
	Anti-Coagulant		Heparin (IV/SQ) Lovenox (SQ)	Heparin Lovenox	*Anemia, thrombocytopenia* **Bleeding**	*Assess for bleeding: tarry black, or maroon stools, nosebleeds, bruising, or hematuria** *Administer SQ in abd, NOT proximal to umbilicus *Pinch abd. fold before/during administration *Assess for decreased platelets (heparin induced thrombocytopenia-HIT)
Analgesic	Narcotics	CNS	Hydromorphone Morphine Oxycodone Codeine	Dilaudid MS Contin Oxycontin Codeine	*Confusion, sedation, hypotension, constipation* **Resp. Depression**	*Assess BP-HR-RR and LOC closely after giving-especially when drug is peaking (this will vary on drug and if given po vs. IV-check your drug book!) *Elderly more sensitive to effects of opiod analgesics and develop SE and resp. complications more frequently *THEREFORE always give LOW range if ordered *Assess bowel function closely due to risk of constipation…determine LBM! *Tolerance develops with long-term use-will need higher doses to achieve adequate pain relief
	Combo	CNS	oxycodone-acetaminophen hydrocodone-acetaminophen codeine-acetaminophen	Percocet Vicodin Tylenol #3	*Confusion, sedation, hypotension, constipation* **Resp. Depression**	*Assess pain relief 1 hour (PEAK) after giving po *Assess BP-HR-R and LOC closely after giving-especially when drug is peaking. *Elderly more sensitive to effects of opiod analgesics and develop SE and resp. complications more frequently *THEREFORE always give LOW range if ordered *Assess bowel function closely due to risk of constipation…determine LBM! *Tolerance develops with long-term use-will need higher doses to achieve adequate pain relief

Category	Class	Body System Impacted	Generic Name	Brand Name	Most Common Side Effects (italics) SEVERE	Nursing Considerations and Vital Assessments
	Non-narcotic	CNS	Acetaminophen Aspirin	Tylenol ASA	**Liver failure, toxicity w/OD or high doses SEVERE**	*Max. daily dose is 4000 mg. Liver damage can result if reaches this level or is malnourished or abuse of ETOH more likely to be toxic *Monitor liver labs (AST-ALT-bili-PT/INR) with Tylenol & Aspirin *Give Aspirin w/food to minimize risk of ulcer/GI bleed
	Non-steroidal anti-inflammatory (NSAID)	CNS	Ibuprofen Indomethacin Naproxsyn Ketorolac	Motrin/ Advil Indocin Aleve Toradol	*Headache, constipation, N&V* **GI Bleeding, Hepatitis**	*Give w/food to minimize risk of ulcer/GI bleed *Assess for GI bleeding: tarry black, or maroon stools, lightheaded, tachycardia *Elderly are at higher risk to develop GI bleeding *Monitor liver labs (AST-ALT-bili-PT/INR) *Assess response to pain med 1 hour after giving *Increases bleeding times. Be sure to DC before surgery. Effects last 24 hours after last dose
Anti-anxiety	Anti-anxiety	CNS	Alprazolam Diazepam Lorazepam	Xanax Valium Ativan	*Dizziness, drowsiness, lethargy*	*Assess closely for dizziness, drowsiness with first doses *CNS side effects increase w/elderly. THEREFORE always give LOW range if ordered
Anti-convulsant	Anti-convulsant	CNS	Carbamazepine Gabapentin Levetiracetam Phenytoin	Tegretol Neurontin Keppra Dilantin	*Drowsiness, ataxia, weakness*	*Neurontin commonly used for neuropathic pain or chronic pain syndromes
Anti-depressant	Selective Serotonin Reuptake Inhibitors (SSRI)	CNS	Citalopram Fluoxetine Paroxetine	Celexa Prozac Paxil	*Drowsiness, headache, insomnia, nervousness, tremor*	*Requires 2 weeks to have physiologic effects when new medication *Assess for increased suicidal tendencies with new therapy
Anti-Parkinson		CNS	Carbidopa-Levodopa	Sinemet	*N&V, involuntary movements*	*OK to give w/food to minimize GI side effects *Assess for Parkinson's effects improving: rigidity, tremors, shuffling gait, drooling

Category	Class	Body System Impacted	Generic Name	Brand Name	Most Common Side Effects (italics) **SEVERE**	Nursing Considerations and Vital Assessments
	Anti-psychotic	CNS	Quetiapine Haloperidol	Seroquel Haldol	*Constipation, dry mouth, blurred vision, extrapyramidal reactions (EPSE)*	*OK to give w/food to minimize GI irritation *Assess mental status (mood-orientation-behavior) before and after giving *Expected effect is DECREASED agitation/restlessness if given prn *Monitor for increased restlessness-agitation after first dose. This is a side effect *Monitor for EPSE-these are Parkinson like: difficulty/speaking or swallowing, loss of balance, pill rolling, rigidity, shuffling gait and tremors *Monitor for dystonic reaction: muscle spasm, especially in neck causing head to stay fixed on affected side, weakness of extremities
Gastric Acid Reducers	Proton Pump Inhibitors (PPI)	GI	Pantoprazole Omeprazole	Protonix Prilosec	*Abdominal pain*	*May give w/without regards to food *Assess frequently for epigastric/abd pain and blood in stool, emesis
	Histamine Blockers (H2)	GI	Cimetadine Famotidine Ranitidine	Tagamet Pepcid Zantec	*Confusion,* **Arrythmias**	*Administer w/food to prolong effects *Assess frequently for epigastric/abd pain and blood in stool, emesis. Given to prevent ulcers. This would be indicative of GI bleeding
Anti-Nausea		GI	Ondansetron Prochlorperazine Promethazine	Zofran Compazine Phenergan	*Headache, constipation, diarrhea, extrapyramidal reactions (Compazine only)*	*With prochlorperazine (Compazine) monitor for sedation and dystonic reaction: muscle spasm, especially in neck causing head to stay fixed on affected side, weakness of extremities *May develop EPSE w/prochlorperazine. Assess for difficulty/speaking or swallowing, loss of balance, pill rolling, rigidity, shuffling gait and tremors
Laxatives		GI	Docusate Sennosides Psyllium	Colace Senokot Metamucil	*Abd cramps, diarrhea*	* Assess GI system carefully for abd distention, presence of bowel sounds, and color, consistency and amount of stool *Hold if has recent pattern of loose stools

Category	Class	Body System Impacted	Generic Name	Brand Name	Most Common Side Effects (italics) SEVERE	Nursing Considerations and Vital Assessments
	Bronchial dilators	Resp.	Albuterol Albuterol-ipatropium	Ventolin Combivent	*Nervousness, restlessness, tremor, chest pain, palpitations*	*Assess breath sounds, pulse and BP before and after giving. Note amount, color and character of any sputum *Inhaled albuterol onsets in 5-15" and peaks in 1 hour *Assess therapeutic benefit of neb in 15"
	Bronch. Dilator & Steroid Combo	Resp.	Fluticasone-salmeterol	Advair	*Headache, nervousness*	*Assess breath sounds before and after giving. Note amount, color and character of any sputum *Because it is a maintenance combination, will not likely see any changes after administration *Rinse mouth with water after use to prevent thrush
	Inhaled Steroids	Resp.	Triamcinalone Fluticasone	Azmacort Flovent	*Headache, pharyngitis, flu like symptoms*	*Monitor resp. status and breath sounds closely *May cause increased serum and urine glucose levels due to steroid effect-monitor as needed
Anti-Infectives	Anti-fungal	Systemic	Fluconazole Nystatin	Diflucan Mycostatin	**Liver toxicity**	*Obtain any specimen cultures before giving first dose *Excreted by kidneys so monitor renal function (creatinine) closely
	Cephalosporin	Systemic	Cephalexin	Keflex	*Diarrhea* **Colitis, seizures**	*Obtain any specimen cultures before giving first dose *Can give w/wo food *Assess for allergic response of any kind (rash-itching-hives-anaphylactic-resp. distress) *Determine if has allergy to penicillin, give w/caution as there is risk for cross sensitivity to penicillin *Continue to assess for response to infection (temp-appearance of wound-WBC/neutrophils)
	Penicillins	Systemic	Amoxicillin Ampicillin	Amoxil Polycillin	*Rashes, diarrhea* **Seizures, allergic reactions, colitis**	*obtain any specimen cultures before giving first dose but do need results *can give w/wo food *assess for allergic response of any kind (rash-itching-hives-anaphylactic-resp. distress) *determine if has allergy to cephalosporins, give w/caution as there is risk for cross sensitivity to cephalosporins *continue to assess for response to infection

Category	Class	Body System Impacted	Generic Name	Brand Name	Most Common Side Effects (italics) SEVERE	Nursing Considerations and Vital Assessments
	Sulfonamides	Systemic	Sulfamethoxazole & trimethoprim	Bactrim	*Epigastric pain, N&V, itching, rash*	*Obtain any specimen cultures before giving first dose *Give on empty stomach with full glass of water *Primarily used for urinary tract infection-assess response (fever-ongoing painful/burning urination) *Assess for allergic response of any kind (rash-itching-hives-anaphylactic-resp. distress)
	Tetracyclines	Systemic	Doxycycline Tetracycline	Doxy Tetracyn	*Diarrhea, N&V, light sensitivity*	*Obtain any specimen cultures before giving first dose *Give on empty stomach with full glass of water *Assess for allergic response of any kind (rash-itching-hives-anaphylactic-resp. distress)
Steroids		Systemic	Dexamethasone Hydrocortisone Prednisone	Decadron Solu-cortef Deltasone	*Depression, hypertension, anorexia, nausea, bruising*	*Give orally w/meals to avoid GI irritation *Causes hyperglycemia-monitor glucose levels closely especially if diabetic *Decreases immune response and WBC count: assess closely for signs of infection *Decreases serum K+ levels and increases Na+. Monitor these labs closely *Assess for signs of adrenal insufficiency that can cause hypotension, weight loss, weakness, N&V, confusion, peripheral edema *Monitor I&O and daily weights for these reasons
Thyroid Hormone		Systemic	Levothyroxine	Synthroid	*Usually seen only when excessive doses cause hyperthyroid symptoms*	*give on empty stomach in the morning *assess apical pulse and BP prior to giving periodically *monitor thyroid function tests (T3-T4-TSH)
Muscle-skeletal Agents	Arthritis	Joints	Leflunomide	Cerebrex	*Dizziness, drowsiness, rash, ataxia*	*assess range of motion and degree of swelling and pain in affected joint
	Gout			Alloprim Colchicine	*Rash-Allopurinol Diarrhea, N&V-colchicine*	*give with meals to minimize gastric irritation *monitor for joint pain and swelling

Category	Class	Body System Impacted	Generic Name	Brand Name	Most Common Side Effects (italics) **SEVERE**	Nursing Considerations and Vital Assessments
	Muscle relaxants	Muscle	Cyclobenzaprine methocarbamol	Flexeril Robaxin	*Dizziness, drowsiness, dry mouth,*	*Assess for pain, muscle stiffness and range of motion before and periodically throughout therapy *Monitor elderly closely for increased sedation and weakness *Administer with caution in combination w/narcotics due to increased sedation with any age
	Electrolyte replacement	Systemic	Potassium Chloride	K-dur	*Abd. Pain, N&V, diarrhea* **Arrythmias (PVC's or V-Tach)**	*Administer w/meals-is very hard on stomach! *Monitor serum K+ closely throughout therapy *Assess for signs of hypokalemia (weakness-fatigue-increased PVC's on cardiac monitor) *Assess for signs of hyperkalemia (bradycardia-fatigue-muscle weakness-confusion)

References

1. Vallerand, A.H., Sanoski, C.A., & Deglin, J.H. (2013) *Davis's drug guide for nurses.* Thirteenth ed. Philadelphia, PA: F.A. Davis Company

Lab Planning: Creating a Plan of Care with a PRIORITY Lab

Lab:	Normal Value:	Clinical Significance:	Nursing Assessments/Interventions Required:
Value:	Critical Value:		

Lab:	Normal Value:	Clinical Significance:	Nursing Assessments/Interventions Required:
Value:	Critical Value:		

Lab:	Normal Value:	Clinical Significance:	Nursing Assessments/Interventions Required:
Value:	Critical Value:		

Lab:	Normal Value:	Clinical Significance:	Nursing Assessments/Interventions Required:
Value:	Critical Value:		

Lab:	Normal Value:	Clinical Significance:	Nursing Assessments/Interventions Required:
Value:	Critical Value:		

Clinical Lab Values & Nursing Responsibilities: ©2013-Keith Rischer/www.KeithRN.com

	Patho	Ranges	Causes	Treatments	Nsg. Considerations
I. Blood Chemistries **Sodium: Hyponatremia** Normal: 135-145 mEq/L	*Most abundant cation in EXTRAcellular fluid *Maintains osmotic pressure of extracellular fluid *Regulates renal retention & excretion of water *Responsible for stimulation of neuromuscular reactions & maintains SBP	Serum below 135mEq/L **Critical RED FLAG: <120**	*Excess sodium loss through N-V-D, skin and kidneys *Excess diuretic dosage *Liver Failure *CHF *Increased hypotonic IV fluids	*Sodium containing IV fluids *Lactated Ringers *NS 0.9% or 3%	**THINK VOLUME** *Monitor electrolytes *Monitor vital signs *Monitor neurological responses *Mental Status *Headaches *Monitor fluids/I&O for overload *Weights daily *Cardiac overload-CHF *Monitor musculoskeletal-cramps/weakness/tremor
Sodium: Hypernatremia Normal: 135-145 mEq/L		Serum above 145 mEq/L **Critical RED FLAG: >160**	*Dehydration-fluid loss through N-V-D (water loss in excess of salt loss) or excessive sweating *Diabetes-DKA *Fever	*Replace fluids *D5% *Diuretics- Excrete excess volume and excrete (sodium is then concentrated with fluid volume deficit)	**THINK VOLUME** *Monitor electrolytes *Monitor vital signs *Mental Status *Weight/I&O *Monitor for seizures
Potassium: Hypokalemia Normal: 3.5-5.2 mEq/L	*Most abundant INTRAcellular cation and is essential for transmission of electrical impulses in cardiac and skeletal muscle *Helps maintain acid-base balance and has inverse relationship to metabolic pH...decrease in pH of 0.1 (acidosis) increases K+ by 0.6 mEq/L *80-90% K+ filtered through the kidney	Serum below 3.5 mEq/L **Critical RED FLAG: <2.5**	*Inadequate intake of K+ *ETOH abuse *CHF/HTN *GI Loss-V&D *Renal Loss *Diuretics-Loop: Furosemide (Lasix) Bumetadine (Bumex)	*Oral or Parenteral Potassium *Diet high in potassium *Balanced electrolyte solutions *Pedialyte *Sports drinks	**THINK ELECTRICITY** *Monitor electrolytes *Monitor vital signs-low BP *Monitor cardiac responses *Irregular heart rate and rhythm for increased ectopy-PVC's/VTach

Clinical Lab Values & Nursing Responsibilities: ©2013-Keith Rischer/www.KeithRN.com

		Ranges	Causes	Treatments	Nsg Considerations
Potassium: Hyperkalemia Normal: 3.5-5.0 mEq/L		Serum above 5.0 mEq/ **Critical RED FLAG: >6**	*Metabolic acidosis *Dehydration *Excess potassium intake *Potassium sparing diuretics *Tissue damage-Burns (K+ goes out of cell) *Renal Failure	*Insulin- Moves K+ into the cell *D50- Prevents hypoglycemia caused by the infusion of Insulin *IV Calcium Gluconate also given at the same time to counteract cardiac effects of potassium *Sodium Bicarbonate-treats the acidosis caused when K+ moves into the cell and pushes hydrogen ions into the serum	**THINK ELECTRICITY** *Monitor electrolytes *Monitor cardiac responses *Monitor musculoskeletal cramps, weakness, parathesias *Peaked T wave/wide QRS *Monitor neurological responses, mental status, headache *Irregular heart rate and rhythm for increased ectopy-PVC's/Vtach
Magnesium: Hypomagnesemia Normal: 1.6-2.6 mg/dL	*Second most abundant intracellular cation *Required for transmission of nerve impulses and muscle relaxation *Controls absorption of sodium, potassium, calcium, and phosphorus *Magnesium.Potassium and Calcium all go low or high together!	Serum below 1.6 mg/dL **Critical RED FLAG: <1.2**	*Chronic Alcoholism *GI Loss-V&D *Impaired absorption *Renal Disease *Pancreatitis	*Treat underlying cause *GI Loss *Give Magnesium replacement	**THINK NEUROMUSCULAR TRANSMISSION THINK CARDIAC RESPONSE** *Monitor electrolytes *Monitor vital signs *Tachycardia *Hypertension *Tremors, tetany, paresthesias *Muscle weakness
Magnesium: Hypermagnesemia Normal: 1.6-2.6 mg/dL		Serum above 2.6 mg/dL **Critical RED FLAG: >6.1**	*Dehydration *Severe metabolic acidosis *Renal Failure *Tissue trauma	*Treat underlying cause *Renal patients treat with dialysis *Monitor cardiac effects of magnesium-increased PVC's-VT *Give Calcium Gluconate	**THINK NEUROMUSCULAR TRANSMISSION THINK CARDIAC RESPONSE** *Monitor electrolytes *Monitor vital signs *Bradycardia *Hypotension *Muscle weakness

Clinical Lab Values & Nursing Responsibilities: ©2013-Keith Rischer/www.KeithRN.com

	Patho	Ranges	Causes	Treatments	Nsg Considerations
Calcium: Hypocalcemia Normal: 8.2-10.6 mg/dL	*Most abundant cation in body and necessary for almost all vital processes *Half of total body calcium circulates as free ions that participate in coagulation, neuromuscular conduction, intracellular regulation, control of skeletal and cardiac muscle contractility *98-99% calcium reserves stored in teeth and skeleton	Serum below 8.2 mg/dL **Critical RED FLAG:** **<7**	*ETOH abuse *Pancreatitis *Chronic renal failure Inadequate intake *Decreased Vitamin D (Sunshine) *Lack of weight bearing *Loop Diuretics *Hypomagnesemia 1q`	Oral Calcium carbonate/gluconate Calcium chloride (more irritating to the vein) Watch for extravasate into subcutaneous tissue	**THINK MUSCLE RESPONSE** *Monitor electrolytes *Monitor vital signs *Cardiac Output decreased *Hypotension *Dysrhythmias *Monitor neuromuscular responses: seizures, tetany, paresthesias, muscle spasms
Calcium: Hypercalcemia Normal: 8.2-10.6 mg/dL		Serum above 10.6 mg/dL **Critical RED FLAG:** **>12**	*Prolonged immobilization *Dehydration *Cancer *Excess Antacid Intake	*Eliminate Calcium through kidneys through IV fluids *Loop diuretic to promote elimination of calcium	**THINK MUSCLE RESPONSE** *Monitor electrolytes *Monitor vital signs Hypertension *Monitor GI: N&V-anorexia *Dysrhythmias
Creatinine Normal: 0.5-1.2 mg/dl	*End product of creatine metabolism which is performed in skeletal muscle *Small amount of creatine is converted to creatinine which is then secreted by kidneys *Amount of creatinine generated proportional to mass of skeletal muscle	Serum above 1.2 mg/dl *Gold standard for kidney function because creatinine is produced in consistent quantity and rate of clearance reflects glomerular filtration	**Decreased in:** Decreased skeletal muscle Inadequate protein intake **Increased in:** CHF Dehydration Acute & chronic renal failure Shock	Correct underlying problem Fluid resuscitation to keep SBP>90 Dialysis	**THINK FLUID BALANCE** *Assess I&O closely *Fluid restriction *Assess for signs of fluid retention/edema

Clinical Lab Values & Nursing Responsibilities: ©2013-Keith Rischer/www.KeithRN.com

	Patho	Ranges	Causes	Treatments	Nsg Considerations
Blood Urea Nitrogen (BUN) Normal: 10-20 mg/dl	*Urea represents end product of protein metabolism performed in the liver *Urea diffuses freely in intra/extracellular fluid and then excreted by kidneys *BUN reflects balance between production and excretion of urea *Ratio to creatinine is 15-24:1 (if creatine 1.0 expected BUN should be 15-24) *Is indirect measurement of renal function but does not reflect glomerular filtration	**Critical RED FLAG: >100**	**Decreased in:** Poor protein intake/malnutrition Liver disease Malabsorption syndromes **Increased in:** Acute renal failure CHF Hypovolemia-dehydration Pyelonephritis Hyperalimentation/TPN	*Fluid resuscitation-HIGH *Dialysis-HIGH *Improve nutritional intake/Failure to thrive-LOW	**THINK FLUID BALANCE** *Assess I&O closely *Fluid restriction *Assess for signs of fluid retention/edema *Assess for agitation, confusion, fatigue, *N&V-HIGH *Assess liver profile labs for correlating liver damage
II.Hematology **Hemoglobin-HGB** Normal: Adult- 13-17 g/dl	*Primary protein of erythrocytes that is composed of heme (iron) and globin (protein) *Carries O2 to cells and CO2 back to lungs *Parallels Hematocrit which is the % of RBC in proportion to total plasma volume *GOLD Standard for evaluating blood/RBC adequacy (anemia, blood loss)	**Critical RED FLAG: <6 or >18** *Range of Anemias:* **Mild** Hgb 10-12 g/dl-asymptomatic **Moderate:** Hgb 6-10 g/dl weakness, fatigue, palpitations, SOB, decreased tol to activity-orthostatic hypotension **Severe:** Hgb < 6 g/dl Hypoxia: confusion, SOB, skin pallor- and MM and nailbeds, dizziness, weakness, tachycardia	**Clinical Uses:** Detect blood loss, anemia and response to treatment Detect any possible blood disorder **Decreased in:** Anemia Cancer Fluid retention/overload Hemorrhage **Increased in:** COPD CHF Dehydration Polycythemia	*Correct underlying problem *Blood transfusions if symptomatic	**THINK BLOOD LOSS/ANEMIA** *Identify early signs of blood loss: tachycardia, then hypotension *Transfuse as needed-assess closely in first 30" for transfusion reactions *Assess for signs of tissue hypoxia (see above)

Clinical Lab Values & Nursing Responsibilities: ©2013-Keith Rischer/www.KeithRN.com

	Patho	Ranges	Causes	Treatments	Nsg Considerations
White Blood Cell Count (WBC) Normal: 4,500-11,000 mm3	*WBC represent primary defense against invading infections *This is a total count of all 5 leukocytes: neutrophils, lymphocytes, eosinophils, basophils, and monocytes *Indicates overall degree of bodies response to pathology, but must be evaluated and correlated through differential count *Elevated WBC due to significant increase in one differential-usually the neutrophil *Physiologic stress or steroids will increase WBC	**Critical RED FLAG: <2500 or >15,000**	**Decreased in:** ETOH abuse Anemia Bone marrow depression Viral infections **Increased in:** Infection Anemia Inflammatory disorders Steroid use (acute or chronic)	*Identify infectious process *Confirm bone marrow depression in chemo/radiation therapy	**THINK INFECTION** *Low or elevated WBC can represent sepsis *Assess closely for hypotension with known infection (septic shock) *Assess closely for any change in temperature trend-hypothermia or febrile can both represent sepsis especially in elderly
Neutrophils Normal: 50-70% of differential	*Most predominant differential WBC- comprise 50-70% of all WBC's *First line of defense against bacterial infection through phagocytosis (think pacman) ***BANDS-** if present on differential-correlate with overwhelming sepsis.Immature neutrophils body is kicking into circulation before they are ready because of the severity of infection/sepsis	**Critical RED FLAG: >80%**	**Increased in:** Infection Acute hemorrhage Physical stress Tissue necrosis/injury **Decreased in:** Bone marrow depression (chemo/radiation therapy) Viral infection (due to increased lymphocytes)	*Identify infectious process *Confirm bone marrow depression in chemo/radiation therapy	**THINK INFECTION** *Low or elevated WBC can represent sepsis *Assess closely for hypotension with known infection (septic shock) *Assess closely for any change in temperature trend-hypothermia or febrile can both represent sepsis especially in elderly

Clinical Lab Values & Nursing Responsibilities: ©2013-Keith Rischer/www.KeithRN.com

	Patho	Ranges	Causes	Treatment	Nsg Considerations
III. Cardiac **Troponin** Normal: <0.05 ng/ml This may vary depending on each hospital lab	*Contractile protein found in cardiac muscle that will be released into systemic circulation with cardiac ischemia or acute MI *Levels will rise 2-6 hours after injury-peak 16-24 hours and then remain elevated for several days *If acute onset CP to r/o MI they will be done every 6 hours x3 to determine pattern of abnormal elevation	**Critical RED FLAG: ANY ELEVATION** If elevated this establishes diagnosis of acute MI *If positive MI, the degree of elevation provides general barometer of degree of heart muscle damage	**Increased in:** Acute MI Unstable angina Minor myocardial damage after CABG or PTCA/stent placement	*Standards of cardiac care include continuous telemetry, b-blockers to decrease cardiac workload, heparin or nitroglycerin gtts. *Definitive treatment of MI includes PTCA/stent or CABG	**THINK CARDIAC-MI** *Assess closely for recurrent or new onset of chest pain *Assess cardiac rhythm for any changes such as PVC's, VTach or atrial fibrillation *Assess HR and SBP carefully to promote decreased cardiac workload (maintain heart rate <80 and SBP <140 *Assess tolerance to activity closely
Brain Natriuretic Peptide (BNP) Normal: <100 ng/L	*Hormone that is stored in the ventricle of the heart *When left ventricle is distended and stretched due to CHF exacerbation BNP is released into circulation Inhibits the release of renin by kidneys which promotes water and sodium loss as well as increases glomerular filtration rate (Body's own ACE inhibitor!)	100-500 ng/L abnormal but not critical for ventricular strain (mild) **Critical RED FLAG: >500** critical for positive correlation of HF exacerbation	*CHF exacerbation *Ventricular hypertrophy (cardiomyopathy) *Severe hypertension	*Aggressive diuresis for fluid overload *May be on NTG gtt or po Nitrates to decrease preload which decreases workload of heart	**THINK CARDIAC-HF** *Assess respiratory status for tachypnea and breath sounds closely for basilar or scattered crackles *Assess HR and SBP carefully to promote decreased cardiac workload (heart rate <80 and SBP <140 *Assess tolerance to activity closely *Assess I&O closely *Assess K+ closely with loop diuretics

References

1. Van Leeuwen, A. & Poelhuis-Leth, D.J. (2009). *Davis's comprehensive handbook of laboratory and diagnostic tests with nursing implications*. Third ed. Philadelphia, PA: F.A. Davis Company.

Clinical Reasoning Questions to Develop Nurse Thinking

(Formulate and reflect before and after report, but **BEFORE** seeing patient the first time)

1. *What is the primary problem and what is its underlying cause or pathophysiology?*

2. *What clinical data from the chart is RELEVANT and needs to be trended because it is clinically significant?*

3. *List all relevant nursing priorities. What nursing priority captures the "essence" of your patient's status and will guide your plan of care?*

4. *What nursing interventions will you initiate based on this priority and what are the desired outcomes?*

5. *What body system(s), key assessments and psychosocial needs will you focus on based on your patient's primary problem or nursing care priority?*

6. *What is the worst possible/most likely complication(s) to anticipate based on the primary problem?*

7. *What nursing assessments will identify this complication EARLY if it develops?*

8. *What nursing interventions will you initiate if this complication develops?*

While Providing Care (Review and note after initial patient assessment)

9. *What clinical assessment data did you just collect that is RELEVANT and needs to be TRENDED because it is clinically significant to detect a change in status?*

10. *Does your nursing priority or plan of care need to be modified in any way after assessing your patient?*

11. *After reviewing the primary care provider's note, what is the rationale for any new orders or changes made?*

12. *What educational priorities have you identified and how will you address them?*

Caring and the "Art" of Nursing

13. *What is the patient likely experiencing/feeling right now in this situation?*

14. *What can I do to engage myself with this patient's experience, and show that he/she matters to me as a person?*

Patient Preparation Worksheet

Time	Meds/Care Priorities	Misc.

Adm. Date_____ Days since adm._____ POD#_____

Chief Complaint/Primary Problem:

Past Medical History

	CV	Resp	Neuro	GI	GU	Skin/Pain	Misc.	VS
Prior Nursing Assessment >>>								
Current Nursing Assessment >>>								

Lab Test	Current	Most Recent
Na+		
K+		
Mg+		
Creat.		
WBC		
Neut. %		
Hgb.		

Allergies_____
Code Status_____
IV site_____
IV Maintenance_____
IV Drips_____
Activity_____
Fall Risk/Safety_____
Diet_____
Bladder/Bowel_____
_____
_____
_____
_____
_____
_____

End of Shift SBAR to Oncoming Nurse

Situation:
Background:
Assessment:
Recommendation:

KeithRN
Clinical Reasoning Resources

Though there is an almost limitless number of topics that could be covered in nursing education, there are fewer concepts that must be mastered to prepare students for professional practice. I have created a workbook with twelve case studies that cover the most important concepts to practice. If your program uses a concept-based curriculum, these 12 case studies serve as examples that will provide the hook of contextualization that students require to acquire deep learning of what is most important. My store has additional clinical reasoning resources to strengthen student learning.

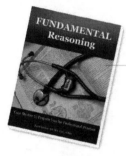

FUNDAMENTAL Reasoning (263 p.)

FUNDAMENTAL Reasoning is a basic introduction to clinical reasoning that is best suited for the fundamental level in registered nurse programs or practical nursing programs. It emphasizes application of the applied sciences of pharmacology, dosage calculation, and F&E. Recognizing clinical relationships and identifying the nursing priority to establish a plan of care are situated with a salient clinical scenario.

RAPID Reasoning (281 p.)

RAPID Reasoning is a "just right" length for most students and educators, best suited for basic med/surg content. Each RAPID Reasoning case study situates essential content to the bedside, and incorporates my step-by-step template of clinical reasoning questions that allows thinking to be practiced in the safety of the classroom.

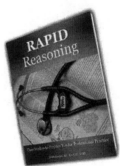

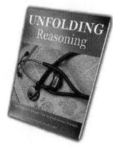

UNFOLDING Reasoning (377 p.)

UNFOLDING Reasoning is an advanced/synthesis level of case studies that contextualizes essential content to the bedside, and incorporates my step-by-step template of clinical reasoning questions. In addition, evaluation is integrated into the scenario with a clinical change of status that must be recognized as the scenario unfolds over time.

Clinical Dilemmas: Case Studies that Cultivate Caring, Civility & Clinical Reasoning (182 p.)

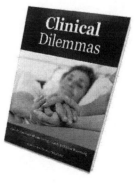

Clinical dilemmas are a series of 15 clinical reasoning case studies that emphasize the "art" of nursing. Each study has an emphasis that integrates aspects of caring, spiritual care, nurse engagement/presence, and ethical decision making and its relevance to nursing practice. Categories include patient, treatment, ethical, and nurse dilemmas that address incivility.